Apraxia

Apraxia
The Cognitive Side of Motor Control

Georg Goldenberg

OXFORD
UNIVERSITY PRESS

OXFORD
UNIVERSITY PRESS

Great Clarendon Street, Oxford, OX2 6DP,
United Kingdom

Oxford University Press is a department of the University of Oxford.
It furthers the University's objective of excellence in research, scholarship,
and education by publishing worldwide. Oxford is a registered trade mark of
Oxford University Press in the UK and in certain other countries

First Edition Published in 2013

Impression: 1

Published in the United States of America by Oxford University Press
198 Madison Avenue, New York, NY 10016, United States of America

British Library Cataloguing in Publication Data
Data available

Library of Congress Control Number: 2013938575

ISBN 978–0–19–959151–0

Printed and bound by
CPI Group (UK) Ltd, Croydon, CR0 4YY

Preface

Apraxia is a fascinating syndrome. Clinical observations of patients who cannot decide whether a fork or a knife is the right instrument for slicing bread, who are unable to replicate the movement of cutting with scissors immediately after they have used them, or whose left hand withdraws objects from the right hand but gives them readily to other persons yield intriguing insights into the fragility of the deliberate control of human action. Apraxia is also a fascinating topic of research. Its scientific exploration has a history of some 140 years and continues to produce novel and exciting insights. The twists and controversies of this long history touch on core issues in our understanding of mind and brain.

The aim of this book is to provide a comprehensive review of history, clinical appearance, and scientific research on apraxia. The review is guided by the hypothesis that apraxia is a disturbance at the boundary between cognition and motor control. Its position on one or the other side of this boundary is a topic of controversy that runs as a central thread through conflicting theories of apraxia. The attraction of apraxia as a field of theorizing and research owes much to this ambiguous position that ultimately refers to a mind–body dichotomy.

I hope that the width of its scope will make the book attractive to readers with backgrounds ranging from therapeutic disciplines, medicine, neuropsychology, and neuroscience to history and philosophy. I tried to write understandably for all of them and to explain terms and facts that are evident for specialists but unfamiliar for readers from other disciplines. Some very basic notions of clinical neuroscience, for example, that lesions of one side of the brain cause motor impairments of the opposite side of the body should suffice for following the course of the arguments. French and German quotes from early work on apraxia have been translated by me. Keeping a balance between literal translation and comprehensibility was sometimes a challenge particularly for nineteenth-century German texts. When comprehensibility was endangered, I supported it by comments on the concepts that underlay the choice of words.

I have researched and published on aspects of apraxia for nearly 30 years. I do not claim exception to the long-standing scientific tradition of considering one's own contributions as being exceptionally important and reliable, but I have made a serious effort to adhere also to the somewhat less universal tradition of giving due space and attention to the work of others. Out of 600 references cited in this book, 51 have been authored or co-authored by me. This is, I would say, a decent proportion. I have strained to discuss controversial results and theories in a fair and balanced way even if one of the controversial positions was my own.

There are many persons who helped me in writing this book. First of all, I want to thank the patients who consented not only to being videotaped but also to the use of these records for cartoons illustrating their problems. For them, apraxia is less a source of fascination than an intriguing assault on lifelong established competency and autonomy. The nurses and therapists of our department gave me precious insights into the consequences of apraxia for daily living and the possibilities and limits of their therapy.

Armin Schnider encouraged me to propose this book to Oxford University Press where a competent team accompanied me from the first synopsis to the final production of the book, and Charlotte Green was always ready to answer my questions.

Paul Eling gave me critical feedback on the historical chapters. Joachim Hermsdörfer and Wolfram Ziegler read single chapters and Joseph Spatt a first draft of the whole book. Discussions with them were extremely helpful for clarification of my own position with respect to the boundary between cognition and motor control. Philippe Peigneux and Andreas Marneros provided me with copies of influential nineteenth-century contributions preceding Hugo Liepmann's seminal first report of apraxia, and Ioanna Athanasoupoulou shed light on the confusing nomenclature of the first modern accounts of intermanual conflicts by Andrew Akelaitis.

Dani Goldenberg drew the cartoons for illustrations and Anna Goldenberg advised me to make sentences short. Their affection is the solid ground on which my life and this book rest.

Georg Goldenberg
Munich, February 2013

Contents

Chapter 1

Apraxia before Liepmann: Mind-palsy, asymbolia, and apraxia

As a first approximation, apraxia can be defined as a disturbance of the mental control of deliberate motor actions. Apraxia is a clinical syndrome with a long history, the beginning of which is usually identified with the seminal writings of the German psychiatrist Hugo Karl Liepmann in the first decades of the twentieth century (Goldenberg, 2003a), but disturbed mental control of deliberate movements had been subject to clinical observation and theorizing before Liepmann. The clinical literature of the late nineteenth century recognized three syndromes characterized by wrong or awkward actions in spite of preserved motor strength and coordination: mind-palsy, asymbolia, and apraxia.

Mind-palsy

Usually, the recognition of new clinical syndromes starts with clinical observations which do not fit in established diagnostic categories. When the reliability of the observation has been established, the next step is a search for underlying mechanisms, possibly supported by experimental studies. Finally, explanations of the syndrome may lead to a revision of basic theoretical assumptions.

The syndrome of mind-palsy developed in the opposite direction. Its starting point was a general theory of localized brain function. The framework of the theory led to the expectation of a hitherto unknown syndrome which was then sought for and allegedly found in animal experiments. Only then were clinical observations adduced, which pointed to the existence of the syndrome in patients with brain damage. We will follow this course and discuss first the basic theoretical model, then the animal experiments, and finally the clinical observations.

Theoretical foundations

The concept of mind-palsy ("Seelenlähmung") was based on an associationist[1] model of brain organization (Figure 1.1), which had been elaborated by the Viennese psychiatrist

[1] This approach to brain functions has also been termed "connectionist" (Caplan, 1987; Eling, 2011). This designation has the advantage of emphasizing the distinction from the British version of associationism that culminated in the writing of John Hughlings Jackson (Young, 1990; see Chapter 3) but the disadvantage that it is still in use in modern cognitive science where it characterizes computerized network models of cognitive functions (McClelland et al., 1986; Fodor & Pylyshyn, 1988). I prefer "associationism" because it is not in common use any more and thus underlines the historical nature of the present discussion.

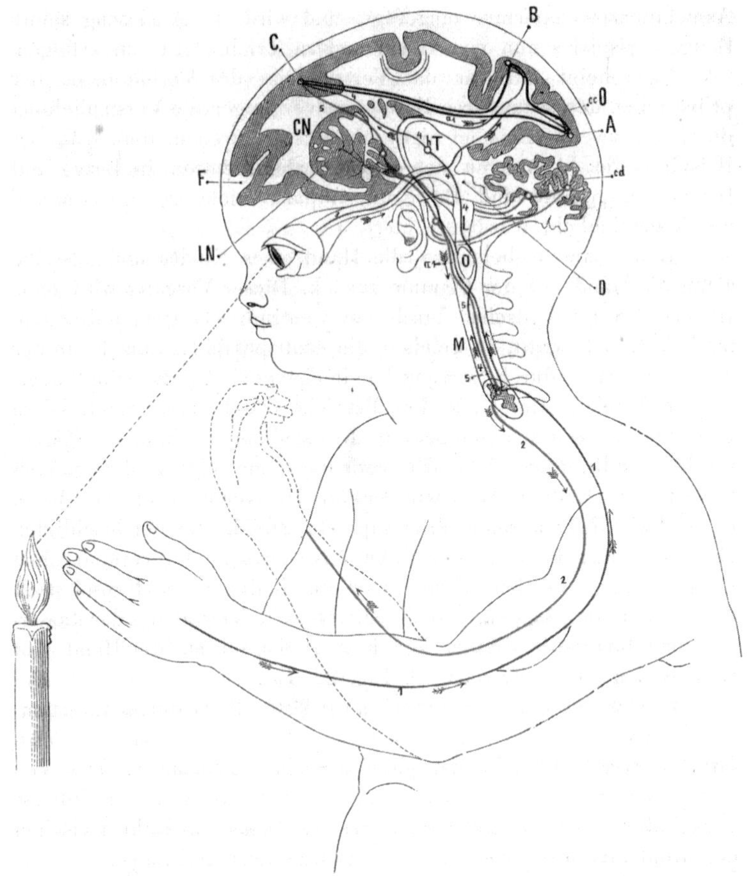

Figure 1.1 An associationist schema illustrating the motor reaction of the hand to the sight of a candle and the sensation of heat. The blue lines indicate centripetal, the red lines centrifugal, and the black lines association tracts. In this schema, neural processing beyond the incoming of sensation and outgoing of motor commands is limited to uninterrupted connections from the cortical end points of the sensation tracts (A and B) to the origin of the motor command (C). A: a point within the visual center; B: a point within the center for cutaneous sensations; C: a point within the territory of innervation sensations; ccO: occipital cortex; F: frontal cortex; 1: tract leading sensations from hand; 2: tract of movement of arm; 4C: tract for sensations of innervation; 5: centrifugal tract originating from C. Reproduced from Meynert, T. *Klinische Vorlesungen über Psychiatrie auf wissenschaftlichen Grundlagen für Studirende und Aerzte, Juristen und Psychologen*, p. 147 © 1889, Wilhelm Braumüller. (See Plate 1.)

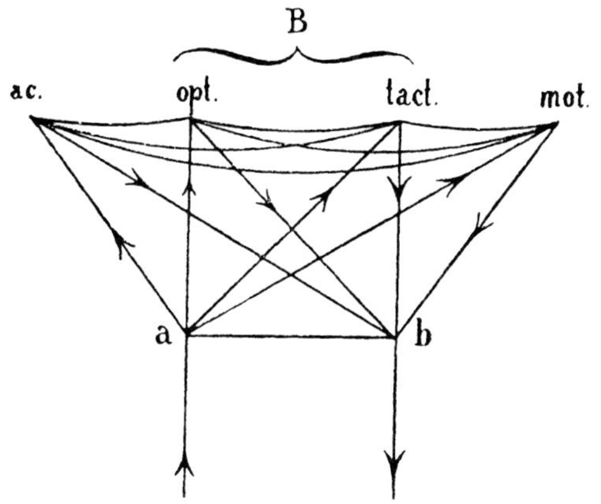

Figure 1.2 Wernicke's (1893, p. 100) schema is primarily concerned with understanding and production of words rather than with the control of limb movements. It is included here to illustrate the generation of psychic processes from associations between multimodal memory images. The elements of the schema are stored memory images. a: acoustic form of words; b: articulatory pattern of words. Ac, opt., tact., mot.: acoustic, optical, tactile, and motoric memory images associated with the perception and manipulation of objects. B: concepts of objects; although the parenthesis encloses only the optical and tactile memory image, the text leaves no doubts that the concept is composed of memory images from all modalities. The connections between the modality-specific memory images form a network which constitutes the neural basis of thinking and consciousness. Since these "intrapsychic" processes emerge from interactions across the whole network, they defy narrow localization of their neural substrate. Reproduced from C. Wernicke, Gesammelte Augsätze und kritische Referate zur Pathologie des Nervensystems ©1893, Verlag von Fischer's Medicinischer Buchhandlung.

and anatomist Theodor Meynert (1874), and applied to the study of aphasia by his disciple Carl Wernicke (1874) (Figure 1.2).

The empirical background for their model of brain function was the discovery that nerves transmitting input from peripheral sense organs, as well as nerves transmitting motor commands to peripheral muscles, are rooted in circumscribed regions of the cerebral cortex. For example, the optic tract brings visual information from the eyes to the occipital cortex, and excitation of motor cortex located in the central cortex triggers movements of the limbs (Fritsch & Hitzig, 1870; Munk, 1881; Young, 1990). The associationist model of brain function assumed that excitation in the cortical end points of afferent nervous tracts does not completely vanish when peripheral stimulation ceases. The remnants of past sensations are stored as "memory images" in cortical areas surrounding the end points. Likewise, movements of the body or the limbs give rise to memory images of the executed movement which are stored near the cortical region where the motor commands are generated. Localization of cerebral function is confined to such simple memory images surrounding the anatomical end point of the nervous pathways carrying sensations to, or movement commands away from, the cortex. These memory images are, however, richly interconnected by fiber tracts. Due to these connections, memory images can be evoked and recombined also in the absence of peripheral stimulation or action. They thus form the substrate of "intrapsychic" processes which defy further reduction to localizable elements:

> Memory images of sensations on the one hand, of movements of the own body on the other, are the elements provided by outer reality for constituting the contents of consciousness. Everything beyond these most simple functions, the combination of different sensations to a concept, thinking, consciousness, are an achievement of the masses of fibres which link the different sectors of the cerebral cortex among each other. (Wernicke, 1874, pp. 4, 9)

Incoming sensations must make connections with corresponding memory images of the same modality in order to be integrated into the multimodal network. If such integration fails, the sensation remains isolated and meaningless. There are thus two ways how cortical lesions can interfere with the perception and comprehension of external stimuli: destruction of the area where the pathways from the periphery reach the cortex would lead to "cortical" losses and destruction of the surrounding memory images to "mind" losses.[2] Depending on the modality of the sensation whose memory images were lost, the theory predicted the existence of mind-blindness, mind-deafness, and mind-numbness (Munk, 1877; Lissauer, 1890). By analogy, a loss of motor memories should result in "mind-palsy."[3]

The search for clinical correlates of these theoretical predictions was conducted in animal experiments before it was applied to clinical observations in humans.

Animal experiments

Berlin around 1870 was a good place for scientists interested in the anatomy and physiology of the human brain but was a bad place for dogs. They were the preferred subjects of experimental studies exploring the effects of stimulation or destruction of circumscribed parts of the brain. They had to sustain stress and pain from surgical procedures, which in the beginning were carried out without anesthesia, and some of them died from bleeding or inflammation of the exposed brain (Fritsch et al., 1870; Munk, 1877). When the experiment was successful, the dogs remained mutilated for the rest of their lives.

---

2 Successful connection of incoming sensations to memory images of the same modality does not necessarily guarantee integration into the multimodal network of memory images, since there can be interruption between memory images of the same modality and associated images from other modalities. Heinrich Lissauer, a disciple of Wernicke, described this possibility for the visual modality and suggested naming it "associative" mind-blindness (Lissauer, 1890).

3 The German expressions were "Seelenblindheit," "Seelentaubheit," "Seelenfühllosigkeit," and "Seelenlähmung." In English literature they have sometimes been translated as "psychic blindness." I prefer the combination with "mind" because "psychic paresis" has a connotation of paresis from non-organic causes like hysteria or conversion disorder. "Mind-palsy" was used by Wilson (1908) in a review of the current state of the art in apraxia. In German, the word "Seele" means both the mind and the immortal soul. Munk, who introduced the terms, addressed possible misunderstandings of "Seele" in a footnote regarding mind blindness ("Seelenblindheit"): "I choose this designation in 1877 after long reflection and I thought to have good reasons for preferring it to 'image-blindness' ('Vorstellungsblindheit') or 'memory-blindness' ('Erinnerungsblindheit'). Since I made clear repeatedly that soul-blindness = absence of mental visual images, absence of memory images of visual perceptions, I felt legitimated to consider the use of the word 'soul' as harmless as if I had used α- blindness or β-blindness." (Munk, 1881, p. 53)

In 1870, the anatomist Gustav Fritsch and the psychiatrist Eduard Hitzig attacked two contemporary beliefs about the cerebral cortex: that it could not be excited by electrical currents and that it had no direct access to motor actions of the limbs (Fritsch et al., 1870). They removed parts of a dog's skull and applied weak electrical currents to the bare surface of the brain. When such stimulation was administered to the anterior part of the brain it elicited contractions of muscles on the opposite side of the body, whereas no such reactions could be obtained by even much stronger currents applied to the posterior part. Further explorations of the effects of weak currents revealed specializations within the anterior part of the brain. There appeared to be fairly constant localizations where stimulation elicited motor twitches of the mouth, the neck, the foreleg, or the hind leg. Fritsch and Hitzig concluded that the cerebral cortex could send motor commands to the muscles, and that the cortical origins of these commands were laid out in a somatotopic map, so that the effects of local stimulation were body part specific.

While these observations had an enormous impact on brain research in Germany and beyond (Young, 1990; Finger, 2000), the results of subsequent excision studies are particularly relevant for the concept of mind-palsy. Fritsch and Hitzig opened the skull on the left side and excised a lentil-sized piece of cortex at the location where stimulation had elicited movements of the right foreleg. The excision did not result in a complete paralysis, but motor actions of this limb became somewhat awkward. During walking or standing the affected limb tended to slide away or to touch the ground with the dorsum instead of the sole. After partial recovery, one of the dogs showed a more spectacular symptom: When he was standing and the experimenter placed his right forelimb into an uncomfortable position, for example, amid the other three legs, the dog would neither protest nor try to bring the foreleg back into its natural position. When, however, the dog started to run, the leg was immediately brought back in its correct position and participated in running. Fritsch and Hitzig denied any deficiency of sensory afferences, but nonetheless concluded that the dog "apparently had only defective awareness of the conditions of this limb. He has lost the ability to form a complete mental image of that limb." (Fritsch et al., 1870, p. 331).

Introducing the parietal lobes

In Meynert's and Wernicke's version of associationism, memory images of sensations and of movements equally contributed to the "contents of consciousness." In the further development of the concept of mind-palsy their equality was replaced by the assumption that only memories of sensations give rise to conscious mental images. According to the "ideo-motor principle," voluntary movements had their origin in mental images of their sensory consequences (Prinz, 1987). The motor mechanisms that bring forward the intended consequences were believed to run automatically outside the realm of consciousness. Translated into anatomy, the "ideo-motor principle" shifted the possible source of mind-palsy from the motor cortex located in the frontal lobes to sensory regions located in the parietal lobe (see Figure 1.3). The further development of the concept of "mind-palsy" reflects this basic shift.

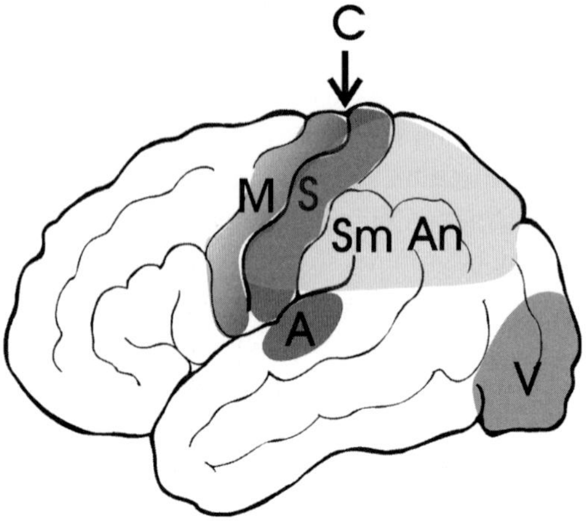

Figure 1.3 A schematic side view of the brain illustrating the anatomical considerations that underlay the discussions about the neural substrate of mind-palsy. According to the associationist model of brain function, memory images are stored close to the location where the original sensations have been received or the original motor commands have been sent out. Motor memories are thus stored in front of the central sulcus, and sensory memories behind it. The postulate that voluntary actions start with a mental image of the sensation of the completed movement and that this sensation is automatically transferred into motor action thus necessitating a stream of association from postcentral parietal to precentral motor areas constitutes a rudimentary form of a posterior to anterior stream of action control (see Chapter 2). A: acoustic cortex; C: central sulcus; M: motor cortex; S: somatosensory cortex; Sm: supramarginal gyrus; An: angular gyrus; V: visual cortex. Blue regions receive sensory afferences from the periphery, whereas the red region sends motor efferences to the periphery. Green denotes the extension of the parietal lobe. (See Plate 2.)

In 1878, the physiologist Hermann Munk (1878) replicated Fritsch and Hitzig's experiments. After excision of only a few millimeters of left-sided cortex, he found impairment of the right forelimb almost identical to the previous description by Fritsch and Hitzig. Munk emphasized the contrast between the lack of isolated deliberate movements of the affected limb and its swift integration into global movement patterns involving all limbs, as, for example, in walking. He referred the leg's immobility to the loss of limb-specific mental images of movements, but specified that these images are not equivalent to stored motor actions. They are sensory images of the tactile or kinesthetic feedback associated with a movement. These movement images elicit execution of the imagined movement, because "the generation of a movement image posits *eo ipso* the corresponding motor action" (Munk, 1878, p. 178). Therefore, the consequences of excisions depended on the affection of sensory areas:

> Within the sensory area of each body part small excisions cause a partial loss of sensory images of that body part, larger excisions a complete loss: mind-palsy of that body part. (Munk, 1878, p. 176)

The assumption that the causal damage in mind-palsy affects kinesthetic memory images of the moving limb rather than the motor cortex directing the movement was foundational for the belief that the crucial lesions for mind-palsy affect the parietal lobes. It was further elaborated in the first descriptions of putative human analogs to the experimentally induced disturbances of motility in dogs.

A human case of mind-palsy

In 1887, the German internist Hermann Nothnagel reasoned that the memory images, whose destruction should give rise to mind-palsy, cannot be stored within or very close to the "motor centra" which transmit motor commands from the cortex to the periphery, because destruction of the motor-centra causes paralysis of the opposite limb but leaves intact the will to execute movements of the paralyzed part. He explained the preservation of the will to move by preservation of the conscious mental image of the intended motor action and concluded that this mental image must have a different neural substrate than the commands directing execution of the movement. Nothnagel suggested that "the field of motor memory images lies in the parietal gyrus. The motor neurons in the paracentral and central region only transmit the motor command" (Nothnagel, 1887, p. 214). Consequently, mind-palsy should result from parietal lesions.

Nothnagel did not support his conclusions with clinical observations of mind-palsy nor did he elaborate on the expected clinical features. The first detailed report of a presumed human case of mind-palsy was published 15 years after Munk's creation of the syndrome, by the Swiss psychiatrist Eugen Bleuler (1893). Bleuler gave a very detailed and lengthy description of aphasia and other symptoms in a patient whose lesions analyzed post-mortem affected, among other regions, left supramarginal and bilateral anterior parietal regions. This patient had an incomplete paresis but a complete sensory loss of his right arm. He could move the shoulders and the upper arm when he was looking at them, but "when the patient does not see his right arm, he is not only unaware of the arm's momentary position, but he is also completely unable to innervate any of its muscles" (Bleuler, 1893, p. 38). Bleuler reasoned that the inability to move the arm without visual control was due to the absence of kinesthetic motor memory images. Referring to Nothnagel, he classified the disturbance as mind-palsy.

From sensory memory images to mental processes

A few years later, but still three years ahead of Liepmann's first paper on apraxia, Ludwig Bruns (1897) contributed a further case report together with an extensive discussion of mind-palsy. The patient was a luetic musician who suddenly developed aphasia, right-sided hemianopia, right-sided hemianesthesia, a mild paresis of the right leg, and a strange motor disorder of the right arm:

> The patient never uses the right arm spontaneously; it lies beside him as if it were completely paralysed. He offers the left hand for greeting, eats with the left hand, takes his pinch (of tobacco) with the left hand, and uses the left hand for blowing his nose. He can be prompted to use the right hand only by long verbal encouragement. It seems that at first he does not understand what he is expected to do and that this irritates him. If one wants him to raise the right hand to his nose, one must withhold his left hand and demonstrate the path of his right hand to the nose by passive movement.

> Then, he will eventually execute the movement himself. In the same way it is possible to finally get him to give the right hand for greeting by withholding the left hand or refusing it repeatedly and asking for the right hand. Likewise, after long encouragement, he leads the spoon to the mouth with the right hand.
>
> The patient is aware that something is wrong with his right hand. He frequently looks at it with astonishment and calls it: "you bastard." (Bruns, 1897, p. 379)

Surprisingly, when actions of the right hand could be induced at all, movement strength was normal and dexterity only mildly reduced. Unlike Bleuler's patient, this patient did not need to look at his hand in order to control it.

This peculiar disturbance of right-hand motor control recovered within a few days and only a slight awkwardness remained. The patient could even play the piano again, although his right hand sometimes missed the keys and hit the edge of the piano. In spite of this amelioration he died a few weeks later. Post-mortem examination revealed a left superior temporal lesion which extended parietally into the angular gyrus and the white matter underlying the supramarginal gyrus.

Bruns followed Bleuler in searching for the source of the problems on the sensory rather than the motor side. His emphasis on the importance of intact sensory representations for deliberate motor control went even further than Bleuler's ideas. Whereas Bleuler had considered only kinesthetic sensations as being crucial for motor actions, Bruns reasoned that connections from all sensory modalities can elicit motor actions. He defended a radical response to the question whether mind-palsy was due to loss of motor or sensory memory images. He emphasized the importance of sensory and downplayed that of motor images:

> Every "deliberate" movement has its source in a stimulus originating from a sensory centre. Intactness of these sensory centres and their connections is as necessary for deliberate movements as is the intactness of the so-called motor centres: After all, these motor centres are nothing more than the point where the sensory part of an intended movement turns into its motor part, and it is impossible to indicate exact borders between them. (Bruns, 1897, pp. 383–384)

Interruption of the connections from these centers deprives the motor centers of sensory stimulations and results in spontaneous disuse of the extremity, as had been observed in the case of the luetic musician.

To clarify the importance of the involvement of multiple sensory centers in the preparation of deliberate movements, Bruns compared them to simple reflex movements like the knee jerk. In these primitive reflexes, one specific sensory stimulus (tapping below the knee) always elicits the same specific reaction (extending the leg), and they are based on direct subcortical or (as in the case of the knee jerk) spinal connections between sensation and motor control. By contrast, for deliberate movements, the path from sensation to motor response travels through the cortex and is modulated by the inclusion of cortically stored memory images. The inclusion of memory images mitigates the tightness of the association between sensation and motor response. External sensory stimuli lose the power to firmly determine the nature of the motor response. They give way to mental processes mediating between stimulus and response:

> Mental processes are based on associations between sensory centres distributed across the whole cortex—therefore mental processes cannot be localized in the same way as their single constitutive parts—they always demand the whole or a great portion of the brain. Mental processes express themselves by muscular actions. Via the association tracts they stimulate motor regions and evoke movements. If these tracts are interrupted the mind cannot influence movements any more—there is mind-palsy: Deliberate movements are absent, while reflexes in a narrow sense come to the fore without restriction. (Bruns, 1897, p. 387)

Since cortical sensory centers are located in the posterior part of the hemisphere and motor centers in the frontal region, the cortical path from sensation to motor action leads from posterior to anterior brain regions. It thus resembles the neural connections underlying the most primitive spinal reflexes, where the nerves carrying sensory stimulation enter the posterior part and those exciting the muscular response originate from the anterior part of the spinal cord.

The alleged dissociation between preserved reflex and defective deliberate movement transgressed the clinical evidence of Bleuler's and Bruns' case reports. No such dissociation had been noted by Bleuler. Bruns adduced as evidence that his patient used the right hand to scratch himself when the left one was restrained. However, restriction of the left hand could also bring forward less reflex-like movements, like greeting (see earlier extract). Arguably, the alleged dissociation between deliberate and reflex movements owed more to theoretical expectations than to clinical observations.[4]

Mind-palsy as a physiological concept

Although it bears the notion of mind and in German even the immortal soul in its name, mind-palsy is essentially a physiological rather than a psychological concept. "Memory images" are traces left by sensations in cortical areas and their connections. Both the generation and the destruction of memory images are completely determined by transformations or destructions of cells and fiber paths. Mental states are thought of as the product and not the cause of physiological changes. The lack of spontaneous movements of the right hand of Bruns' patient was not attributed to deficient understanding or unwillingness or any other mental state, but to destruction of either sensory centers or fibers connecting them with motor centers. It is significant that the syndrome was described in dogs before it was searched for in human beings. While it is reasonable to assume that the physiology of sensation and motor control is similar in humans and other animals, it would seem harder to argue that the mental capacities of dogs are a good model for understanding human behavior.

An important argument in favor of the physiological nature of mind-palsy was its body part specificity. Mind-palsy affected only the limbs on the side opposite to the lesioned hemisphere, and the animal experiments even suggested that it could be restricted to only one part of the limb. The explanation for this body part specificity was sought in the

[4] The opposition between propositional and automatic movements was central to the writings of John Hughlings Jackson. We will come back to his influence on the science of apraxia in Chapter 3.

somatotopy of the motor cortex rather than in differences between the mental processes associated with movements of different body parts.

The literature on the anatomical substrate of mind-palsy did not consider possible differences between the hemispheres. In the cases reported by Bleuler and by Bruns, the lesions happened to be in the left hemisphere and mind-palsy affected the right limbs, but in their presentations there is no hint of a suspicion that right-sided lesions would not cause the same kind of mind-palsy of the left limbs. The indifference to laterality is remarkable, because in the last decade of the nineteenth century the left hemisphere's dominance for speech was already firmly established. It was, however, consistent with the associationist doctrine that the cortical end points of nerves leading to the periphery are the firm poles determining the extension of associative fiber networks. The layout of the cortical origins of sensory and motor nerves does not differ between hemispheres. This symmetry was considered to be more relevant for understanding functional divisions of the brain than the strikingly different effects of right- and left-hemisphere lesions on speech and language.

The legacy of mind-palsy

From the point of view of modern neuropsychology, Bleuler's case would probably be classified as an instance of "kinesthetic ataxia" (alternative terms are "afferent apraxia," "tactile apraxia," and "parietal hand"; Luria, 1980; Freund, 1987; Goldenberg, 2003c), and Bruns' case as motor neglect (Laplane & Degos, 1983; Coulthard et al., 2008). Possibly, they were the first detailed descriptions of these disorders, but their historical importance lies elsewhere. In Chapter 2, I will argue that Bruns' interpretation of mind-palsy came as close as possible within a strictly associationist framework to Liepmann's analysis of ideo-kinetic apraxia.

Before we leave mind-palsy let me briefly sum up features of this syndrome which recur in Liepmann's elaboration of apraxia.

There is a stream of action control from posterior to anterior brain regions in which the parietal lobe plays a central role. Along this stream, sensory images of the intended actions are transferred into motor commands which produce a muscular expression of the sensory image. Interruption of the conversion of sensory images into motor commands causes a body part-specific inability to perform voluntary actions.

Asymbolia

In his seminal report of aphasia following a left frontal lesion, Paul Broca (1861) classified the patient's disorder as a selective loss of articulated speech with preservation of other mental functions. He remarked, however, that "unable to manifest his ideas or his desires other than by movements of his left hand, he frequently made incomprehensible gestures," and that "some questions to which a man with normal intelligence would have found a mean to respond by gesture remained unanswered."

Nearly ten years later, the German psychiatrist Carl Maria Finkelnburg (1870) criticized the tenet that aphasic patients had a selective loss of speech and expanded on their defective production and comprehension of non-verbal conventional signs. He had observed an aphasic musician who could no longer read musical notes, a salesman who confused the values of different coins, and a government official who could not distinguish rank signs and who had forgotten how to behave during Mass. The problems were not confined to interaction with external signs or rules but also concerned the patients' gestural expressions. Thus, an aphasic woman "who had been raised as a devout catholic never made the sign of the cross at the common grace. When asked by her surrounding to make it, she hesitantly reached sometimes behind the ear, sometimes to the neck until it was demonstrated to her. Then she imitated it correctly." The salesman's "mimic expression during speaking was exaggerated and gross, his gestures awkward and sometimes completely incongruent to what he wanted to express" and in another patient "mimic expression and gesticulation become gross and incomprehensible, and the comprehension for pantomimes made by other persons diminished."

Finkelnburg concluded that the term "aphasia" was ill-chosen because the language disturbance was only one of several manifestations of a general "asymbolia," that is, "a pathological disturbance of function where the ability to understand or express concepts by means of learned signs is partially or completely abolished."

> Obviously the deficiency of word production represents only an aliquot—though the one interfering most with the living conditions and the most conspicuous for the surrounding—part of the total disturbance which extends more or less to all brain processes mediating the manifestation of conceptual ideas by learned sensory signs of any kind—symbols. (Finkelnburg, 1870, p. 461)

Finkelnburg invoked philosophy as support for the existence and importance of symbolic abilities:

> The important and independent role of symbolic abilities for the reproduction and combination of mental images has long been acknowledged by philosophical schools of thought. Kant, for example, calls this ability, to which he dedicates a whole section of his *Anthropology*, as "facultas signatrix" and its accomplishments as "symbolic cognition." (Finkelnburg, 1870, p. 461)

Concerning the cerebral substrate of asymbolia, Finkelnburg referred to Meynert's anatomical findings and reasoned that the central part of the hemisphere, would be the most likely seat of responsible lesions, because of the plenitude of fibers connecting it with many different sectors of the cortex and multiplying their interactions.

Finkelnburg also discussed the laterality of lesions. Not surprisingly, all but one of his aphasic patients had left-sided lesions as manifested by their right-sided motor symptoms. Finkelnburg complained that the reasons for the asymmetry of lesions causing aphasia or, respectively, asymbolia had not yet been elucidated. He discussed but dismissed the possibility that due to asymmetry of vascular anatomy the left hemisphere is more likely to be the target of brain damage than the right, but he also refused the "paradoxical idea of French authors that as a rule the organ of language competence becomes functional only on the left side, analogue to the right hand, and that in left handed persons the right speech centre is filled with learned contents" (Finkelnburg, 1870, p. 461).[5]

Motor asymbolia

Finkelnburg's argument that lesions in the central part of the hemisphere are most likely to cause asymbolia because they interrupt the interactions between multiple regions paid lip service to cerebral localization of functions but implied that asymbolia cannot be ascribed to dysfunction of any single narrowly confined brain region. Asymbolia could be reconciled with Meynert's and Wernicke's anatomical schema at best by identifying it with a disturbance of the whole network of association fibers connecting the cortical end points of peripheral afferences and their surrounding memory images. However, these anatomical considerations were not constitutive for asymbolia. The concept of asymbolia was derived from the psychology of thought and language and not from the anatomy of its neural substrate.

Wernicke (1874) ignored this derivation from the physiological approach to mental functions and equated asymbolia with a loss of memory images. A logical consequence of this interpretation was that, in addition to a general asymbolia where all images are erased, there can be modality specific "asymbolia" which, in the end, is nothing else than the mind losses of functions conceptualized a few years later and without reference to asymbolia by Munk (1877, 1878).

In a series of lectures published in 1889, Theodor Meynert did not mention Finkelnburg but declared:

> Wernicke calls the manifestations of the combined loss of memory images as well in the optical as in the acoustical sense and in most cases also in the tactile sense, asymbolia. (Meynert, 1889, p. 224)

In a later lecture, he elaborates the effects of selective asymbolia affecting memory images of motor actions:

> Different areas of the cortex contribute distinguishing features for one and the same object, and the object becomes object of consciousness by their combined sensory stimulation. The loss of each of these distinguishing features is called asymbolia. With regard to the motor modality the distinguishing feature of object recognition is associated with the use of the object. Asymbolia will be revealed by the patient's inability to make proper use of the object. For motor asymbolia it suffices that a softening in the middle portion of the central regions makes the innervation images of the upper extremity inaccessible. (Meynert, 1889, p. 270)

The term "motor asymbolia" found little recognition and soon vanished from the literature, but it left a footprint in the history of apraxia: it figured as a parenthesis in the title of Liepmann's seminal first paper on apraxia (Liepmann, 1900). In later writings, Liepmann recognized "motor asymbolia" as a precursor of "limb-kinetic apraxia" (Liepmann, 1908).

[5] The formulation "paradoxical idea" for the refusal of French ideas sounds rather sharp for a scientific lecture. Finkelnburg's lecture was published in September 1871 and had probably been held shortly before. It may be relevant that the Franco-Prussian War had only ended in May 1871. Finkelnburg had participated in it and had returned "decorated with the iron cross" (Lent, 1896). Apparently the lecture demonstrates his patriotism as much as his clinical astuteness.

Asymbolia and mind-palsy

After the digression to Wernicke's attempt to reconcile asymbolia with his associationist model of brain function, we return to Finkelnburg's original concept of asymbolia. Although Finkelnburg briefly considered the possible anatomical substrate of asymbolia, the concept itself was grounded in psychological or even philosophical considerations rather than in the physiology of brain function.

In contrast to mind-palsy, asymbolia was not meant to be modality specific. It affected production and comprehension of visual and acoustic signs as well as motor actions. Aberrant, awkward, and incomprehensible gestures were symptoms of the general degradation of symbolic aptitudes. Deficient motor control did not contribute to their incomprehensibility. Consequently, the somatotopy of the motor cortex was irrelevant and there was no body part specificity of deficient motor actions. Finkelnburg did not consider the possibility that the woman who was unable to make the sign of the cross with the right hand would succeed when using the left hand.

Apraxia

The first printed appearance of the term "apraxia" was in a book published by the German linguist Chaim Steinthal (1871). Steinthal gave examples of the diversity of clinical manifestations of aphasia, emphasizing that it is not a unitary disorder but a combination of preserved and disturbed verbal and non-verbal capabilities. As an example for non-verbal impairment he reported the observation of an aphasic composer who wrote notes awkwardly, placing the head of quarter-notes to the right instead of the left side of the stem. He continued the discussion of this case:

> The patient had been aphasic and anarthric; yet he had remained intelligent. But when he was asked to write, he grasped the pen upside-down; he also took hold of spoon and fork as if he had never used them before. He asked for his violin, but gripped it so awkwardly that it was impossible to play on it. These symptoms are not equivalent to anarthria but to aphasia, specifically to the confusion of words; because it is not the movement of the limbs which is inhibited, but the relationship between the movements and the object used. The relationship between the mechanism and its purpose is disturbed.
>
> This apraxia is an obvious amplification of aphasia. In another direction aphasia extends to a general inability to comprehend sign, asemia. (Steinthal, 1881, p. 458)

Steinthal then listed examples of "asemia." They were taken from Finkelnburg's paper and made clear that Steinthal considered "asemia" as being synonymous with Finkelnburg's "asymbolia." He did not elaborate on the definition of apraxia. The term was introduced in passing as if it were already in common use. However, this passage is generally acknowledged as being the first printed appearance of the word "apraxia."[6]

[6] I am citing from a reprint of the second edition of Steinthal's book. This second edition was published in 1881, ten years after the first, but the preface of the editor of the reprint states that there were only minimal changes between the first and the second edition.

A psychological approach to brain functions

Steinthal defied the belief in the power of physiology for explaining mental functions (Hitzig et al., 1874; Jacyna, 1999; Eling, 2006). He stated: "Psychology is the indispensable prerequisite for a physiology of the brain" (Steinthal, 1881, p. 473) and accused the prevailing associationist model of cerebral function of overstretching the explanatory value of associations:

> Our medical doctors apparently have not yet realized the insufficiency of the category "association." Neither words, nor kneeling and making the sign of the cross, nor coins or insignia of military ranks are mere associations. Those are certainly present; but they are only the prerequisite for mental processes. And in the same way it is not just due to the inefficiency of associations if someone has forgotten how to use the pen or spoon and fork or to correctly position the bow upon the violin. (Steinthal, 1881, p. 469)

The first sentence of this quote points to another aspect of the debate between proponents of the physiological and the psychological approach to brain function. While physiology was a domain of medical doctors, psychological arguments were brought forward mainly by graduates of humanities (Hitzig et al., 1874; Jacyna, 1999). The division was not strict, however: Finkelnburg, whose proposal of asymbolia clearly belongs to the psychological camp, was a medical doctor. Nonetheless, it may be more than accidental coincidence that Hugo Liepmann, whose model of motor control united both approaches, had graduated in both fields (Goldenberg, 2003a).

Apraxia and asymbolia

Steinthal refused to relate the distinction between apraxia and asymbolia to the existence of different brain centers supporting the comprehension of signs and the use of objects. He wrote:

> The seat of symbolic action must not be separated from that of practical actions. To the machine the meaning of a movement is completely irrelevant. The meaning associated with a movement cannot make a difference to the physiological mechanism, and one and the same movement may sometimes be symbolic and sometimes practical. It cannot make a difference to the physiological mechanics whether I lift an arm for greeting or for working, whether I kneel in the service of god or for doing craftwork. (Steinthal, 1881, p. 468)

The argument that both aptitudes must have a common cerebral substrate because they exert commands of the same motor mechanisms is not necessarily compelling, but it illustrates Steinthal's refusal of cerebral localization as an explanation for dissociations between psychological entities. Instead, he offered a purely psychological explanation for dissociations between disturbed use of symbols and of objects. It started from the observation that disturbances of symbolic abilities are present in many patients and can be associated with only mild degrees of brain damage, whereas defective use of objects occurs only in severe cases in combination with aphasia. Furthermore, object use recovers earlier than symbolic aptitudes. If both abilities were supported by anatomically distinct substrates there would be no obvious reason why one of them should be more vulnerable to brain damage than the other, and there should be cases where use of objects is affected more severely and recovers later than use of symbols. The assumption that the decisive difference concerns psychological mechanisms rather than cerebral locations can offer a better explanation:

> For a purely psychological theory, the milder brain damage and later recovery of symbolic function than of object use are easily comprehensible. Associations which are based on connections of arbitrary and immaterial, purely subjective, features (and symbols belong to this category) have only little power and get more easily into confusion than associations based on objective relationships. (Steinthal, 1881, p. 471)

It is somewhat confusing that in this quote Steinthal uses the very term "association" that he criticized as being insufficient for understanding mental processes, but there are obvious differences to its use in the associationist model of brain functions. Firstly, it refers only to relationships between mental entities and makes no reference to fiber connections between areas of the brain and, secondly, the coupling of associated entities is modulated by meaningful properties like, in the given example, the arbitrariness of their connection.

The first 30 years of apraxia

Nearly 30 years elapsed between the first edition of Steinthal's book and Liepmann's report of the imperial counselor (see Chapter 2). The term "apraxia" survived this gap although the number of publications referring to it seems to be rather limited. Those I could locate[7] (Kussmaul, 1885; Laquer, 1888; Starr, 1888; Lepine, 1897; Pick, 1898) used the term apraxia to denote wrong use of tools and objects and distinguished apraxia from general dementia, aphasia, and asymbolia, but none of them considered the possibility of a link between apraxia and mind-palsy or other motor disturbances. The source of errors was sought in recognition of tools and objects rather than in motor execution of their use. For example, Kussmaul described an aphasic patient whose speech was characterized by semantic paraphasias and paragrammatism and who:

> calculated correctly, was polite, greeted, and knew the sign of the cross. But he urinated into the washbasin, bit into the soap and did more of such actions which must be referred to misrecognition of objects. He made wrong actions and suffered from what is usually designated as apraxia. It is clearly to see, that in this case the misrecognition of objects which underlies apraxia was much more severe than the misrecognition of expressive signs. (Kussmaul, 1885, p. 199)

In this quote, Kussmaul described examples of misuse that are inextricably linked to the body part involved. One can bite only with the mouth. However, the accusation of defective recognition as being the source of errors left no place for the anatomy of the motor cortex to play a decisive role for the genesis of symptoms which would manifest itself by body part specificity of errors. Provided that the patient was not hemiplegic (Kussmaul did

[7] In 1876, Hughlings Jackson described a woman with a large right-sided tumor who "Now and then would do odd things, she would put sugar in the tea two or three times over, she made mistakes in dressing herself; put her things on wrong side before, and did little things of that kind." He did not, however, use the term "apraxia" for these disturbances (Jackson, 1873/1932c). Jackson's influence on theories of apraxia will be discussed in Chapter 3.

not comment on this aspect of the case), it seems very likely that he carried the soap to the mouth, regardless of whether he had grasped it with the right or the left hand.

Parakinesia

One year before Liepmann's seminal first paper on apraxia, the Belgian neurologist David de Buck published a paper on "parakinesies" (de Buck, 1899). It started with a description of "synkinesies," that is, involuntary movements of one body part accompanying either deliberate or reflex movement of other body parts. This phenomenon is quite common in hemiplegic patients. For example, the paralyzed arm raises involuntarily when the sound arm is raised or when the patient yawns or sneezes. The major part of the paper, however, was devoted to a more exceptional observation which de Buck classified as an instance of "parakinesia." He presented the case of a 40-year-old woman who, half a day after her fifth childbirth, suddenly had the sensation that "something wanted to get out of her genitals." She retained no memory of the subsequent events but her family reported that she fell into a coma which lasted for three weeks. During that time she was nursed by her family, and de Buck remarks that he could not obtain medical reports because she was rarely, if at all, seen by medical doctors. The coma cannot have been complete as she must have been capable of swallowing food and fluid.

When she awoke, her whole body was flaccidly paralyzed and insensitive to pain, and she did not speak. Within two months mobility and speech returned but they remained abnormal. Speech was fluent and well articulated but distorted by repetitions of letters, syllables, and sometimes whole words, and she did not always find the right word to express her ideas. The most remarkable symptoms concerned the posture and mobility of her body and her limbs. De Buck described her appearance:

> Stout woman with the appearance of good physical health. But what's striking the examiner is her posture. Regardless of whether she is sitting or standing, she never displays the usual posture of rest with both upper limbs hanging down or resting on the knees. They are in demi-flexion crossed one over the other before her chest. Her gaze is directed downwards and her face expresses melancholy. The posture frequently has a cataleptic appearance. (de Buck, 1899, p. 366)

She seemed to be unable to perform even the simplest actions and replaced them by rather bizarre movements which were performed with much apparent effort. For example:

> When asked to raise her right arm, she makes energetic efforts, the right hand crosses the trunk and is placed in the left armpit and the left hand extends backwards. Then the left hand tugs with effort her skirts. (de Buck, 1899, p. 366)

Generally, her movements deteriorated when she was asked to pay attention to them. The dependence of the severity of disturbance from the context of examination went even further:

> when she believes that she is not observed but left on her own in solitude, she executes swiftly quite complex movements like scratching her face or the hair. If she is asked shortly afterwards to execute the same movements, she is totally unable to make them but replaces them by series of substitute movements. (de Buck, 1899, p. 372)

Clinical wisdom says that a disorder which vanishes when the patient believes they are unobserved does not, or at least not only, have an organic cause. But rather than embarking on a psychiatric diagnosis, de Buck proposed an explanation in terms of motor control. He postulated that:

> our patient has the idea of her actions, but does not arrive at evoking the corresponding kinetic images. There is a rupture between the centres of movement and the area of ideation . . . The perturbation that gives rise to the parakinesie takes place in the transmission from the mental sphere to the sphere of motor images. (de Buck, 1899, p. 373)

This explanation leaves open the question why the transition from the idea to the execution of voluntary actions depends on whether the patient believes herself to be observed. Nonetheless, it merits David de Buck's admission into the hall of fame of apraxia. He had arrived at almost exactly the same ideas, and used nearly identical formulations for describing them, as Liepmann in his seminal first paper on apraxia which appeared only one year later.

Chapter 2

Hugo Karl Liepmann

Since the beginning of the twentieth century, clinical diagnosis and research of apraxia has been dominated by the writings of the German neuropsychiatrist Hugo Karl Liepmann (Goldenberg, 2003a) (Figure 2.1). Liepmann was born in Berlin in 1863, the son of a cultured and wealthy Jewish family.[1] He studied philosophy and acquired a PhD with a thesis on the mechanism of Leukipp–Democrit's atoms, but then entered university again to study medicine and acquired his MD in 1895. In the same year he started as an assistant to Wernicke in Breslau where he stayed until 1899. He then returned to Berlin and took a post at the municipal welfare for the mentally ill. He was first assistant, then consultant in the psychiatric hospital of Dalldorf (known today as the Karl Bonhoeffer Psychiatric Clinic, Berlin-Lichtenau) and from 1915 director of the psychiatric hospital in Herzberge (today Berlin-Lichtenberg).

The imperial counselor

In Liepmann's times, a substantial portion of patients in psychiatric hospitals were afflicted by dementia caused by general paralysis of the insane, a late manifestation of syphilis infection. On February 10, 1900, one such patient was admitted to the psychiatric hospital of Dalldorf where Liepmann had only recently started to work. The patient was a 48-year-old engineer who had worked in the imperial patent office. Since he was employed as an official he was qualified to bear the proud title of an "imperial counselor," but he had almost certainly never given advice to the German Emperor. He had acquired syphilis some ten years ago. His present illness had begun suddenly two months ago with a state of confusion accompanied by aphasia and agitated depression.

Liepmann described his first encounter with the patient, one week after his admission:

> I saw the patient for the first time on February 17. He was asked to point to certain objects and to carry out certain hand movements. He failed in almost everything, handling objects quite absurdly. At first sight it appeared as if the patient did not understand—that he was cortically deaf, possibly also cortically blind. However, I noted certain bizarre and distorted movements which he made during the course of the examination; they were confined to the right upper extremity which the patient used exclusively during the period of observation. This peculiar motor behaviour made me wonder if his incorrect responses reflected a basic lack of comprehension or, rather, faulty

[1] A substantial portion of the German clinicians and scientists contributing to the early development of apraxia were Jews, although partly converted to the Christian religion. I have indicated only their civic nationality because I think that this corresponds better to their own attitude versus religion and nation.

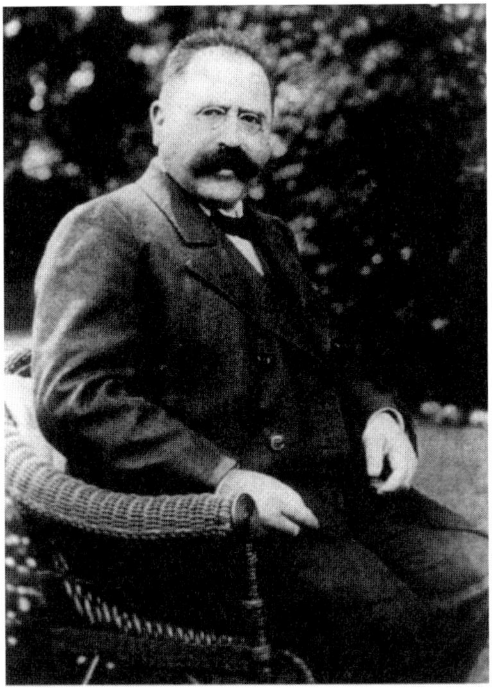

Figure 2.1 Hugo Karl Liepmann.

> motor execution . . . To resolve this question I held on to the patient's right hand and forced him to use his left hand. Now, all of a sudden, the picture changed. With his left hand he immediately selected the card that was asked for from among five cards laid out in front of him. The same test repeated with the right hand led in general to faulty responses. I then established that the situation was the same as regards his lower extremities. The patient could imitate movements of my foot with his left foot but failed altogether with his right foot. Thus, it was established that the patient had neither word-deafness nor mind-blindness. Reproduced from Liepmann, H., Das Krankheitsbild der Apraxie (motorische Asymbolie) auf Grund eines Falles von einseitiger Apraxie. Monatschrift für Psychiatrie und Neurologie, 8, p. 19 © 1900, Karger, with permission.

This quote is from the fourth page of the first paper devoted to the "imperial counselor." Others were to follow. In the end, Liepmann's reports of this single case had given rise to 137 printed pages distributed on a tripartite paper (Liepmann, 1900) and another two-part paper (Liepmann, 1905a, 1906) reporting the subsequent clinical course, death, and post-mortem of the patient.

I will try to briefly summarize the main findings of Liepmann's extensive and methodically ingenious examinations:

Spontaneous speech was restricted to a small repertoire of exclamations like "yes" "oh God," "no," and he was unable to repeat any words. Comprehension of spoken commands varied according to which body part was addressed. He promptly followed commands for moving the whole body like standing up or going to a window, but was unable to follow commands for even simple movements of the head, the mouth, or the tongue. Whereas verbal commands were executed promptly using the left hand and named objects could be selected from an array, the right hand acted as if he could not understand anything at all.

The same pattern of preserved and disturbed compliance applied to written commands and also to imitation: he correctly imitated movements with the left leg and the left hand, but not with the right limbs, the head, mouth, and tongue.

Writing to dictation with the right hand produced a regular sequence of up and down strokes interspersed with single recognizable letters which had no relationship to the target word. On first sight, his left-handed writing looked completely aberrant, but on close inspection it turned out that the left hand produced mirror writing. The letters were drawn awkwardly and irregularly, and some of them were completely wrong, but the intended words were always recognizable. The left hand could also compose words out of single anagram letters whereas this task gave rise only to meaningless letter sequences when tried by the right hand.

When he was asked to point blindfolded with one hand to the location where the other hand had been touched, he failed in both directions though with somewhat different kinds of errors. The right hand did not follow the command at all, whereas the left hand tried to comply but made gross spatial errors. These errors were particularly impressive when single fingers of the right hand had been pricked. Then the left hand would search for the location of the prick on the forearm, while the right hand made small movements with the pricked finger as if it wanted to help the other hand finding the right place.

Unimanual use of objects was normal with the left hand. By contrast, the right hand committed impressive errors. For example, when given a comb the right hand stuck it behind the ear like a pen. The right hand used a toothbrush like a pen on one occasion and put the handle into the mouth on another. On a third trial the right hand took the toothbrush like a spoon, shoveled with it, and finally put it into the mouth.

Generally right-hand performance was better when the required actions were embedded in their natural context rather than being asked for in an examination, and there were a few activities in which the right hand nearly always succeeded. One such activity was smoking a cigar and another, that Liepmann considered particularly important for his interpretation of the imperial counselor's apraxia, was buttoning:

> The patient is always capable to button and unbutton. However, this happens virtually never after a first request, and sometimes much exhortation is necessary to get him to begin the action. But once the fingers have touched the button, the remainder of the action is performed with considerable deftness, even when the eyes are closed. (Liepmann, 1900, p. 32)

Bimanual coordination varied across different tasks. Seated before a piano, he placed both hands correctly and played simple recognizable melodies, though with errors. By contrast, he was unable to cooperate with both hands to spread butter on a slice of bread or to make a knot in a scarf. Sometimes the right hand interfered with unimanual left-hand activities:

> He is asked to pour water from a jug into a glass. The left hand takes the jug and wants to pour, but at the same time the right hand leads the empty glass to the mouth. If one holds onto the glass and thus enables the left hand to pour, it succeeds without further problems. (Liepmann, 1900, p. 35)

Figure 2.2 shows a snapshot of this episode and a similar observation made some 80 years later (Goldenberg et al., 1985).

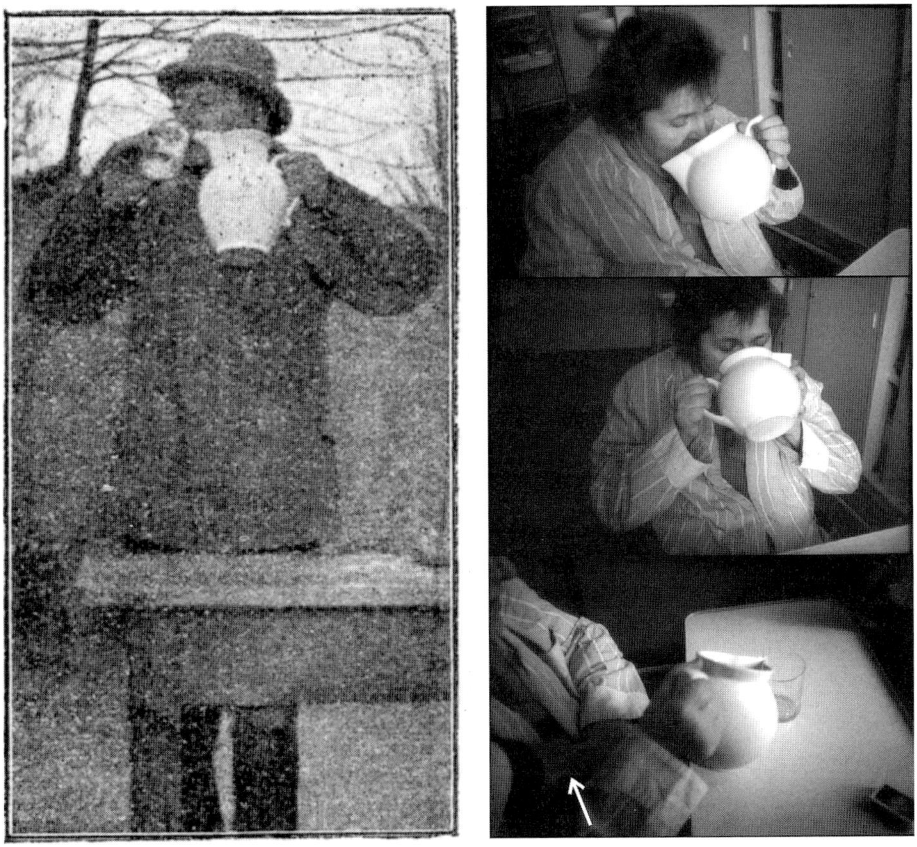

Figure 2.2 Left: The imperial counselor was asked to pour water from a jug into a glass with the left hand. The right hand interfered and took the glass to the mouth. The left hand followed with the jug. Reproduced from Liepmann, H. (1900). Das Krankheitsbild der Apraxie (motorische Asymbolie) auf Grund eines Falles von einseitiger Apraxie. *Monatschrift für Psychiatrie und Neurologie*, *8*, p. 34 © 1900, Karger, with permission. Right: A very similar observation made some 80 years later. In this patient with callosal disconnection the left hand was apraxic. Reproduced from G. Goldenberg, A. Wimmer, F. Holzner, and P. Wessely. Apraxia of the left limbs in a case of callosal disconnection: The contribution of medial frontal lobe damage. Cortex. 21, pp.135–148 © 1985, Elsevier. She was asked to pour water from a jug into a glass. *Top*: when the handle was on the left side the left hand took the jug and led it to the mouth for drinking. *Middle*: when the handle was on the right side, the right hand took it, but the left hand touched the other side of the jug and both together led the jug to the mouth. *Bottom*: when the examiner's hand (arrow) touched the patient's left hand and thus prevented its interference, the right hand poured water into the glass. Note that in both observations the conflict between both hands was brought forward by the similarity of their movements. The imperial counselor raised both hands toward the mouth, and our patient's right hand followed the intention of the left hand to raise the jug to the mouth as long as the left hand was not retained from the space of action. We will come back to this aspect of intermanual conflict in Chapter 14.

The patient reacted to his deficiencies with shame and depression, but retained not only his well-educated and polite manners but also the patriotic convictions appropriate for a German official:

> It has already been mentioned that the patient could reproduce some familiar melodies on the piano, albeit rather primitive for a proficient piano player which he allegedly was. By contrast he could join in singing melodies without errors. When singing "Hail thee in the victor's wreath"[2] he even articulated sounds with some resemblance to single vocals of the text. Having sung several songs in this way he was presented the Marseillaise. He joined in but then suddenly stopped, without doubts because he considered the performance of this song improper for a person of his rank. (Liepmann, 1900, p. 41)

It seems difficult, if not impossible, to explain all of these observations by one common mechanism and to guess the location of the causal lesions, but Liepmann met this challenge. He proposed that there must be several lesions which together isolate the left central sensorimotor region from the remainder of the brain. The preservation of right-handed buttoning was a central argument for this interpretation since it proved the intactness of fine graded motor coordination and tactile sensation of the right hand. The direct connection between them constituted a "short circuit" from local sensation to motor commands which enabled performance of a limited repertoire of highly practiced actions but failed when appropriate action required connections to visual information or verbal commands or to any other function located in other brain regions. Similarly, the short circuit between kinesthetic feedback from, and motor commands to, the leg enabled walking but did not suffice for imitation of visually presented leg movements. Even the severe reduction of verbal output could be accommodated by this mechanism. The intactness of sensorimotor coordination of the oral muscles was proven by intact chewing, moving of the bolus by the tongue, and swallowing. This sufficed for production of a few high-frequency words, but the disconnection from the acoustic images of words as well as from visual images of objects prevented the use of the intact articulators for more differentiated speech. "The aphasia shown by our patient is apraxia of the motor apparatus of speech" (Liepmann, 1900, p. 129).

Liepmann admitted that the disconnection of sensorimotor coordination of right limbs and bilateral speech muscles from the remainder of the brain could not be absolute. For example, buttoning could be induced by repeated verbal commands, and the involuntary grasping and leading to the mouth of a glass would be impossible without visual perception of the glass. Joining in a song requires a connection of acoustic input with motor control of the articulators, and its interruption when the song offended the patient's patriotism testifies of an intervention by brain mechanism transgressing the motor coordination of speech.

---

[2] "Heil dir im Siegerkranze." Though not a national anthem in the strict sense, this song praising the power and wisdom of the German Emperor Wilhelm was sung at festive opportunities particularly if they were related to Germany and its Emperor.

The observations reported in the first series of papers had been collected from February to June 1900. In 1905 and 1906, a further two-part paper (Liepmann, 1905a, 1906) reported the subsequent course and the results of the post-mortem examination. In the second half of 1900 the imperial counselor showed some improvement, particularly of speech, but then he suffered repeated strokes and finally died on April 8, 1902. Post-mortem examination[3] was compatible with Liepmann's predictions. The corpus callosum, that is, the big fiber bundle connecting the cortex of both hemispheres, was atrophied along its full length with the exception of its most posterior portion connecting the visual areas. In addition there were large subcortical infarctions beneath the left parietal and the left frontal lobes. Liepmann concluded:

> Summing up the major findings, both left central gyri prove to be deprived of many connections to the frontal cortex by the subcortical frontal focus, disconnected from the occipital and the temporal lobe by the parietal subcortical focus, and completely disconnected from the whole right hemisphere by the atrophy of the corpus callosum. (Liepmann, 1905a, p. 310)

This summary demonstrates quite clearly that Liepmann's interpretation of the anatomical findings was "hodological" (Catani & ffytche, 2005; ffytche & Catani, 2005): it considered lesions of the fiber tracts connecting brain areas as equally or even more relevant than lesions to the cortical areas themselves. In this respect Liepmann remained faithful to Wernicke's and Meynert's associationist dictum that only the cortical insertions of sensory afferences and motor efferences are narrowly localized whereas their "combinations to concept, thinking, consciousness, are an achievement of the masses of fibres which link the different sectors of the cerebral cortex among each other" (Wernicke, 1874). Liepmann corroborated this stance in a later paper:

> I do not believe at all that there is a praxis centre, let alone that it is, as I have occasionally been misunderstood, in the supramarginal gyrus. I never proposed that the apraxia of the imperial counsellor was caused only by the focus in the supramarginal gyrus. I postulated a separation of the sensorimotor region of the right limbs from cortical areas of both hemispheres and believed that this was achieved by interruptions in the white matter of the supramarginal gyrus and of callosal connections to the other hemisphere.
>
> I have argued that eupractic action is bound to the cooperation of multiple cerebral territories with the hand centre, and that lesions of the involved cortical territories and particularly their connections with the hand centre can destroy eupraxia. (Liepmann, 1908, p. 77)

We will interrupt the discussion of the case history at this point. It is beside the point whether or not Liepmann's account of this particular case remains convincing when confronted with our current knowledge about brain mechanisms of motor control. There are reasons to doubt, but they do not invalidate the historical significance of Liepmann's single case report. It provided the empirical material upon which he built the foundations of a comprehensive theory of apraxia.

---

3 Liepmann himself did not perform pathological examinations. The post-mortem examination of the imperial counselor was done by Oscar and Cecilie Vogt.

Theoretical foundations of apraxia

A large part of Liepmann's reports of the imperial counselor were devoted to discussion of theoretical foundations of apraxia. Combining critical discussion of the previous literature on mind-palsy, asymbolia, and apraxia with relevant observations of his own case study, Liepmann developed a coherent conceptual framework for apraxia. We will first consider his discussion of the previous literature.

Mind-palsy

Liepmann reduced mind-palsy to a loss of limb-kinetic memories which are stored within the sensorimotor region. He argued that such memories are limited to a few highly over-learned motor actions of that limb: "kinetic—(innervatory)—kinaesthetic memory images within the central region can be assumed only for relatively simple and excessively practiced movements, like walking or knitting etc" (Liepmann, 1905a, p. 240). Their loss could not account for the ubiquitous difficulties of the imperial counselor. On the contrary, highly practiced routine actions like buttoning which should be the first victims of such loss of limb-specific memories stood out as islands of preserved motor aptitudes.

Liepmann recognized, however, that "Bruns' lucid exposition has put mind palsy on another anatomical basis which has much in common with the anatomical basis on which I have put apraxia," but dismissed it nonetheless because in Bruns' case mind-palsy was associated with absent rather than deviating actions and thus "with a clinical presentation which differs widely from the clinical picture of apraxia" (Liepmann, 1905a, p. 243).

Asymbolia

Liepmann recognized that the term "asymbolia" had originally been introduced by Finkelnburg to characterize "all forms of disturbed production or comprehension of signs" but had received a different interpretation as "loss of memory images" in Wernicke's and Meynert's concept of "motor asymbolia." In the 1900 part of his paper "motor asymbolia" appeared as a parenthesis in the title. In the 1905 part it had vanished. Liepmann commented on the deletion:

> In my first publication I related in dutiful reverence to Meynert's "motor asymbolia," but now I must emphasize the important differences between this syndrome and my motor apraxia. Meynert places the seat of motor asymbolia in the central region, whereas I locate that of my apraxia in the connections between the central region and the rest of the brain. He assumes that the "innervation images" of the extremities have been lost, whereas I assume that they are dissociated from the entirety of the psychic life. Meynert's innervation images are identical to what I have designated as possession of the sensori-motor region, as limb-kinetic images. Just this possession of the sensorimotor region was preserved in the imperial counsellor. He could walk, button, point etc. (Liepmann, 1905a, p. 235)

The critiques of mind-palsy and of motor asymbolia limited the role of "limb kinetic memories" to swift performance of a few highly practiced motor acts. Liepmann distinguished these limited local "possessions" of the central regions from the associative network supporting consciousness and psychic functions. This separation severed the continuity of neural networks connecting motor control with mental processes and called for the introduction of an anatomically and functionally distinct connection bridging the cleft.

Liepmann did not discuss Finkelnburg's original conception of asymbolia in the papers on the imperial counselor but returned to it later when he had found out that apraxia is predominantly linked to left hemisphere damage and in most cases is accompanied by aphasia.

Apraxia

Liepmann was unaware of Steinthal's contribution when he wrote his report of the imperial counselor The first time he mentioned Steinthal was in 1920, in a book chapter, where he credited him with having introduced the term "apraxia" and with having used it in the same sense as he had done, but noted that this had only recently been discovered (Liepmann, 1920).[4] In the papers devoted to the imperial counselor, the discussion of apraxia referred to contemporary authors using this diagnosis for disturbances of tool and object use. Liepmann made the criticism that they had explained faulty use of objects mainly by misrecognition of objects: "Apraxia was in this sense a disorder of recognition, an agnosia" (Liepmann, 1905a, p. 238). By contrast, he sought the source of faulty object use not in the perceptual access to knowledge about objects and their use but in the translation of this knowledge into appropriate motor actions:

> The case described in this work reveals something new: it is possible that one recognizes an object, knows how to use it, his limbs may be freely movable, even the innervation images in the limb centres may be preserved, and yet he is unable to use the object with certain limbs. (Liepmann, 1905a, p. 238)

We now see the theoretical importance of Liepmann's insistence on a discontinuity between local limb-kinetic memories and the neural basis of mental processes. This discontinuity created the need for a distinct connection between functionally and anatomically separated areas and hence the possibility that such a connection could be destroyed without major damage to the connected parts themselves.

In order to emphasize the difference between his new interpretation of apraxia and that of previous authors, Liepmann called his new version of apraxia "motor apraxia" or, in later papers, "ideo-kinetic apraxia."

The multimodality of the movement formula

Liepmann's idea that all but the most highly practiced movements of the limbs are directed by connections from widespread cortical areas to the central region was not meant to imply that "kinetic–kinesthetic images" of the required movements were sent from their

[4] Wernicke had mentioned Steinthal's work, though not explicitly his use of the term apraxia in his thesis (1874). However, Liepmann joined Wernicke only 20 years later and it is plausible that Wernicke did not find it worthwhile to alert his disciples to Steinthal's treatise which defended ideas opposite to his own.

original storage place to the central region. He rather conceived of the original representation as multimodal images specifying the intended body configuration or the intended effect of the action upon the external world. He named these images "movement formula." He thought that they were dominated by the visual modality. For example, "in combing the sequence of single movements is maintained by the influence of visual images of the comb, the head, and the hairs" (Liepmann, 1900, p. 123). The predominance of vision is, however, not obligatory. For example, when playing a musical instrument, the movements are guided by acoustic images of the intended melodies, and when scratching oneself by the somatosensory image of the itching body part. These multimodal images are preserved in motor apraxia but their disconnection from the central motor region deprives them of the power to control the sequential flow of local kinetic–kinesthetic images.

From anatomy to psychology

Liepmann's "dutiful reverence" to Wernicke and Meynert influenced not only the choice of the title but also the style of his papers. He adhered quite strictly to the language of anatomy and physiology and mostly avoided terms referring to mental contents such as, for example, consciousness or will. When he could not resist the temptation to rise above the strictly organic level into the realm of mental life (remember that he was a doctor of philosophy!) he mitigated this deviation by pretending that he was just translating his scientific discoveries into the language of "popular psychology":[5]

> The clinical picture which we have demonstrated and analyzed is a further step on the way paved by Broca, Wernicke and others. These scientists have proven that certain "abilities" of the mind[6] as they are assumed by popular psychology get lost after damage to circumscribed parts of the brain. Damage of one defined territory destroys one defined ability like the linguistic expression of thought, and damage of another the comprehension of language, while comprehension of visual, acoustic, tactile entities depends on intactness of still other parts of the brain.
>
> Apraxia adds to these partial diseases of the mind caused by circumscribed brain damage a new one. Damage to a part of the brain destroys what popular psychology calls the government of the limbs by the mind. Moreover, it appears that this government can be abolished independently for only the right or the left side of the body. Popular psychology would explain this condition by saying that the will has lost control of the right half of the body although the movement apparatus is intact. (Liepmann, 1900, p. 191)

Later, when Liepmann had become an authority himself, he did not need to disguise his excursions into psychology with reference to "popular psychology" any more. Nonetheless he used the same expressions for explaining the psychological side of motor apraxia:

> The kinematics of the limbs must be set in cooperation with the whole cerebral cortex. Psychologically this means communication of kinematics with optics, acoustics, with all contents of the mind, and hence the government of the limbs by the mind. (Liepmann, 1913, p. 489)

[5] Liepmann spoke of "Populäre Psychologie." "Popular psychology" is the literal translation but presumably "folk psychology" would better correspond to our understanding of the term.

[6] In German "Seele" which means both the mind and the immortal soul.

A further excursion into the psychological side of brain function concerned the conscious nature of multimodal and limb kinetic movement images:

> The word "movement image" needs a clarification. Is it really an image, a distinct content of consciousness, a clear memory of all sensations which accompanied previously executed movements? This can be admitted without restriction for the optical component, but not for the kinaesthetic one. How my motorium selects the muscles it has to innervate, the strength and the sequence of single impulses: Nothing of this comes into my consciousness. However, although the memories of previous kinaesthetic sensations are represented in consciousness only very incompletely, they must have a material (nervous) equivalent; because "learning" by practice presupposes that the repeated execution of movements leaves permanent changes in the nervous system which cause what we call: to know a movement.
>
> If one talk about a movement image one should be aware that for the kinaesthetic part the word "image" does not apply in a strict sense; it serves only a short summary of the entirety of the permanent material traces of previous centripetal stimuli. It designates not a psychological but a physiological concept. (Liepmann, 1900, pp. 121–122)

Translated into modern terms, this rather complicated passage opposes procedural motor learning to the conscious representation of actions and characterizes the former as "physiological" and the latter as "psychological." Apart from its genuine historical interest as an early formulation of the nowadays widely recognized distinction between procedural and declarative, or implicit and explicit, learning and memory (Tulving, 1985; Squire et al., 1993), the distinction emphasizes once again that to Liepmann the flow from widespread cortical areas to the sensorimotor region was more than just a displacement of motor images from one area of the brain to another. It was associated with the transformation of conscious, multimodal mental images of intended actions into a sequence of motor commands inaccessible to introspective consciousness, or, in Liepmann's nomenclature, a translation from the psychological to the physiological side of motor control.

Liepmann's fame

Liepmann's reports of the imperial counselor were received enthusiastically by the scientific community. Karl Heilbronner, another disciple of Wernicke who had worked on "motor asymbolia," began the first paper he wrote after the publication of Liepmann's report: "Liepmann's fundamental study has obtained a permanent residence in neurology for apraxia" (Heilbronner, 1905, p. 161). Arnold Pick, whose contribution to "ideational apraxia" will be discussed later in this chapter, started a case report published in 1902: "Liepmann's fundamental study of apraxia has provided a decisive insight into the mechanics of the relevant processes" (Pick, 1902, p. 994). The British neurologist Kinnier Wilson characterized the case report of the imperial counselor as a "classic case of apraxia, which will remain a monument of clinical insight and examinational ingenuity" (Wilson, 1908, p. 166).

At the end of Chapter 1 I referred to the Belgian neurologist De Buck who had used formulations very similar to those of Liepmann to characterize "parakinesia" consequential to interrupted transmission from the mental sphere to the sphere of motor images (de Buck, 1899). De Buck's article appeared 1899 in the September issue of the *Belgian*

Journal de Neurologie, that is, about four months before Liepmann's first examination of the imperial counselor. Presumably Liepmann had not read De Buck's paper when he wrote the case report of the imperial counselor. In any case he did not mention it. He referred to it only in a much later review (Liepmann, 1920) as "having remained hidden for a long time"[7] and acknowledged that De Buck's "dissociation between idea and movement corresponds to ideo-kinetic apraxia, provided that de Buck's centre of ideation is translated into a multitude of cerebral regions" (Liepmann, 1920, p. 17).[8]

It is unlikely that the similarity between Liepmann's and De Buck's formulation indicates plagiarism. It rather demonstrates that the underlying assumption of two hierarchically ordered levels of motor control was already in the air and ready for being spelled out. Indeed, variants of this dichotomy can be identified in Munk's distinction between cortical paresis and mind-paresis, in Meynert's and Wernicke's opposition of localized motor memories to the associative network connecting them with other modalities, and in Finkelnburg's and Steinthal's defense of the importance of psychological analysis, since this defense aimed at limiting the explanatory power of low-level physiological processes but did not deny their existence. The expectation that brain damage could interrupt the control of the lower level by the higher one was a logical consequence of this basic dichotomy. It was explicitly formulated first by De Buck and then, independently, by Liepmann.

Doubts upon the priority of Liepmann's basic concepts should not detract from the originality and profoundness of his work. They underline, however, that Liepmann's ideas were successful not only because of their novelty but also, and perhaps even more, because of their familiarity to a scientific community coming to grips with the division between the mental and the bodily side of action control.

Apraxia and hemisphere dominance

The imperial counselor had apraxia of the right hand while the left one acted normally. For Liepmann, the unilaterality of the disorders was crucial for the diagnosis of motor apraxia, but side did not matter. A disconnection between sensorimotor cortex and the rest of the brain would have been equally credible for unilateral left-sided apraxia. Nor was laterality a central issue for Meynert's and Wernicke's associationist approach which derived localization of cortical functions mainly from the anatomy of afferent and efferent connections to the periphery which do not differ between right and left hemisphere. Nonetheless, Liepmann undertook a systematic study of the differential effect of right and left brain damage. Perhaps he wanted to explore whether the degradation of expressive gestures, described by Finkelnburg as an obligatory accompaniment of aphasia, could be a manifestation of apraxia.

[7] Arnold Pick cited De Buck's article in 1905 (Pick, 1905b).

[8] Liepmann did not comment on the difference between circumscribed organic brain damage of his case and the possibility of a psychiatric illness in De Buck's patient. Indeed, he did not consider this as a sharp and insurmountable distinction. In another section of the paper he even proposed that in hysteria the "interruption is located at the same part of the psyche" as in apraxia, since in both of them "the will has lost his dominance over the apparatus" (Liepmann, 1900, p. 197).

Between 1900 and 1905 Liepmann performed a "mass study" of apraxia. Since at that time there were no means to directly assess the laterality of brain damage, it was inferred from the clinical symptoms. Right-sided hemiparesis and aphasia were taken to indicate left brain damage, and left-sided hemiparesis right brain damage. Liepmann examined 42 patients with left-sided and 41 with right-sided hemiparesis as well as five aphasic patients without hemiparesis with a collection of tests for apraxia. In order to clearly separate apraxia from paresis, he always examined the hand ipsilateral to the lesion, that is, the right hand in patients with left-sided paresis and vice versa. He asked patients first to perform a number of "expressive movements" like threatening, beckoning, military salute, or swearing, and then to pretend the performance of object-related "transitive" movements like knocking, pulling the door bell, catching a fly, turning a barrel organ, etc. Furthermore he tested the actual manipulation of objects, like combing, brushing the examiner's sleeve, sealing a letter, etc. Finally, he "never missed letting them imitate movements" (Liepmann, 1908).

The results were clear-cut: in patients with left-sided paresis, there were rare instances of difficulties with single items, but generally they performed flawlessly. "Their examination was astonishingly swift; their movements went like clockwork." The same applied to an additional control group composed of non-paretic senile and demented patients. By contrast, 20 of the 41 patients with right-sided hemiplegia, and three of the seven non-paretic aphasic patients committed many errors. Liepmann noted no difference between the severity of errors for expressive and transitive movements on command. Twenty of the 23 patients who had problems with movements on command had difficulties also with their imitation, whereas manipulation of real objects was disturbed in only six of them.

Six apraxic patients had no aphasia and four aphasic patients had no apraxia. From this double dissociation Liepmann concluded that aphasia and apraxia are independent symptoms of left brain damage.

Callosal apraxia

A few years after completion of the group study a series of single case studies endorsed the left hemisphere dominance for action control. Together with the neurologist Otto Maas, Liepmann published a short report of a right-handed patient who had suffered a stroke rendering the right limbs plegic (Liepmann & Maas, 1907). He had no aphasia, but was completely unable to write, to copy letters, or to compose words from anagram letters with the left hand. The left hand was skillful for everyday actions like buttoning, eating, or drinking from a glass, but committed gross errors when confronted with less routine tasks. For example, when a pince-nez was handed to him, he:

> brought it to the mouth, sticked out the tongue and tried to put the pince-nez on the rolled up tongue. Given a matchbox and asked to light a match, he brought the box to the mouth, took out two matches with the tongue, put one of them on the table, and kept the other in the mouth as if it were a cigar (Liepmann & Maas, 1907, p. 217).

He also committed gross errors when verbally asked to make left-hand movements. He died before more extensive examinations could be performed. Post-mortem examination displayed two lesions. One was in the brainstem while the other, much larger one, destroyed the anterior and middle portion of the corpus callosum. Liepmann and Maas referred the paresis of the right limbs to the brainstem focus and reasoned that agraphia and apraxia of the left hand were due to callosal disconnection depriving the right-sided motor cortex from its connections to the left hemisphere (see Figure 2.3).

Soon after Liepmann and Maas' publication a number of case reports by other authors supported and complemented the proposal that destruction of the corpus callosum causes apraxia of the left limbs (Hartmann, 1907; Maas, 1907; Van Vleuten, 1907; Goldstein, 1908, 1909; Kroll, 1910). These reports demonstrated that left-hand apraxia in patients with extensive callosal lesions is not restricted to defective writing and defective execution of verbal command but can also affect imitation of gestures and, like in Liepmann and Maas' own case, the actual use of objects. Kurt Goldstein, another disciple of Wernicke, provided an impressive description of conflicts between the patient's conscious intentions and the actions of her left hand in a woman whose corpus callosum and adjacent right medial frontal lobe had been destroyed by ischemic stroke:

> The patient complained that her left hand refused to obey her and did what it wanted. Once it had seized her throat and choked strongly. It could be detached only by force. Likewise, it had torn to pieces the bed linen against the patient's will. When the left hand had grasped something it would not let it go again; "when I am drinking and it gets hold of the cup, it does not let it go but pours out the fluid. I hit it and say: my little hand, be quiet. There must be a bad spirit in this hand." (Goldstein, 1908, p. 170; see also Chapter 14, this volume)

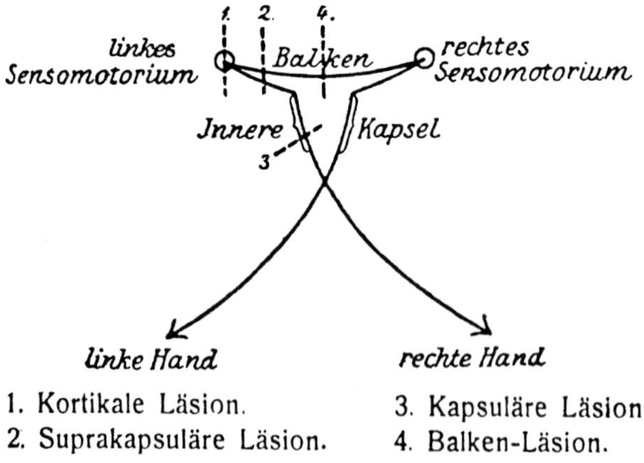

Figure 2.3 The "vertical schema" illustrates the putative anatomical basis of unilateral left-sided apraxia. Linkes/rechtes Sensomotorium: left/right sensorimotor regions; Balken: corpus callosum; Innere Kapsel: internal capsule; Linke/rechte Hand: left/right hand; Kortikale Läsion: cortical lesion; Suprakapsuläre Läsion: supracapsular lesion; Kapsuläre Läsion: capsular lesion; Balken Läsion: callosal lesion. The left sensorimotor region commands the right hand via the internal capsule and the left hand via the corpus callosum. Isolated callosal lesions (4) cause only apraxia of the left hand, whereas isolated capsular lesions (3) cause only paresis of the right hand. Lesions in 1 or 2 combine both. The combination may also arise from two lesions, one in 4 and one in 3. This was assumed to the case in Liepmann and Maas' patient. Reproduced from Liepmann, H. (1908). *Drei Aufsätze aus dem Apraxiegebiet*, p. 59 © 1908, Karger, with permission.

Revisiting the imperial counselor

The demonstration of unilateral apraxia after destruction of the corpus callosum was at the same time a confirmation of, and a challenge to the validity of Liepmann's analysis of the imperial counselor. It confirmed that destruction of the corpus callosum can render one side of the body apraxic, but it challenged the laterality of the imperial counselor's apraxia, because in his case the right rather than the left hand bore the sequels of disconnection. Since the right hand is commanded directly by the left hemisphere, its callosal apraxia implied that disconnection from the right hemisphere had rendered it apraxic, and that consequently the right hemisphere was dominant for deliberate movement control. Liepmann was aware of this contradiction and proposed two possible explanations (Liepmann, 1908). Firstly, he noted that, although the imperial counselor was a right-hander, he usually played out cards with the left hand and speculated that he might have had some degree of ambidexterity. Since Liepmann believed that the cerebral lateralization of apraxia was closely linked to handedness (see Chapter 12), he considered deviant lateralization in an ambidextrous patient as conceivable. Secondly, Liepmann now emphasized that the imperial counselor's left hand had performed voluntary actions much better than the right but not faultlessly. The dramatic difference between left and right hand had concealed the minor degree of apraxia of the left hand.

Seen from a distance of more than 100 years and from the top of the large mountain of studies on apraxia accumulated since then, the case of the imperial counselor still remains somewhat of a riddle. To my knowledge there has been only one further report of callosal apraxia of the right hand but this patient was completely left-handed (Poncet et al., 1978). The quest for replication or re-interpretation of Liepmann's seminal case is still open.

Apraxia, language, and handedness

In right-handers the leading role of the left hemisphere for praxis coincides with left-hemisphere dominance for speech and with motor control of the dominant right hand. As we have already mentioned in the discussion of his group study, Liepmann dismissed a strong link between apraxia and aphasia because of their double dissociation[9] in patients with left-hemisphere damage. He recognized a correspondence between apraxia and degraded gestural expression in aphasic patients, but in contrast to Finkelnburg he considered the degradation of expressive gestures as a symptom of apraxia rather than of general asymbolia. He argued that the feature which made expressive gestures vulnerable to left brain damage was the need to perform them "purely from memory" without support from

[9] "Double dissociation" is a central concept in neuropsychology. It is diagnosed when opposite relations between preserved and defective abilities, so that the ability that is preserved in one of them is impaired in the other and vice versa. It is taken as proof that the abilities are supported by different neural substrates. In modern neuropsychology this conclusion can be endorsed by the demonstration of different locations of underlying lesions (Shallice, 1988).

manual interaction with external objects.[10] Again, this contention was supported by his group study where nearly all patients who failed on expressive and transitive gestures to command failed also on imitation which does not put particularly high demands on "symbolic function," whereas only a minority failed on real object use.

Liepmann believed that the left-hemisphere dominance for praxis is closely related to handedness:

> Right-handedness means that the right hand can do many things which the left cannot. Our results show that even that what the left hand can is to a large part not it's (respectively the right hemisphere's) property, but is borrowed from the right hand (respectively, the left hemisphere). The right sided hand centre which in most cases has learned all higher achievements only after the left one, remains lifelong to some degree dependent on the left hemisphere. (Liepmann, 1908, pp. 34–35)

The hypothesis of a close functional link between laterality of lesions causing apraxia and handedness makes the testable prediction that in left-handers apraxia should invariably be associated with right brain damage. I will come back to this prediction (Chapter 12), but conclude at this point that the choice of handedness rather than language or symbolic functions as the decisive feature of hemisphere asymmetry is equivalent to a preference of motor skill over mental aptitudes or, respectively, physiology over psychology for explanation of cerebral function.

A posterior to anterior stream of action control

In the following years Liepmann elaborated a general model of voluntary action control which served as a basis for the classification of different variants of apraxia. The center of this model was the "government of the limbs by the mind," that is, the conversion of images of the intended action into motor commands which is disturbed by "ideo-kinetic apraxia." Figure 2.4 shows one early and two later variants of his model. Liepmann distinguished three elements acting together in the voluntary control of actions:

1 the movement formula
2 the ability to transform it into motor innervations
3 for a limited number of movements a kinetic memory. (Liepmann, 1908, p. 44)

The movement formula is a multimodal, predominantly visual, mental image of the intended action. In the first version of the diagram the movement formula is a product of the whole cortex, whereas in the later versions it originates mainly from the left hemisphere. Moreover, the later versions shift the region of origin posteriorly into occipital

[10] Liepmann extended this argument to left-hemisphere dominance for speech. He speculated that the "motor act of speaking is also a movement without objects. Tongue, mouth, and palate move only relative to each other, similar to the hand in expressive gestures or miming of object use. The control exerted by the ear during speaking is not equivalent to the guidance which hand and eye receive from manipulated objects" (Liepmann, 1908, p. 49). This hypothesis is, however, called into doubt by the results of Liepmann's own group study: the double dissociation between apraxia and aphasia contradicts not only a causal role of aphasia for apraxia but also the reverse causality of apraxia for aphasia.

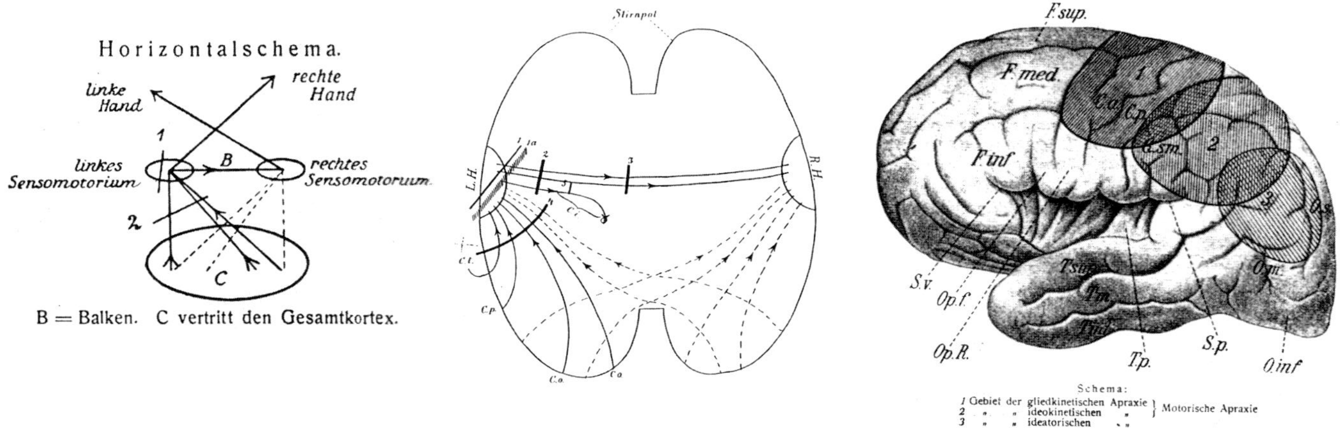

Figure 2.4 Left: Liepmann's first "horizontal schema" depicts the conversion of mental images into motor commands. The anatomical designations are the same as in Figure 2.3. The caption says "C stands for the entire cortex." The dominance of left-hemisphere motor control arises only from the asymmetry of connections between the entire cortex and the sensorimotor regions. They lead predominantly to the left sensorimotor region. Lesions in 2 cause bilateral apraxia because they interrupt these connections. Reproduced from Liepmann, H. (1908). *Drei Aufsätze aus dem Apraxiegebiet*, p. 76 ©1908, Karger. Middle: In this late version of the diagram (Liepmann, 1920, p. 413) the origin of the fibers connecting the entire cortex with the motor region has become asymmetric as well. They now arise predominantly from the left hemisphere. Moreover, their origin has now been assigned a distinct anatomical location within the hemisphere: They come exclusively from posterior regions, mainly in occipital ("C.o."), but to a minor degree also in posterior parietal (C.p.) and temporal (c.t.) regions. Right: The confinement of the crucial tracts and regions to the left hemisphere makes it possible to show them in a lateral view of the left hemisphere. The convergence of fibers from the entire cortex to the left sensorimotor regions turns into a posterior to anterior stream of action control. The caption clarifies that "1" is the region of limb-kinetic apraxia, "2" that of ideo-kinetic apraxia, and "3" that of ideational apraxia. Note that whereas the lines marking the lesions in the two horizontal versions indicate quite unequivocally that the lesions exert their effects by section of fiber paths, the areas indicated on the lateral view are more ambiguous. They could also indicate the localizations of cortical centers devoted to the compromised functions. Reproduced from Liepmann, H. (1920). Apraxie. In H.Brugsch (Ed.), *Ergebnisse der gesamten Medizin* p. 413, © 1920, Urban & Schwarzenberg.

cortex. This shift reflects the predominance of visual images in the movement formula. According to the associationist theory, visual memory images should be located in the vicinity of the primary visual cortex which receives the optical input from the eyes. This visual cortex is located in the occipital lobes.

"Kinetic memory" consists of motor traces of frequently practiced actions which can be executed without intervention of the multimodal movement formula. It is located in the central region very close to, or even within, primary motor cortex and directs actions of the opposite limbs.

The transformation of the movement formula into innervations is achieved by fiber tracts from other cortical areas to the central region. They converge predominantly, though not exclusively, to the left central region. This asymmetry is the anatomical substrate[11] of left-hemisphere dominance for the guidance of movements "fully from memory." It justifies the third schema which shows the three elements of voluntary motor control only within the left hemisphere and demonstrates their posterior to anterior sequence. Since they are anatomically separated, brain lesions can selectively disturb one of them while sparing the others. Such selective damage gives rise to three syndromes: (1) posterior parieto-occipitial lesions interfere with generation of the movement formula and cause "the localizable component" of ideational apraxia; (2) inability to transform the movement formula into motor innervations is the core of ideo-kinetic apraxia; (3) loss of kinetic memory results in limb-kinetic apraxia.

Before we discuss the clinical reality of these theoretically posited syndromes, it is worthwhile taking a critical look at the development of this posterior to anterior stream of voluntary action control. In the early version of the schema the movement formula is a product of the whole cerebral cortex. Its translation into motor innervations is thus equivalent to a transition from non-localizable to localizable brain function, which in turn corresponds to a transformation of conscious, multimodal mental images of intended actions into a sequence of motor commands inaccessible to introspective consciousness, or, to put it another way, a transmission from the psychological to the physiological side of motor control. The schema thus illustrates no less than the "government of the limbs by the mind." By contrast, in the later versions the origin of the movement formula has been shifted to the posterior part of the left hemisphere. The stream of action control now flows from a localized origin to a localized target. The reference to non-localizable psychological processes has been eliminated and the stream of action control appears to be completely embedded in anatomy and physiology. Indeed the side view presented in the third schema looks very much like a reflex arch in which sensory input elicits motor reactions (see Figure 1.1). There is, however, a crucial difference between this posterior to anterior stream of deliberate action control and the mundane anatomy of sensorimotor reflexes.

[11] Note that Liepmann did not provide any direct anatomical evidence for the postulated asymmetry of fiber tracts. The anatomical asymmetry was deduced from the very asymmetry of function that it was purported to explain. We will come back to this problem of Liepmann's models in the discussions of "diagram making" (Chapter 3) and of alternative accounts for the asymmetry of apraxia (Chapter 15).

The origin of deliberate action control is an internally generated mental image of the intended action and not the perception of an external stimulus eliciting a reflex response. Apraxia disturbs the guidance of movements by this mental image but not the adaptation of movements to external constraints. Thus, the posterior to anterior stream of motor control remains recognizable as depicting the governance of the limbs by the mind. The schema is ambiguous: it looks like an instance of the mundane brain mechanism of reflex responses to sensory stimuli but it depicts the supremacy of psychology over physiology.

Classification of apraxia

Liepmann considered the description of "motor" or, respectively, "ideo-kinetic" apraxia as his own major contribution to the clinical diagnosis of apraxia. His model of action control predicted the existence of at least two other variants caused by destruction of either the posterior or the anterior pole of the stream of action control. Liepmann named the destruction of the posterior pole "ideational" and that of the anterior pole "limb-kinetic" apraxia. For their clinical description he relied mainly on contributions of other authors. The main source for the description of ideational apraxia was Arnold Pick (1905b), and for "limb kinetic apraxia" Karl Heilbronner (1905) and Karl Kleist (1907/1934).[12]

Ideational apraxia

Arnold Pick was professor of psychiatry at the German University of Prague. Similar to Liepmann, Pick's clinical practice was mostly concerned with demented patients. Extensive observations of these patients' difficulties with manipulation of objects and the completion of everyday chores led him to propose a more differentiated view of their difficulties than proposed either by Liepmann or by preceding authors (Pick, 1905b). Like them he noted instances of gross misuse of single tools and objects evoking a suspicion of misrecognition. For example, a patient grasped scissors correctly but tried first to brush and then to write with them (p. 105). Another patient used a piece of bread for wiping his eyes (p. 59). A female patient used a cloth brush for wiping her hands. When asked to clean the examiner's trousers she laid down the brush and stroked the trousers with a grater (p. 83). The same patient could correctly name a comb but held it before her eyes commenting: "this is for the eyes" (p. 84). There were many more such observations. However, Pick found that a significant proportion of errors concerned the coordination of the multiple steps necessary for obtaining the final goal of multistep action sequences above and beyond the faulty use of single tools and objects. He described different varieties of such errors. One was the confusion of actions related to multiple objects involved in the multistep task. For example, a patient put the pipe in his mouth and took a match out of the box, but then replaced the pipe with the match and made smoking movements as if the match were a

[12] Kleist published a description and analysis of limb kinetic apraxia in 1907 with the title: "Kortikale (innervatorische) Apraxie" in a journal named *Jahrbuch der Psychiatrie*. Liepmann referred to this publication. I was not able to retrieve a copy of it and cite from Kleist's later treatment of the subject in his book *Gehirnpathologie* (1934).

cigar, commenting: "That does not work" (p. 18). Another frequent type of error was perseveration. For example, a patient who had drunk milk from a pot and was then handed a slipper repeated the same drinking movements with the slipper (p. 28). Another type of error specific to multistep tasks were "short circuits" due to omission of single steps. For example, a patient who was asked to seal an envelope pressed down the gummed margin of the lid without having moistened it (p. 103). Finally, the chain of action petered out without attaining its goal. For example, a patient asked to light and smoke a pipe put it in his mouth, took a match out of the box and lit it but then let the match burn down in his hand without making any attempt to light the pipe (p. 106).

Pick identified a deficiency of attention as the common denominator of such errors:

> I want to emphasize a factor which has not been sufficiently appreciated in the theory of motor apraxia: The importance of attention for the correct performance of voluntary action. Clarity of consciousness or, more precisely, attention and its distribution are certainly of outstanding importance among the aetiological moments of apraxia. The maintenance of the image of the final goal keeps the subordinate actions together and arranges them to a regular sequence, whereas otherwise they disintegrate in single actions which trigger one another arbitrarily. (Pick, 1905b, p. 4)
>
> A failure of attention disturbs the relationships between the single intermediate images and the image of the ultimate goal. (Pick, 1905b, p. 106)

He proposed to designate the apraxia caused by such a general disorder of attention as "ideo-motor apraxia" to indicate that it derives neither from insufficient perceptual recognition of objects nor from insufficient motor execution of their use.[13] Pick left no doubt that the mechanisms of his new variant of apraxia belonged to the realm of non-localizable intrapsychic processes and should be analyzed in psychological terms. His observations proved to him that "in the analysis of voluntary movement one must again and again ultimately return to psychic factors like attention, sensory threshold, etc." (p. 121).

Liepmann changed the name from "ideo-motor" to "ideational" apraxia. He subscribed to Pick's conclusion that this variant of apraxia is generally due to "a mental insufficiency which manifests itself in the domain of action but has its roots in deficits which are not specific for action" (Liepmann, 1929), but he repeatedly mentioned that parieto-occipital lesions might be of particular importance because they destroy the neural basis of mental visual images of the intended actions.

Limb-kinetic apraxia

Limb-kinetic apraxia was the last descendant of Meynert's and Wernicke's "motor asymbolia" and, in further lineage, of Munk's original concept of mind-palsy. Like its predecessors it was a theoretical postulate searching for clinical reality. Theoretically it should result from a loss of kinetic memories which are stored in the central regions and enable swift execution of highly routinized skills by the opposite limb. One might expect that such loss would lead to a dissociation between disturbed routine and

[13] Pick did not comment on the homonymy with the "ideo-motor" principle that formed part of the discussions on mind-palsy.

preserved non-routine movements, but there was no convincing proof for the clinical reality of this dissociation (Heilbronner, 1905). The empty space left by the absence of a clinical correlate to the theoretically defined disorder was filled by another disciple of Wernicke, Karl Kleist. He emphasized that in contrast to other variants of apraxia the manifestations of limb-kinetic apraxia depend on the motor complexity of the intended movements:

> We find a slowing and stiffness of movements, a difficulty of isolated movements and a tendency to synergistic and associated movements and a particularly severe loss of fine graded and structured movements. The simultaneous as well as the sequential coordination of single movements is disturbed. The higher the demands on innervatory combinations, the more severe are the deficits of manual skills. By contrast, actions like clapping hands, praying, catching a fly, which are less finely tuned, are successful. (Kleist, 1934, p. 458; see also Figure 3.1, this volume)

Kleist's confirmation of the clinical reality of limb-kinetic apraxia was associated with abandonment of the idea that it was due to a loss of "kinetic memories" and hence confined to frequently practiced routine actions. He believed that "the ability to combine or isolate single innervations is only partly acquired by practice. To the other part it is based on inborn capacities of the motor cortex, particularly of (Brodman) area 6" (Kleist, 1934, p. 503; see also Figure 3.1, this volume).

Liepmann agreed with Kleist on the close similarity between limb-kinetic apraxia and incomplete paresis of the affected limb. He stated that limb-kinetic apraxia "stands between paresis and apraxia" and acknowledged its inclusion only into an "enlarged concept of apraxia" (Liepmann, 1908).

Variants of apraxia

Table 2.1 gives an overview of the defining features of Liepmann's three variants of apraxia. Body part specificity is most marked for limb-kinetic apraxia which is strictly confined to the limb opposite to the damaged central region. Ideo-kinetic apraxia results from interruptions of fibers ending in somatotopically ordered central motor cortex. Circumscribed lesions can affect the connections to limited sectors of the central region and cause body part-specific symptoms. For example, apraxia may be confined to voluntary movements of the tongue, the mouth, and the head and spare the limbs, or vice versa. Liepmann

Table 2.1 Variants of apraxia

	Limb-kinetic	Ideo-kinetic	Ideational
Body part specificity	+	+	–
Task specificity			
Imitation	–	+	+
Emblematic gestures and	+	+	–
pantomime of tool use	+	+	–
Use of tools and objects	+	–	+

also mentioned that the severity of apraxia could vary between hands, legs, and trunk. The fact that each motor region commands the limbs of only the contralateral side of the body is a further source of body part specificity. Liepmann maintained that although ideo-kinetic apraxia from left-sided lesions is bilateral, it affects the right more than the left limbs because there are weak connections from the remainder of the cortex also to the right central region. The most impressive demonstrations of body part specificity resulting from the anatomy of fiber tracts were the unilateral apraxia of the imperial counselor and other cases of callosal disconnection. By contrast, ideational apraxia affects actions of all body parts equally.

The severity of symptoms in limb-kinetic apraxia depends on the motor complexity of movements but not on the task they are needed for. Task specificity of errors in ideo-kinetic apraxia follows from the postulate that the essence of the disorder is the breakdown of the "government of the limbs by the mind." Consequently apraxia should manifest itself most distinctly when movements are directed by mental images of intended actions rather than by material interactions with external objects. Liepmann reasoned:

> The great support provided by seeing and feeling the object—in many cases the hand is directly guided by the object, as by scissors, barrel organ, coffee mill, key in the keyhole—permits passable completion of the task. Only if the patient is deprived of the help by objects and is requested to make movements wholly from memory, the insufficiency of the right hemisphere becomes conspicuous. The guidance of the left hand by mental images of the shape of the movement is disturbed. In the majority the disturbance becomes manifest only if they are required to imitate or to make expressive movements or manipulations without object.[14] (Liepmann, 1908, p. 49)

Liepmann emphasized in particular the disturbance of imitation, because in this task the mental image of the intended movement is provided by the demonstration so that errors are an unequivocal proof of the inability to translate such mental images into appropriate motor actions. By contrast, in ideational apraxia imitation should be preserved as long as the required movements are not "too long and intricate." Liepmann did not comment on the ability of patients with ideational apraxia to show emblematic gestures or pantomimes of tool use. However, from his assumption that ideational apraxia is most marked for multi-step actions involving several tools and objects one might deduce that the performance of single gestures without objects might be affected less.

What was new in Liepmann's theories?

Liepmann's writings are generally recognized as laying the ground for the future development of research and theorizing on apraxia. His fame has extinguished the memory of

[14] In today's terminology, Liepmann's expressive gestures are referred to as "symbolic," "emblematic," or "intransitive," and manipulations without objects as "pantomime of tool use" or "transitive gestures." In this book the designations "emblematic gestures" and "pantomime of tool use" are preferred.

precursors like Munk, Bruns, de Buck, Steinthal, and Finkelnburg. However, as this and Chapter 1 have amply shown, central tenets of Liepmann's theory had been formulated before. The reliance of action planning on sensory, particularly visual, mental images and the possibility of apraxia resulting from disruption of their connection to motor regions, as well as the posterior to anterior direction of the stream of action control had been developed in the framework of mind-palsy. The dominance of the left hemisphere for action control had not been formulated explicitly, but was implicit in Steinthal's and Finkelnburg's insistence on the obligatory association of apraxia and asymbolia with aphasia. As I have argued in the section on de Buck, even the necessity and the vulnerability of transmission from the mental sphere to the sphere of motor images had been considered before. It thus seems appropriate to ask what, if anything, was really new in Liepmann's writings on apraxia.

I propose that the novelty of Liepmann's contribution was the comprehensive integration of the anatomy and physiology of motor control into the context of mind–body relationship. As I have argued in Chapter 1, earlier authors had subscribed to two opposing approaches. The proponents of mind-palsy based their theories on physiology and anatomy and avoided the introduction of philosophical or psychological explanations. By contrast, asymbolia and apraxia were psychological concepts defined without recourse to their anatomical underpinning. Liepmann combined them in an ingenious way. Rather than opting for one or the other, he accepted both and made their conflict the driving force of his theory of action control. The posterior to anterior stream of action control described both the anatomy of fiber pathways from posterior brain regions to the motor cortex and the conversion of conscious mental images into the physiology of motor commands. It led from the realm of psychology to that of physiology or, expressed in a more principled way, from the mind to the body. Liepmann's statement that apraxia interrupts the governance of the limbs by the mind expresses this core of his theory cogently.

The mind–body dichotomy underlies not only the posterior to anterior stream of action control but also the left hemisphere dominance for action control. Liepmann related the association of apraxia with left brain damage to the left hemisphere's unique ability to perform "movements wholly from memory," that is, without material interaction with external objects. Arguably, this definition reflects the basic dichotomy between an immaterial mind and the solid body. Only the latter is spatially extended and can interact with external objects. Actions wholly from memory are excluded from this interaction and depend exclusively on mental images entertained by the ethereal mind.

Liepmann recognized both sides of the mind–body dichotomy as necessary for explaining motor control and apraxia, but his sympathies were clearly on the body side. He subscribed to the materialist endeavor to replace the immaterial mind by the mechanics of brain functions. The body part specificity of ideo-kinetic apraxia was precious to him because it revealed the confines which the anatomy of motor cortex put upon the government of the limbs by the mind.

Liepmann expressed this consequence of body part specificity of symptoms in a discussion of the unilaterality of the imperial counselor's apraxia (Liepmann, 1905b). He argued that the preservation of left-handed skills excluded a loss of general psychic abilities, and continued:

> This forced us to release his one and only psyche from any culpability for the disturbance. It must, so to speak, be exempted from prosecution, and we were urgently reminded to look for the culprit not in the spaceless properties of the mind, but in definite places of the brain. The disturbance turned out to be localizable. (pp. 37–38)

Chapter 3

The decline of diagrams

The enthusiasm for Liepmann's schema of apraxia did not remain unquestioned. The combination of a dynamic posterior to anterior stream of motor control with distinct locations for different variants of apraxia was attacked from two sides. It was accused of rendering too much importance to the interplay of widespread brain regions and, conversely, of undue belief in narrow localization of function. The first of these mutually exclusive reproaches was presented by Karl Kleist who had already contributed to the definition of limb-kinetic apraxia (see Chapter 2). Kleist disapproved of Liepmann's contention that parietal lesions cause apraxia because they interrupt the connection between posterior brain regions creating mental, predominantly visual, images of the intended action and the sensorimotor regions commanding the execution of movements. Kleist argued that such a disconnection account would also predict ideo-kinetic apraxia after loss of mental visual images caused by posterior lesions, but that "loss or weakening of optical mental images in mind blindness does not cause apraxia." He wrote:

> I suppose that a higher, mnestic-associative device is located in the anterior parietal lobe, where kinaesthetic movement engrams are combined with movement directives coming from optical and acoustic territories. This territory should consequently be regarded as the location of complex engrams of single actions. Liepmann's apraxia results from a more or less complete loss of these engrams and not from their psychological or anatomical dissociation from other brain functions. (Kleist, 1934, p. 465; see also figure 3.1)

This argument turned the parietal lobe into the "apraxia center" which Liepmann himself had rejected. Curiously, when contempt of diagrams eventually ended and associationism came to the fore again, it was Kleist's and not Liepmann's interpretation of parietal lesions that was revamped and believed to express Liepmann's own ideas (see Chapter 4).

The opposite line of critique argued that the assignments of distinct kinds of apraxia to distinct locations drew artificial boundaries between syndromes which are in reality only variants of one multifaceted disorder (Marie, 1906a; von Monakow, 1914). A vigorous formulation of this critique was brought forward by the French neurologist Pierre Marie. Marie's vigorous assaults on generally accepted notions on the location and nature of aphasia had earned him the epithet "iconoclast." He believed that aphasia is not a disturbance of language but a manifestation of a general loss of intelligence (Marie, 1906a, 1906b), and that lesions in Wernicke's area are responsible for this intellectual decline. He illustrated the alleged loss of intelligence with the observation of an aphasic cook who, led into the hospital kitchen and asked to prepare a fried egg, emptied the egg into the pan without caring about breaking the yolk, added the butter on top of the egg, salted and peppered the mixture, and put it on the stove. Marie concluded: "No need to say that the meal was absolutely not presentable, which, by the way, did not seem to touch our patient" (Marie, 1906a, p. 242). In a footnote Marie mentioned Liepmann's finding that errors of motor actions were frequent in patients with right-sided hemiplegia. He accepted the validity, but not the interpretation of this observation:

> The distinguished professor from Berlin thinks that these difficulties indicate a special role of the left hemisphere for movements of both the left and the right limbs, and he invokes for this effect the intervention of a special fibre tract and a participation of the corpus callosum. I don't think that this view is correct. To my view, if right hemiplegics are incapable of performing some acts with their left hand, this depends not at all on an affection of the motility of their left limbs, but on the seat of their lesions in that zone of the left hemisphere that is called an area of language, but is indeed a sphere of intelligence. The difficulties which these patients present are a consequence of their intellectual deficit. (Marie, 1906a, p. 242)

Liepmann's refusal of this interpretation of apraxia was quite severe:

> All is put into one pot and becomes evidence of the great general disorder of intelligence from which these patients suffer, and which explains all their behaviour. It is astonishing that Pierre Marie does not realize that it is precisely the removal of aphasia and apraxia from the undifferentiated slime of the concept of dementia which constitutes a progress. (Liepmann, 1908, p. 71)

A French turn

In spite of such harsh arguments, Marie remained interested in apraxia. In 1914 he and his disciple Charles Foix published descriptions of two patients with Wernicke aphasia, that is, aphasia with fluent or even logorrheic speech distorted by paraphasia and neologism and resulting from lesions to the posterior third of the upper temporal convolution. Both patients could correctly execute simple orders but failed when confronted with complicated tasks which necessitated "reflections and memory." For example, when asked to light a cigarette, they would rub the cigarette rather than the match on the match box. Marie and Foix insisted that these problems were manifestations of a general intellectual decline but conceded that, "if one wants, one may call this intellectual deficit ideational apraxia." They even acknowledged that in clinical practice "search for the phenomena which are called ideational apraxia constitute a valuable means for revealing conditions of intellectual decline and disorientation" (Marie & Foix, 1914, p. 277).

In a later paper Foix (1916) also re-established Liepmann's distinction between ideational and ideo-kinetic apraxia, albeit with two major revisions. The first concerned the nomenclature: the name of "ideo-kinetic" apraxia was changed to "ideo-motor" apraxia.[1] With few exceptions (e.g., Goodglass & Kaplan, 1963) this term has been preferred by most authors until today. The second revision was theoretically more important. Foix rejected the continuity of both variants of apraxia as affecting sequentially ordered steps in

[1] Neither Foix nor his disciple Morlaas who explicitly commented on this change of nomenclature (Morlaas, 1928, p. 19) brought forward any theoretical reasons for this change.

the conversion of ideas of intended actions into their motor execution (see Chapter 2). He insisted that:

> One must absolutely separate ideational and ideo-motor apraxia. There is no parity between them. If they occur quite frequently together in the same patient, this is because the lesions determining one of them are not far away from those provoking the other. (Foix, 1916, p. 284)

He reiterated the postulate that ideational apraxia is a manifestation of general intellectual decline and accepted only ideo-motor apraxia as a "true" apraxia, that is, a disorder of motor control. He presented five patients with left-sided lesions encroaching upon the parietal lobe. They produced hesitant, awkward, and spatially wrong movements when asked to produce emblematic gestures (e.g., beckoning, making a military salute) and pantomimes of tool use (e.g., demonstrating the use of scissors) or to touch distinct body parts (e.g., putting the index on the nose). Use of objects was somewhat clumsy but with few exceptions ultimately successful. Apraxia was distinctly more severe for the right hand in three, and for the left hand in two patients. Foix concluded:

> In sum, we think that an isolated left sided lesion may cause bilateral apraxia, but that this apraxia predominates on the right side, and may be absent on the left. If apraxia predominates on the left side, this may be because there is also an important lesion of the corpus callosum, or, which is perhaps more frequently the case, an additional lesion of the right brain. (Foix, 1916, p. 296)

In comparison with the clinical evidence accumulated over nearly 100 years since Foix's study, the prevalence and strength of the asymmetry of apraxia in Foix's patients seems unusual and raises a suspicion that unilateral "limb-kinetic apraxia" or, respectively, sensory deficits and mild pareses of the affected limbs (see Chapter 2) contributed to their awkwardness. For the historical development of the concept of apraxia, however, the important point is that Foix considered a difference between the severities of symptoms in right and left limbs as a constitutive feature of ideo-motor apraxia. Although he did not comment on the reason for this asymmetry, it is quite evident that it is grounded in the anatomy of motor control. Because the left and the right limbs are controlled separately by their opposite hemispheres, lesions of one hemisphere affect the opposite more than the ipsilateral limb.

At this stage it is worthwhile to pause and compare Foix's views to Liepmann's model of the conversion of mental images into motor acts. Arguably, the postulated absence of any parity between ideational and ideo-motor apraxia divides the mental from the motor side of apraxia. Ideational apraxia is conceived as a manifestation of global mental deterioration totally independent from motor control or body parts. By contrast, ideo-motor apraxia is firmly anchored in the anatomy of motor control, and its manifestations are body part specific. Foix's conception of apraxia agrees with Liepmann's by distinguishing between a mental and a motor side of action control, but differs in the absence of a mechanism for the conversion of one into the other. Ideational apraxia is a disorder of the mind, and ideo-motor apraxia of the body. The only link between them is the proximity of the cortical areas whose damage gives rise to them.

The turn of theorizing initiated by Pierre Marie and continued by Charles Foix was completed by a doctoral thesis of Foix's disciple Joseph Morlaas (1928). Before we discuss in detail this seminal work we should briefly consider another contribution of Pierre Marie that pre-dated and influenced it.

Planotopokinesia

In 1922, Pierre Marie and coworkers published a case report of a patient who had suffered an episode of paresis of his right limbs and mild aphasia (Marie et al., 1922). He passed "classic tests of apraxia," that is, performance of emblematic gestures and of pantomimes of tool use flawlessly, but had difficulties which "evoke, if one refers to German authors, a suspicion of apraxia" with everyday chores. Most spectacular were his difficulties with dressing:

> He takes his shirt up slowly but without dropping it. He knows very well which use he should make of it, but seems to be totally disoriented. He successively takes up each of its ends, examines them, hesitates, and turns the shirt in all directions; only after several minutes he lifts it to his head. In most trials he does not succeed to pass it over his head, and he blinds himself with the flapping ends of the shirt while fighting to disentangle himself.
>
> In spite of a long re-education and of his evident efforts this man has never succeeded in putting on his shirt correctly and rapidly. (p. 508)

This patient's problems were not restricted to dressing. He also was unable to orient himself on a map of Paris or to find familiar routes when walking. Writing was linguistically correct but the lines were oblique, the distances between them irregular with collisions between subsequent lines. He also turned out to be unable to imitate finger postures. The authors concluded that the difficulties of their patient did not fulfill criteria for ideational or ideo-motor apraxia, but that he had a problem with spatial representations and their connection with the execution of deliberate movements. They proposed calling this disorder "planotopokinesia,[2] that is, a failure of execution of movements on the basis of spatial representations."

Joseph Morlaas

Like his teacher Foix, Morlaas insisted on the complete separation of ideational and ideo-motor apraxia. He postulated that they affect different domains of actions and are caused by different underlying mechanisms. Ideo-motor apraxia concerns gestures made without implement. It is caused by "spatial dyskinesia." Ideational apraxia is a disorder of tool and object use resulting from "agnosia of utilization."

Spatial dyskinesia

Morlaas classified ideo-motor apraxia as a disturbance of "gesture per se," that is of motor acts which do not involve external objects. Although such gestures are produced mainly

[2] From Greek: plan-: roaming, elusive; topos: place.

for "symbolism," ideo-motor apraxia is not restricted to gestures with symbolic content. Meaningless gestures like, for example, forming an "8" with the fingers of both hands or snapping fingers below the chin, may be even more severely affected than gestures transmitting symbolic contents. Difficulties are not restricted to performance of the gesture on verbal command but are at least as severe when the patients are asked to imitate the gesture.

The main mechanism underlying ideo-motor apraxia is:

> a spatial dyskinesia that is an incorrect movement of the gesture leading to a wrong final position (e.g., hand covering the eye for the military salute, thumb in mouth for thumbing one's nose): such errors are due to the loss of the intuitive correspondence between the movement of the hand searching for its final position and the own body. They are comparable to those which we commit when we try to arrange our hairs without the help of a mirror. The spatial dyskinesia explains the impossibility of imitating demonstrated gestures. It is the counterpart of planatopokinesia: there can be planotopokinesia without spatial dyskinesia, spatial dyskinesia without planotopokinesia, or both together. (Morlaas, 1928, p. 222)

Morlaas gave vivid descriptions of the behavior of patients during the examination of ideomotor apraxia:

> The patients seem to be lost, they frequently ask: Is it like that, is it good? Rarely do they stop after the first posture, they spontaneously attempt corrections, try other postures. Their mimical expression is questioning; they wait for advice. Sometimes they will succeed a correction, at other times they immobilize the hand in a wrong position, believing, as it seems, to have succeeded. (Morlaas, 1928, p. 47)
>
> It is as if the patients had lost the intuitive sense for the relative disposition of different segments of their body. (pp. 47–48)

The disorder is confined to the context of examination when the target of the movement is the production of the gesture itself rather than its role in the context of everyday life. Thus, a patient who during the examination is totally incapable of making the sign of the cross either on verbal command or in imitation may make it without effort when entering a church. Likewise, meaningless gestures are particularly vulnerable to ideo-motor apraxia because

> they do not evoke in the patient any natural motive for making them. Perhaps this emptiness, where nothing opposes the deficit, explains that their execution is nearly always impossible or at least very poor. (p. 56)

In contrast to Foix, Morlaas did not give much weight to asymmetry of the manifestations of apraxia. He noted that he had not encountered comparable degrees of following hemispheric lesions, but he conceded the reality of unilateral apraxia and intermanual conflict after callosal damage like in Liepmann's imperial counselor.

Agnosia of utilization

Morlaas acknowledged that attentional problems might augment the severity of "ideational apraxia," that is, defective manipulation of objects, but he rejected Pick's proposal that insufficient attention is the main cause of defective object use. He insisted that errors were not confined to multistep actions but also occurred in the simplest actions if they require the manipulation of objects. He also opposed Marie's and Foix's claim that ideational apraxia is an expression of general intellectual decline. He related examples of patients who struggled with the use of single objects displaying both attention to the task and a critical attitude toward their failure. For example:

> A lady with Wernicke's aphasia was presented with a pen holder and asked to write down her name. She asked for ink and dipped in the pen, but then tried to write with the pen-holder upside down. She put on her glasses and tried to find out why the pen did not write; but although she inspected the pen-holder carefully, she could not correct her error. (Morlaas, 1928, p. 31)

Like Marie and Foix, Morlaas considered ideational apraxia as an intellectual rather than a motor disorder, but in contrast to them he considered intellect not a unitary and indivisible entity. He postulated that it consists of multiple functions which can be disturbed independently from each other. One of them is knowledge about the correct use of objects:

> To know how to use and to construct objects is a specialized function, isolated and independent from other specialized functions.

This knowledge is based on recognition of the pragmatic significance of objects:

> The nature of a work of art is to be beautiful; it has no value except its aesthetic significance which offers itself to the purely speculative activities of the intellect. It is deprived of any pragmatic significance. Thus it is out of the reach of gestures. In contrast to this class of objects are objects which have value only by their pragmatic capacities. This practical, pragmatic significance is gestural. The match reveals its significance only if I rub its inflammable end on the appropriate side of the matchbox, which is matchbox only because of its practical property of containing matches. Its significance does not exceed this truism. (Morlaas, 1928, p. 43)

Recognition of the pragmatic significance of objects can be lost although recognition of other aspects of the object is preserved. Morlaas illustrated this selectivity with the example of driving an automobile, a skill not yet ubiquitous in 1928:

> Let us assume that I have never before conducted an automobile and that I do not know how it works. If nonetheless I can name that vehicle an automobile, I have not yet identified it. By designating it as an object devoted to auto-locomotion I possess a rough understanding which prevents me from confusing it with a horse drawn carriage, but not more.
>
> If you ask me to utilize it, that is to produce the gestures giving to the vehicle its veritable significance, which is to progress by its own power without additional traction, I become an ideational apraxic. Because I do not understand its mechanism I produce gestures out of their proper order. I slow down when I should accelerate; I push back when I should move forward, and because of my ignorance I am unable to establish a schema for my actions.
>
> A driver who has some mechanical understanding would identify the object. Even when confronted with an unfamiliar type of machine, he would by applied reasoning succeed to establish the plan of the mechanism.
>
> The apraxic cannot accomplish such pragmatic identification by means of reasoning. He is locked out from this compartment of intellectual activity: He is stuck by agnosia of utilization. (Morlaas, 1928, p. 43)

Anatomy and psychology of apraxia

Morlaas started the discussion of the anatomical basis of apraxia with a faithful account of Liepmann's proposals that lesions causing ideational apraxia are located posteriorly to those causing ideo-motor apraxia, and that lesions of the corpus callosum cause unilateral left-sided apraxia. He then reported post-mortem findings of a series of 19 patients whom he had examined for the presence of apraxia and discussed them in relation with similar published cases. He concluded that ideational apraxia was regularly associated with lesions of the most posterior portion of the left inferior parietal lobe and the adjacent portion of the superior temporal gyrus. In patients with ideo-motor apraxia, left parietal lesions prevailed too, but they were not regularly confined to a distinct portion of this quite extensive area, and there were also cases of bilateral ideo-motor apraxia caused by left frontal and right parietal lesions. These results gave only limited support to Liepmann's speculation about the sequential arrangement of lesions causing ideational and ideo-motor apraxia along the posterior to anterior stream of action control. The other key element of Liepmann's anatomical speculations, the role of the corpus callosum, was supported by one patient in whom destruction of the corpus callosum had led to ideo-motor apraxia of only the left limbs.

Morlaas emphasized that in the majority of patients the lesions were due to vascular infarctions and that consequently their extent and distribution were determined by the anatomy of vascular territories. In contrast to Marie and Foix, he related the frequent association of ideational apraxia with Wernicke's aphasia to irrigation of the responsible cortical areas by the same branch of the middle cerebral artery and not to their common nature as expressions of general intellectual decline.

Morlaas' revision of Liepmann's theories

Morlaas adhered to Liepmann's distinction between ideational and ideo-motor apraxia, and also followed him in classifying ideational apraxia as a "purely psychic" and ideo-motor apraxia as a "psycho-motor" disorder. Like Liepmann, he distinguished the manipulation of real objects from actions with empty hands and considered disturbances of the latter as the core feature of ideo-motor apraxia. Beneath this superficial agreement, however, there were substantial differences between their concepts of ideational and ideo-motor apraxia. For Liepmann, the two variants affected sequential steps in the conversion of mental ideas into motor actions. For Morlaas, they emerged from two independent functional disturbances.

Morlaas also agreed with Liepmann in ascribing a central role for apraxia to left parietal lesions, but again the agreement conceals fundamental differences. To Liepmann anatomy was an explanatory concept: Mental images of intended actions are created in the most posterior regions of the brain because this is the location where the optical tract ends and where memories of visual perceptions are stored. Parietal lesions cause apraxia because the parietal lobe is located between the posterior visual and the central motor region of the brain, so that a lesion there interrupts the stream from visual mental images to motor control. In this line of reasoning the anatomical layout of the responsible lesions is congruent with a model of the symptoms they cause.

Morlaas did not search for anatomical and physiological mechanisms underlying the locations of responsible lesions, and he did not postulate congruence between anatomy and function. On the contrary, he argued that anatomical proximity between responsible lesions can fake relationships between symptoms. Thus, the vicinity of the parietal regions where lesions cause ideational apraxia and superior temporal regions where lesions cause Wernicke's aphasia leads to their frequent co-occurrence and conceals that they are independent disturbances.

I have argued in Chapter 2 that Liepmann subscribed to the materialist endeavor of replacing the immaterial mind by the mechanics of brain functions. To fulfill this purpose, cerebral localization must provide not only a place for the unfolding of psychological processes but a mechanism which explains them by reference to anatomical structures and physiological functions. By contrast, Morlaas' analyses of spatial dyskinesia and agnosia of utilization were based on putative subdivisions and functions of the mind rather than on brain mechanisms. He replaced simple associations between modality-specific memory images by sophisticated psychological models. The interpolation of these psychological models disrupted the congruence between anatomy and symptoms of brain lesions.

Morlaas' thesis was finished in 1928, five years after Liepmann's death.[3] At that time his adherence to Liepmann's basic schema was already more exceptional than the replacement of associationist diagrams by more sophisticated psychological theories. Morlaas' attempt to develop a psychological account of apraxia without abandoning the framework of Liepmann's classification was overtaken by theories proposing a more radical break with associationist theories and diagram making. This may be one reason why Morlaas' work found rather limited resonance by contemporary writers.[4]

As we will see in Chapter 4, the decline of Liepmann's model of apraxia was not irrevocable. Interestingly its comeback was followed by a resuscitation of Morlaas' concepts of agnosia of utilization (De Renzi & Lucchelli, 1988) and of spatial dyskinesia (Goldenberg, 1995). Again, Morlaas' ideas paved the way for transition from the sequential ordering of ideational and ideo-motor apraxia to more sophisticated accounts of the psychological mechanisms at stake in different variants of apraxia.

Reshuffling apraxia

As we have outlined in Chapter 1, Liepmann's schema of apraxia was rooted in the associationist model of brain function proposed by Meynert and Wernicke. The originality and

[3] Liepmann had committed suicide because he was suffering from Parkinson's disease and feared mental decline of which he believed he had noticed the first signs (Goldenberg, 2003a).

[4] Another obstacle for international recognition was the publication of his thesis in a French monograph hardly accessible for students outside France. To my knowledge it has never been translated into English. Morlaas continued to be cited by French authors (e.g., Lhermitte & Trelles, 1933; De Ajuriaguerra & Hecaen, 1960) but was hardly recognized outside France.

inherent dynamics of Liepmann's model transgressed the simplicity of these predecessors but bore unmistakable signs of their paternity. The insufficiency of associationist explanations of aphasia and related symptoms had already been noted in the last third of the nineteenth century (Steinthal, 1874; see Chapter 1), but until the first third of the twentieth century associationism could defend its dominant position. Then, however, the Zeitgeist changed. It no longer encouraged the reductionist division of the mind into a multitude of associations but favored the liberation of mental processes from anatomical determination, providing the stage for the unfolding of holistic and psychodynamic speculations (Harrington, 1996). In the middle of the twentieth century the Meynert–Wernicke tradition of associationism seemed to be finally reduced to a historical reminiscence, ironically referred to as the epoch of the "diagram makers" (Head, 1921). The British neurologist McDonald Critchley (1953) summarized the then current views:

> The conventional association psychology is no longer proving adequate or satisfying. The stage has therefore been set for a different orientation in neurology. A more holistic conception seemed to answer better some of the problems encountered at the bedside. An increasing sympathy with the ideas expressed by configurational or Gestalt psychology has developed in many centres. (p. 419)
>
> Some writers have claimed that no compromise whatsoever is possible between the two schools of thought, organismic and associational, as they present opposite poles in ideology. (p 420)

As we have seen in the previous chapters, the definition and diagnosis of apraxia depend crucially on theoretical considerations which, in their predominant formulation by Liepmann, were anchored in the Meynert–Wernicke tradition of associationism. Doubts about this theoretical fundament resulted in dissolution of the unifying concept of apraxia. Two prominent French neurologists, Theophile Alajouanine and Francois Lhermitte (1960) wrote:

> The term apraxia is ill chosen: On the one hand, the disorder it defines is not related to motor control; on the other hand, it suggests that there is a function of eupraxia, but this is not the case.
>
> Apraxia is not a functional entity. (pp. 628–629)

Skepticism concerning the theoretical unity of apraxia did not, however, abolish the reality of its symptoms. They continued to be discussed, though partly under new headings and in combination with symptoms which had not been classified as belonging to apraxia before. The dissolution of the traditional unity of apraxia prevented the petrifaction of Liepmann's dominant schema and opened the view on neglected relationships with other symptoms of brain damage.

Voluntary and automatic actions

Liepmann's model of action control and apraxia had been founded upon the associationist theories of Meynert and Wernicke. Neurology in the mid-twentieth century attributed a similar founding role to British nineteenth-century neurologist John Hughlings Jackson. A comprehensive discussion of the philosophical fundaments and clinical elaboration of Jackson's ideas is beyond the competency of this author and the scope of this book (see Harrington, 1987; Young, 1990; Jacyna, 2000).[5] We will concentrate on sections of his writings on aphasia with direct relevance for apraxia.

Jackson emphasized that aphasic patients have not completely lost verbal abilities. He claimed that even patients who are unable to express their thoughts by words understand what is said to them and may utter single words or stereotyped short phrases under excitement. They are, however, unable to repeat the same utterances on command. He concluded that only the voluntary use of language is abolished, whereas the automatic use is preserved and referred this dissociation to the division of the brain in two hemispheres. While the voluntary use of language is a domain of the left hemisphere, automatic use can also be supported by the right hemisphere. Consequently, in aphasia following left brain lesions:

> The law, I believe, is that the most voluntary and most special processes suffer first and most. It is only the complementary expression to say that by lesions of the cerebral division of the nervous system, the patient is reduced to a more automatic condition. (Jackson, 1874/1932a, p. 133)

A further passage from the same article suggests that the position of different kinds of gestures along the voluntary–automatic dimension varies, but that generally gestures are more automatic than regular speech:

> There is loss of the most (special) voluntary forms of language (speech) without loss of the more automatic (emotional manifestations). The patient smiles, laughs and varies the tone of his voice, and may be able to sing. We find that pantomime which stands half way suffers little, and gesticulation not at all. (Jackson, 1874/1932a, p. 134)

In another paper Jackson applies the voluntary–automatic dichotomy directly to motor control (Jackson, 1878/1932b). He observed aphasic patients who were unable to stick out their tongue on command, although they understood the command as shown by attempts to put the fingers in the mouth to help the organ out. The same patients did, however, move the tongue freely for eating and drinking or for automatic utterance of swears or "more innocent ejaculations as 'Oh dear!'" (p. 153). Likewise:

> Some people are unable to draw in their breath when told to do so during stethoscopic examination; we have to tell them to cough. It is next to impossible to get some patients to frown (as in suspected one-sided facial paralysis) even if we make a frown for them to imitate. (p. 154)

Although Jackson did not use the term "apraxia," these examples paved the way for applying the dichotomy of voluntary and automatic control to the domains of action which had been considered by Liepmann and the associationist tradition of apraxia. A straightforward

[5] The opposition between German "associationism" and Jackson' concepts is admittedly an oversimplification. The philosophical concept of associationism was developed mainly by British philosophers and provided the basis for Meynert and Wernicke as well as for Jackson's theories (Buckingham, 1984; Young, 1990). However, in the way that Jackson's ideas were defended by Head and other followers in the middle of the twentieth century, this origin was much less conspicuous than it had been in the writings of Meynert, Wernicke, and their followers. Head denied the importance of modality-specific mental images derived from memory traces of previous sensations whose existence was a central tenet of the Meynert–Wernicke version of associationist psychology.

application was to interpret apraxia as "a disorder of voluntary movement contrasting with preservation of reflex and instinctive activities" (Lhermitte & Trelles, 1933, p. 416; Critchley, 1953), but the voluntary–automatic dichotomy gave also rise to more sophisticated interpretations of apraxia.

A new variant of body part specificity

The Prague neurologist Otto Sittig[6] was a great admirer of Jackson whose writings he had translated into German. He believed that apraxia affects predominantly voluntary, and spares automatic movements (Sittig, 1928; Maas & Sittig, 1929). His arguments blended Jackson's functional consideration with a localizing approach. He reasoned that the importance of voluntary control of movements increases with the complexity and diversity of possible movements, which are generally higher for the hands than for legs and trunks. Consequently, the cerebral regions devoted to control of arms and hands are larger than those for legs and trunk. Their extension increases the probability of being affected by brain damage. That is why manifestations of apraxia are usually more severe for manual movements than for whole body or leg movements as required, for example, for walking or sitting down.

Sittig's proposal that apraxia affects predominantly distal and spares axial movements seems not have had much influence on his contemporaries, but recurred some 40 years later in the writings of Norman Geschwind who, however, explained this dissociation solely by anatomical consideration and without reference to a division between voluntary and automatic control (see Chapter 4).

Revival of asymbolia

The British neurologist Henry Head (1920, 1921, 1926) was a fervent critic of the associationist approach to aphasia and related disorders. He opposed to the explanatory validity of diagrams showing connections between localized centers (see figures in Chapters 1 and 2) and coined the contemptuous designation "diagram makers" for their authors.

He agreed with Jackson's dichotomy of voluntary and spontaneous use of language but gave it a somewhat different interpretation and nomenclature. He wrote:

> An organic lesion disturbs certain physiological processes which are necessary for the complex acts which underlie the use of language. Words, numbers, pictures, and every function which depends upon the use of these symbols in constructive thought may be affected. Any mental process is liable to suffer which demands for its performance exact comprehension, voluntary recall, and perfect expression of symbolic representation. I have therefore suggested that the various functions disturbed in aphasia and allied conditions might be spoken of as "symbolic thinking and expression," because it is mainly the use of words, numbers, and pictures which suffers in these disordered states. (Head, 1921, p. 404)

Head, a competent speaker of German (Brain, 1961), mentioned the "remarkable paper read in 1870 by Finkelnburg before a provincial medical society" (Head, 1926, p. 64) as a

[6] Otto Sittig was Jewish. He did not succeed in escaping from the German occupation of Czechoslovakia and was deported first to Theresienstadt and then to Auschwitz where he was murdered in 1944.

predecessor of his theory, but he emphasized other aspects of symbol use than Finkelnburg. Whereas Finkelnburg postulated a general inability to understand or produce symbols, Head believed that difficulties depend on the conditions of symbol use:

> It is symbols used in a particular manner which suffer in these disorders and not all symbolic representations.
>
> The more nearly the symbolic action approximates to a perfect proposition, the greater difficulty will it present, and the patient will probably fail to execute it correctly. Conversely the more closely it corresponds to matching two sensory patterns, the less likely is it to be disturbed. (Head, 1921, p. 404)

Surprisingly, Head did not include Liepmann in his list of notorious diagram makers. He accepted the clinical reality of Liepmann's different types of apraxia but asserted that "it is the act itself which is disturbed and not its intellectual content" (Head, 1926, p. 96). He considered apraxia as a purely motor disorder which he distinguished sharply from the impact of defective symbolic thinking on manual actions of aphasic patients:

> There are certain differentiating characters which serve to reveal the presence of apraxia. Asked to imitate a simple movement such as touching the nose or scratching the head made by the observer, the patient is unable to do so or may fail with one hand although he succeeds with the other. On the contrary, the aphasic can imitate even complex movements made before him provided they do not necessitate the employment of some formula of internal speech such as the differential designation of right and left. (Head, 1926, p. 97)

It is interesting to note that Head considered defective imitation and body part specificity of errors as proof for the purely motor character of apraxia. However, the relegation of apraxia to a purely motor disorder left open the question as to how the alleged disturbance of symbolic thinking and expression influences motor acts of aphasic patients. Head addressed this question, without reference to apraxia, by the "Hand, Eye, and Ears Test."

The power of verbalization

The "Hand, Eye, and Ears Test" was devised for demonstrating the disturbance of symbolic thinking in patients with aphasia. The examiner sat opposite the patient, and demonstrated a series of simple movements which consisted in touching an eye or an ear with one or the other hand. Crucially, the patient was expected to move and touch body parts on the nominally same side of the body as the examiner. When the examiner touched his right ear with the left hand, the patient should do the same although his own left hand was located at the same side as the examiner's right hand. Then the patient was placed in front of a large mirror, and was asked to imitate the reflected movements of the examiner standing behind. In this condition the corresponding body parts of examiner and patient appeared on the same side of external space. Finally, the same movements were elicited by a verbal command to move right or left hand to right- or left-sided body parts. Head observed difficulties and errors of aphasic patients only in the first condition, when they had to transpose the laterality of the examiner's body parts into the laterality of their own body parts.[7] Head reasoned that "there is a natural tendency to select the hand opposite to that used by the observer" (Head, 1920, p. 103). Healthy subjects overcome this tendency by internal verbalization, which is one instance of symbolic thinking. They covertly name the laterality of the examiner's body part involved in the gesture and move the nominally same parts of their own body for imitation. Aphasic patients fail because their "power of verbalization" is defective. The seemingly conflicting finding that they carry out the gestures correctly on verbal command narrows down the deficit to the active evocation of the verbal designation of laterality: "If the word is given, it can be matched to the object, but the adequate symbol cannot be called up at will" (Head, 1920, p. 158).

A mirror of male superiority

The idea that mirroring the lateralization of body parts is more primitive than transposition of their laterality to the nominally matching laterality of the own body supplied the basis for a developmental study. Gordon (1922) tested imitation of raising the right hand by children and adolescents. The examination started with a verbal command to raise the right hand. Then, the examiner turned his back to the child, raised the right hand and said "Do exactly what I do. Hold up this hand." These two preliminary tests were passed flawlessly by virtually all children. The examiner then turned round again and repeated the procedure while facing the child. If the child raised the right hand in spite of seeing the examiner's right hand on their own left side, the response was considered correct. The proportion of correct response was less than 10% for eight-year-olds and increased steadily with increasing age, reaching some 50% in 13-year-olds. Boys surpassed girls in all age groups except the youngest. From the strong prevalence of mirror imitation in the younger children Gordon deduced that the "very strong tendency to 'direct' imitation" is "an inherited automatic action, in which the 'higher centres' are not involved. The stimulus has merely excited a lower, primitive, inherited psycho-physical mechanism not involving the 'higher centres'" (p. 298). Application of this reasoning to the superior performance of boys led to a conclusion which is hardly compatible with today's developmental psychology: "Since the boys do better than the girls at every age it follows that in the case of the boys the higher nerve centres become involved and assume ascendancy at an earlier age than in the case of the girls" (p. 298).

The autonomy of human action

The dichotomy of voluntary and automatic or, respectively, high-level and primitive, mechanisms of action control can be translated as a distinction between autonomy of action and environmental dependency. From this point of view the loss of high-level action

7 Head's patients were mainly soldiers who had suffered gunshot wounds (Jacyna, 2000). Head does not report whether they had motor deficits. If they had, this should have limited the possibility of exploring the laterality of their movements, since only the non-affected hand could be tested. The observation that Head, who was, however, a clinical neurologist, considered a report of the motor deficits of his patients unnecessary illustrates his sole concentration on the "higher level" of action control.

control in apraxia can be conceived as a loss of autonomy rendering the patient a helpless victim of external stimuli. A very influential proponent of this view was the German, later American,[8] neurologist Kurt Goldstein. Like Liepmann, Goldstein had been an assistant of Wernicke. In 1908 he had published a case report of unilateral apraxia caused by damage to the corpus callosum which supported Liepmann's contention that interruption of fiber tracts can lead to dissociations between actions commanded by different parts of the brain (see Chapter 2). Later he became skeptical of the clinical validity of localizing isolated symptoms of brain damage. He now emphasized that the symptoms of brain damage must be understood as reactions of the whole organism to local damage rather than as direct expressions of the local loss of function (Goldstein, 1928, 1948, 1995; Harrington, 1996; Goldenberg, 2002). In particular, he argued that the organism reacts to brain damage by abandoning the "abstract attitude" necessary for liberating thinking and action from their embedment in the present situation.

He applied this theory to aphasic patients' inability to pantomime the use of objects:

> It can generally be said that the patients' efficiency depends on being directly anchored in reality. They are not able to imagine fictional events, nor can they fake actions. It has been known since long time how badly apractic patients pretend the execution of actions which they carry out promptly with an object. This inability to pretend actions is not—as has frequently been assumed—a particular symptom of apraxia, but demonstrates a general change of behaviour which in apraxia comes to the fore particularly clearly. (Goldstein, 1928, p. 238)

This interpretation denies apraxia the status as an independent symptom and reduces it to one of many manifestations of the general loss of abstract attitude. The resulting dependency from the concrete context reduces the autonomy of thinking and action.

Abram Grünbaum's apractagnosia

The Russian–Dutch psychologist Abram Grünbaum (1930) rejected Liepmann's assumption that motor actions start with a mental image of the desired outcome which is then converted into motor acts. He argued that frequently the target of the action derives from recognition of possible motor interactions with objects. For example "recognition of a chair means knowing that it is for sitting." Faulty use of objects can result from the inability to recognize such action related object properties. It should be named "apractagnosia" rather than apraxia to emphasize that the cause of misuse is misrecognition.

The similarity between Grünbaum's apractagnosia, Morlaas' agnosia of utilization, and Meynert's original conception of motor asymbolia is striking, but Grünbaum cited neither Morlaas nor Meynert and thus seemed to have arrived at his proposal independently.

In the last part of his paper Grünbaum introduced an aspect of faulty object use that had been mentioned in some of Pick's descriptions of the errors of demented patients (see

8 The time covered in this chapter includes World War II. As already mentioned, a substantial proportion, if not the majority, of the German scientists working on apraxia and other neuropsychological disturbances were Jewish. Their emigration first from Germany and then also from Austria ended the leading role of German language and German science in the field of brain and behavior, but brought their views and methods to Great Britain and America.

Chapter 2) but had not been explicitly appreciated in the literature. He argued that lack of recognition of functionally important features of objects is not the only possible source of faulty use of objects. Errors could also arise from the opposite deviation which is the "compelling direction of action by exhortation from optical and physical features of the objects." For example, a patient could, on request, first put a ring on his finger and then a cigar in his mouth. When, however, both objects were presented together and the patient was asked to perform the same actions again, he would rather put the cigar into the ring. Grünbaum likened this behavior to forced grasping of visually presented objects in patients with dementia or frontal lesions (Adie & Critchley, 1927; De Renzi & Barbieri, 1992). In both instances the recognition of possible motor actions triggers their execution in spite of diverging instructions. The compelling dependency of actions from stimuli in the immediate environment can be seen as another instance of loss of the autonomy of action control.

Denny-Brown's multiple apraxias

The topic of externally triggered motor actions that conflict with the patient's intentions recurred in an influential paper on apraxia by the neurologist Derek Denny-Brown (1958).[9]

Denny-Brown distinguished five variants of apraxia: The first is ideational apraxia deriving mainly from diffuse lesions as, for example, in pre-senile dementia. Its leading symptom is dissociation between propositional and spontaneous performance of motor actions:

> The defect is first seen in relation to complex movements performed by request of the examiner. The more hypothetic the nature of the request, the more imaginary the circumstances, and the more the requested movement is a mimesis of the real thing, the more vulnerable it is to such disease. The patient is unable to pretend to drink from a glass of water, or even to pretend to drink from an empty glass, yet can perform without difficulty when presented with a glass with water in it. (Denny-Brown, 1958, p. 10)

It is noteworthy that in this classification ideational apraxia affects mainly gestures made without a real implement. This corresponds to Goldstein's dictum that aphasic patients are unable to fake actions but contrasts with Liepmann's original proposal that the predominant affection of gestures made without external objects is the hallmark of ideo-kinetic rather than ideational apraxia.

The second variant is called "adextrous apraxia." This entity includes different conditions where:

> the propositional, purely ideational objective of a motor performance is completely dissociated from the physiology by reason of management ("dominance") by different hemispheres. (p. 13)

Among the instances of adextrous apraxia are cases of inability to play an instrument with preserved comprehension of notes, or of disturbed writing with preserved reading. Denny-Brown mentions that "such disturbances have in the past been attributed to loss of association pathways, notably the corpus callosum" but rejects this possibility because

---

9 I have refrained from assigning a nationality to this prominent and influential neurologist, because he was born in New Zealand, and made successful careers first in London then in Boston.

"Akelaitis[10] has shown that apraxia does not follow division of the corpus callosum" and "whatever the corpus callosum contributes, it is not in the coordinated action of both limbs in the synthesis of a motor act" (p. 13).

The most original part of Denny-Brown's new classification of apraxia is the introduction of two "kinetic" apraxias:

> Apraxia that is independent of conceptual function (kinetic apraxia) can be traced to the abnormal operation of released sensory factors that direct the physiological aspects of behavior. (p. 31)

Denny-Brown distinguished a "magnetic" and a "repellent" variant of kinetic apraxia. Both are unilateral, affecting the limbs opposite to the lesions. They are characterized by aberrant motor actions but reflect more general behavioral tendencies.

Magnetic apraxia is caused by frontal lesions. Its core symptom is forced grasping of objects which happen to be in the vicinity of the hand (Adie & Critchley, 1927), but "forced grasping is only one aspect of a total change in behavior, towards a compulsive exploration of the environment" (p. 17). Magnetic apraxia also affects the feet which in reaction to touch may show a "foot grasp" and which are "glued to the floor" when the patients attempts to walk,[11] and the mouth which tends to approach and to suck objects brought near to it.[12]

Repellent apraxia is caused by parietal lesions. It is characterized by a retraction from environmental stimuli. The hand tends to be overstretched and draws back from objects when the patient is expected to grasp them. When the patient attempts to write, contact is made with the paper only for brief periods, and the hand intermittently withdraws from the paper. Again the disorder is not confined to the hand. When stimuli approach the mouth the patient diverts the face and when he is fed he may refuse chewing and swallowing. Gait is disturbed by hyperflexion of the hip raising the leg high from the ground where it is held for several seconds before being lowered to the ground again.

Finally, there are subcortical apraxias due to a malfunction at the thalamic level. They are characterized by dystonic movements and muscular hypertension. As in kinetic apraxia there are two variants, dystonic grasping and dystonic withdrawal, but in contrast to the kinetic apraxias, the dystonic movements persist when the external objects triggering them are no longer present.

On first glance Denny-Brown's system of apraxia appears as a collection of motor abnormalities that impress the clinician and may be useful for diagnosis of the causal disease but have no theoretical communality. On scrutiny, a common thread shines through. Governance of the body by the mind is subdued to governance by the environment. The sequence

[10] We will come back to Akelaitis' studies (1942, 1945) of apraxia (not) following callosotomy later in this chapter.

[11] The Viennese, later American, neurologists Gerstmann and Schilder coined the term "apraxia of gait" to characterize the gait disorder resulting from bilateral gluing of the feet to the floor in patients with bilateral extensive frontal lobe damage (Gerstmann & Schilder, 1926; Della Sala et al., 2004).

[12] In the modern literature the French neurologist Francois Lhermitte has taken up and further developed Denny-Brown's "magnetic apraxia" widening it to include forced utilization of objects (Lhermitte, 1983; Shallice et al., 1989; De Renzi et al., 1996).

from ideational to kinetic and subcortical apraxias corresponds to an increasing loss of autonomy of action. In ideational apraxia environmental dependence shows up only when patients are requested to demonstrate imaginary actions. In kinetic apraxia the external reality forces patients to approach or avoid surrounding objects and in subcortical apraxias movements occur completely out of voluntary control.

Competition and collaboration of two levels of action control

A comparison of the mid-twentieth century accounts of apraxia with Liepmann's model reveals fundamental differences but also striking similarities. With the exception of some parts of Denny-Brown's system of apraxia, the post-Liepmann authors did not care much about the location of responsible lesions and made no attempt to relate symptoms directly to neural mechanisms. Their approach was not physiological but psychological, and their psychological reasoning was mainly "holistic," seeking for overarching effects of brain damage rather than dissecting symptoms into independent components. In contrast, Liepmann had based his model directly on anatomical considerations and had fervently defended the analytical dissection of symptoms as a necessary prerequisite for determining their anatomical and physiological fundaments.

The striking communality between Liepmann and the post-Liepmann authors is the assumption that action control has a high and a low level. The distinction is explicit in Jackson's opposition of voluntary and automatic action, in Head's and Gordon's conclusion that in healthy subjects "higher nerve centers" overcome "primitive, inherited psycho-physical mechanism," and in Goldstein's distinction between the abstract attitude and the subjugation of action to its concrete context. It is implicit in Grünbaum's and Denny-Brown's analyses of externally triggered actions, since their suppression in healthy subjects presupposes a higher level of action control suppressing the influence of the environmental triggers. In Liepmann's model the lower level is constituted by the central region issuing motor commands, and the higher by the mental image of the intended action.

A crucial difference between Liepmann and the holistic authors concerned the interaction between the two levels. The holistic accounts assume competition between them. If the high level is too weak to suppress the low level, the low level will take the lead and produce actions which correspond to the low level's inherent tendencies but are in conflict with high-level intentions. By contrast, in Liepmann's model, the "government of the limbs by the mind" depends on a translation of high-level mental images of intended actions into low-level motor commands. Such a translation necessitates the collaboration between both levels of action control rather than the suppression of one by the other. The power of high-level control depends on the connection between both levels. If it fails, the execution of high-level plans will be impossible even if they are themselves intact.

Constructional apraxia

Constructional apraxia was a temporary lodger in the house of apraxia. It started its residency as an offspring of associationist diagram making but soon changed and became a favorite topic for psychological analyses of spatial transformation and action. Theories of constructional apraxia did not, however, participate in the holistic attempts to distinguish the autonomy of action from dependency on external influences. Perhaps it was its resistance against hierarchical models of action control that eventually led to the separation of constructional apraxia from theorizing about apraxia. The term "constructional apraxia" is not widely used any more today. The symptoms subsumed under this heading are rather classified without reference to apraxia as visuo-spatial or visuo-constructional deficits (Trojano & Conson, 2008).

The origins of constructional apraxia

The German neuropsychiatrist Walter Poppelreuter (1917, 1990) was head of a rehabilitation unit for soldiers with head wounds from World War I. Training in craft skills was a central constituent of the rehabilitation program. Poppelreuter observed patients with posterior brain lesions whose performance of these skills was awkward, clumsy, and sometimes grossly deviating. He argued that classification of such difficulties into the Liepmann dichotomy of ideo-kinetic and ideational apraxia was very difficult in individual cases and did not accurately express the essence of the syndrome which is the dependence of problems on the need for "visual guidance or control over the execution of movements." He insisted that such problems can occur in patients whose perceptual abilities are sufficient for recognizing the objects which they are unable to handle appropriately[13] and suggested classifying them as "optic apraxia." Since there is a wide variety of manual actions requiring visual control, the scope of optic apraxia was also very wide:

> Optic apraxia becomes evident in all actions that require visual guidance or control over the execution of movements, for walking to a goal, touching, grasping, eating, dressing, and especially for the movements of a craftsman. (Poppelreuter, 1990, p. 193)

This definition included disturbances of grasping, pointing, and navigation in space which had been considered to be intact in all previous elaborations of apraxia. Karl Kleist and his disciple Hans Strauss (Strauss, 1922; Kleist, 1934) adopted the delimitation of a distinct variant of apraxia contingent upon the need for visual control of actions but renamed it "constructional apraxia" and narrowed down the range of its manifestations:

> If one beckons, or blows out a candle, the spatial form of the action is exhausted by the action itself, and there remains no permanent form. By contrast, if I write or draw, form a figure from clay, if the carpenter makes a table or the child arranges the bricks of a construction kit according to a model, their movements create a lasting, spatially formed product.

[13] Poppelreuter illustrated the dissociation between preserved recognition and disturbed manipulation of objects with a schema which showed two routes originating from Vision. One, pointing downward leads to "intellectual processes" and the other, pointing upward, to "motility" (Poppelreuter, 1990, p. 193). The similarity to modern accounts of the "dual route" model of visual perception (Mishkin et al., 1983; Goodale & Milner, 1992) is striking. Although Poppelreuter did not comment on the anatomy of both routes their arrangement on the diagram strongly suggest that the route to "intellectual processes" leads to the temporal, and that to "motility" to the parietal lobe.

> Ideo-kinetic or limb-kinetic apraxia would interfere with the execution of the movements of hammering, carving, moulding, but nonetheless the result could be an awkward but recognizable work. On the other hand, there are disturbances of action which I would call "constructional (optical) apraxia" in which the spatial form of the work is failed although there is no apraxia of the single movements. (Kleist, 1934, p. 483)

Refurbishing the posterior to anterior stream of action control

Kleist had opposed Liepmann's contention that parietal lesions cause ideo-kinetic apraxia, because they interrupt the connection between posterior brain regions producing a predominantly visual mental image of the intended actions, and the central region commanding their motor execution. Instead, he had proposed that the left parietal lobe stores "complex engrams of single actions which combine kinesthetic engrams with movement directives coming from optical and acoustic territories" (Kleist, 1934, p. 465). In the discussion of constructional apraxia, however, he simplified these "complex engrams" to plain "kinesthetic engrams." In order to make space for an anatomical substrate of defective linking between optical brain regions and kinesthetic engrams, he emphasized the division of the inferior parietal lobe into the more anterior supramarginal gyrus (Brodman area 40) and the more posterior angular gyrus (area 39). He confined the territory of kinesthetic engrams to the supramarginal gyrus. Optical processing was assumed to be localized in visual cortex of the occipital lobe. Consequently:

> The centre for constructional apraxia has to be sought in the intermediate territory between anterior parietal lobe and visual areas, that is, in the posterior parietal lobe. Area 40 in supramarginal gyrus would be the organ of the kinaesthetic engrams responsible for ideo-kinetic apraxia, while area 39 on the angular gyrus would be devoted to optic–kinaesthetic coupling, damage to which leads to constructional apraxic disturbances. (Kleist, 1934, p. 489)

Kleist's postulate that in constructional apraxia "the spatial form of the work fails although there is no apraxia of single movements" would also apply to many examples of misuse of tools and objects that had been described under the heading of "ideational apraxia." For example, patients rub the match on the top rather than the striking surface of the match box, lead the toothbrush to the chin rather than the teeth, or put the wrong end of the cigar into the mouth. The motor actions leading to these errors were swift and secure, but they were executed in a wrong section of space and resulted in wrong spatial relationships. Kleist concluded that the loss of optic-kinesthetic coupling that causes constructional apraxia makes also a major contribution to ideational apraxia. Therefore lesions causing ideational apraxia usually extend more posteriorly than those causing only ideo-motor apraxia.[14]

Figure 3.1 sums up Kleist's proposals for the localization of lesions causing constructional, ideo-kinetic, and limb-kinetic apraxia. The similarity to Liepmann's "lateral view" (see Figure 2.4) is striking, particularly considering that for Kleist constructional apraxia

---

[14] Kleist proposed a further variant of apraxia which he called "frontal apraxia of action sequences" and ascribed it to lesions of prefrontal Brodman area 10. Its leading symptom is loss of drive and neglect of the ultimate goal of action sequences. Kleist's descriptions of this putative variant are, however, not easy to discern from Pick's description of ideational apraxia in demented patients (see Chapter 2).

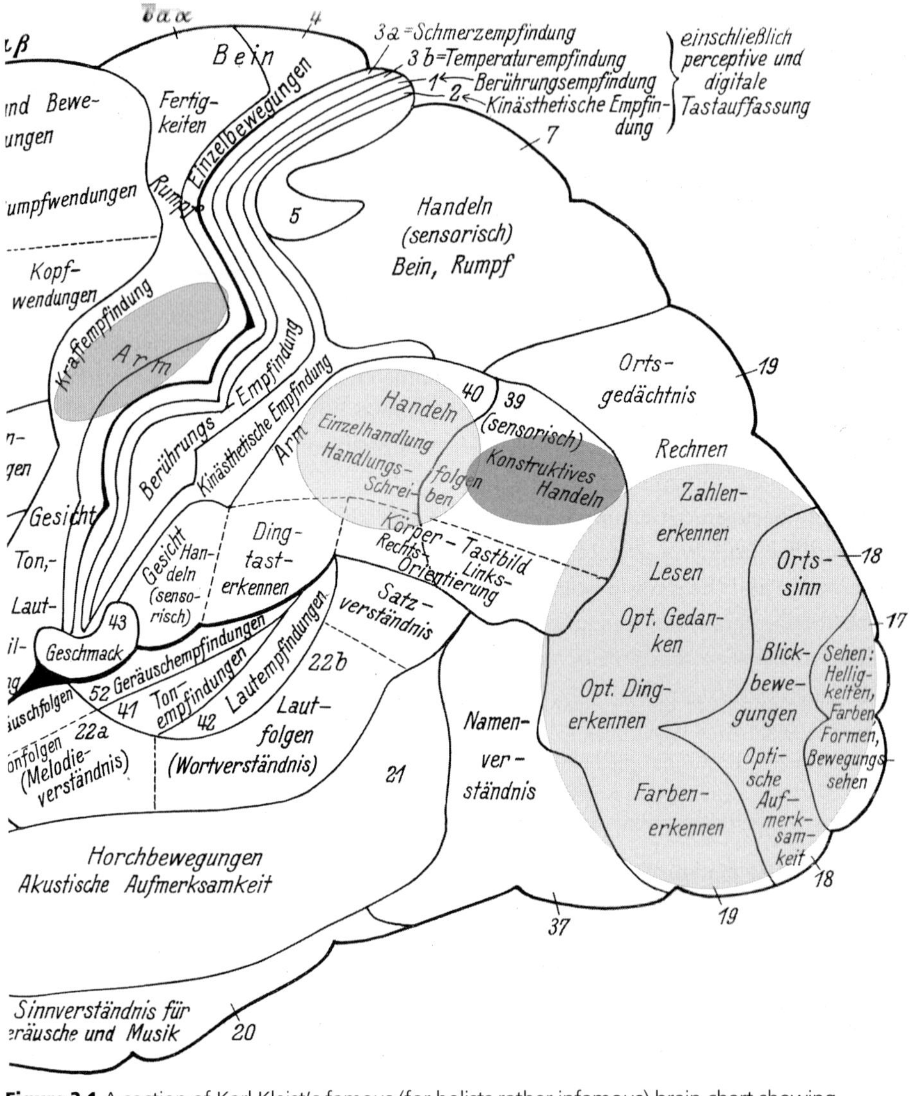

Figure 3.1 A section of Karl Kleist's famous (for holists rather infamous) brain chart showing the putative assignment of functions to Brodman areas of the cerebral cortex. The inscriptions describe functions of intact areas rather than symptoms of their damage, but in the text the clinical symptoms of their damage are elaborated. The colored field indicate the location of lesions causing limb-kinetic apraxia (orange; Brodman area 6a), ideokinetic apraxia (yellow; Brodman area 40), and constructional apraxia (green; Brodman area 39). Area 6a: *Rumpf*: trunk; *Arm*: arm (obviously including hand); *Gesicht*: face. Area 40: *Handeln*: action; *Einzelhandlung:* single action; *Handlungsfolgen:* action sequences; *Schreiben:* writing. Area 39: *Konstruktives Handeln*: constructional action. Ideational apraxia results from damage extending across the whole inferior parietal lobe. These lesions combine the disturbance of action sequencing with defective kinesthetic–optic coupling which is conceived as being at the core of constructional action. The section of Kleist's map is reproduced with kind permission from Springer Science+Business Media: *Zeitschrift für die gesamte Neurologie und Psychiatrie*, Bericht über die Gehirnpathologie in ihrer Bedeutung für Neurologie und Psychiatrie, *158*, 1937, p. 163, K. Kleist. (See Plate 3.)

was a major component of ideational apraxia which was thus located posterior to ideo-kinetic apraxia by both authors.

The similarity between Liepmann's and Kleist's version of the posterior to anterior stream of action control should not distract from their crucial discrepancy. For Liepmann, supramarginal lesions interrupt the translation of mental images into motor commands, whereas for Kleist they destroy kinetic engrams.

Spatial transformations

Kleist's concept of constructional apraxia as a disorder of optic-kinesthetic coupling is easily recognizable as an example of the German associationists' emphasis on associations between basic sensory and motor modalities. It did not find many followers. One possible reason for this neglect was its late appearance. When Kleist and Strauss proposed their model of constructional apraxia, the popularity of the German variant of associationism was already in decline.[15] But while Kleist's anatomical speculations fell into oblivion, constructional apraxia itself participated in the rising interest in psychological models of thinking and action. In this new context the interest was less on the transfer from the visual to the motor modality than on the spatial transformations implied by such a transfer.

McDonald Critchley gave a succinct definition of spatial transformations involved in constructional apraxia:

> The defects which characterize constructional apraxia involve essentially those movements which are directly concerned with space per se, i.e. manipulation of the three dimensions of space, and particularly the translation of an object from one spatial dimension into another. (Critchley, 1953, p. 191)

Constructional apraxia thus joined a family of symptoms concerned with spatial relationships which attracted increasing interest in the middle third of the twentieth century. We have already encountered them in Marie's description of planotopokinesia (Marie et al., 1922), but Marie's pseudo-Greek name did "not receive the impress of neurological recognition" (Critchley, 1953). Subsequent authors referred to disorders of "spatial thinking" (Lhermitte et al., 1928; Lhermitte & Trelles, 1933), "spatial sense" (van der Horst, 1934), or "visual space perception" (Paterson & Zangwill, 1944), to name just a few of the various names given to this family. Among their established members were restrictions of the field of visual attention rendering the afflicted patients unable to simultaneously appreciate multiple objects and their spatial relationships, shifts of visual attention to one side causing neglect of stimuli on the other side, confusion of the right and left side of the patient's own and another person's body, confusion of fingers, topographical disorientation rendering patients unable to find their way and to orient themselves on maps, and defective estimation of positions, angles, and distances.

Ideally constructional apraxia should differ from other members of this family by the confinement of spatial errors to tasks which demand the motor production of spatially

[15] Kleist himself abandoned research on localization of functions after the completion of his monumental book on "Brain Pathology" and dedicated his further scientific work to clinical psychiatry (Kleist, 1937; Neumärker & Bartsch, 2003).

organized representations such as, for example, writing, drawing, or assembling of bricks or sticks into two- or three-dimensional objects. Critchley characterized this peculiarity:

> patients with constructional apraxia have some type of defective orientation in space, but a defect which may not emerge until a motor task is attempted within the visual sphere. (Critchley, 1953, p. 190)

Empirical support for the existence of this dissociation between intact perceptual apprehension and defective motor reproduction of spatial relationships was derived from patients who could name but not copy geometrical figures or found their way in the surroundings in spite of their inability to draw a map (Strauss, 1922; Lhermitte et al., 1928; Critchley, 1953).

The restriction of symptoms to tasks requiring motor production of spatial relationships had been central to Kleist's associationist account of constructional apraxia, but the authors in the middle of the twentieth century reasoned that this apparent modality specificity of errors could also be referred to the particular demands of motor production on spatial thinking. A plausible candidate for such particular demands was the decomposition of spatial entities into their constituents:

> The patients are quite unable to abstract salient spatial relationships in the model and reproduce them consistently from the given elements. (Paterson & Zangwill, 1944, p. 355)
>
> In constructional apraxia, there is undoubtedly a specific impairment of visual spatial cognition, which can be characterized as an inability, when given a real or imaginary visual pattern as a whole, to analyse it piece by piece, in order to construct it, piece by piece. (Critchley, 1953, p. 199)

It seems plausible that extraction of salient spatial constituents is a necessary prerequisite for the stepwise manual construction of complex objects, whereas it is dispensable for tasks which are solved by a single perceptual evaluation of the entire stimulus such as, for example, the comparison of angles and distances, or the naming of geometrical figures.

The laterality of constructional apraxia

Although all of their patients had bilateral lesions, Kleist and Strauss believed that constructional apraxia is, like Liepmann's apraxias, a symptom of left brain damage. The further accumulation of clinical evidence was in favor of a predominance of right-sided lesions although it remained beyond doubt that the most impressive cases were due to bilateral damage. Critchley summarized the laterality of lesions causing constructional apraxia:

> Some would associate this symptom more closely with lesion of the subordinate parietal lobe. It is probably more accurate to say that constructional apraxia may occur with lesions of either hemisphere: that it is seen in its most florid style with bilateral lesions and least clearly with lesions of the dominant hemisphere. (Critchley, 1953, p. 393)

Further clinical observations revealed qualitative differences between constructional apraxia from left- and right-sided lesions (Paterson & Zangwill, 1944; Critchley, 1953; Duensing, 1953; McFie & Zangwill, 1960; Piercy et al., 1960).

They were most conspicuous in copying of complex drawings (see Figure 3.2). Copies by patients with left brain damage (usually accompanied by aphasia) were placed at an

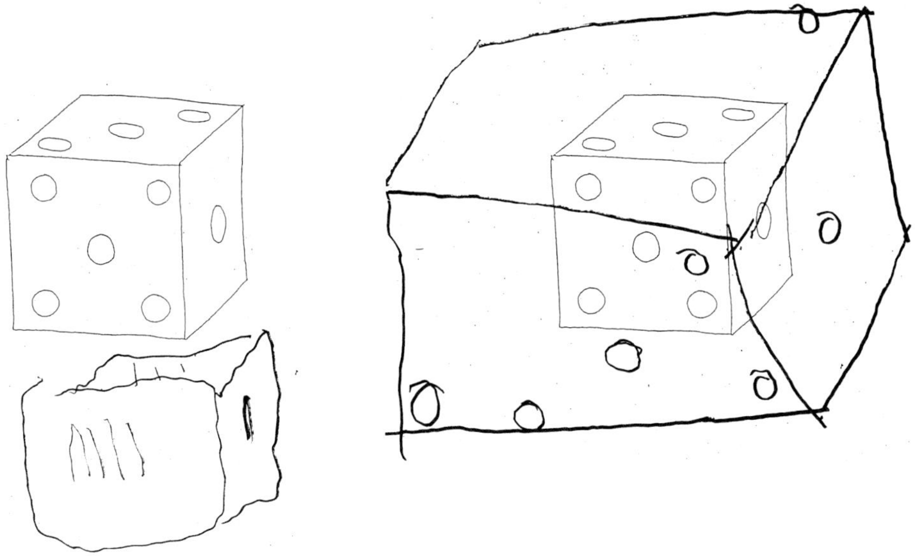

Figure 3.2 Right: Copy of a cube by a patient with right temporal bleeding. The copy is ill placed and "closes in" on the model. The angles of the contours are distorted. The left-sided dots on the upper face are omitted. Those on the front and on the right lateral side are complete but displaced. Left: Copy of the same cube by a patient with a left temporal bleeding. The copy is placed at an appropriate distance below the model and the orientation of the contours is fairly correct though straight lines and angles tend to be rounded. The most conspicuous deviation concerns the dots: linear marks indicate their numbers correctly, but neither their positions nor their forms are reproduced. Both examples are clinical observations of the author.

appropriate distance to the original drawing and preserved its global orientation and outlines, but were impoverished by lack or simplification of details. By contrast, copies by patients with right brain damage were frequently ill placed and overlapped with the original drawing, a phenomenon designated as "closing in" (Mayer-Gross, 1935). Horizontal and vertical axes were frequently distorted. Details were faithfully reproduced and sometimes even overemphasized by multiplication of strokes, but the global structure was broken, distorted, or completely lost. Finally, while both groups of patients tended to neglect parts of the model on the side contralateral to their lesions, the asymmetry was more marked for right than for left brain damaged patients.

Since Liepmann's "mass study" it had been taken as established that bilateral apraxia from unilateral lesions is bound to lesions of the left hemisphere. The discovery that right brain damage can cause at least one variant of bilateral apraxia, and that this apraxia is not just a milder form of apraxia from left brain damage but disrupts autonomous functions of the right hemisphere was a seminal contribution to the further development of research on apraxia.

The absolute dominance of the left hemisphere for apraxia was not the only established finding called into doubt by observations of constructional apraxia. They provided counterexamples to central arguments of the holistic writers and opened alternative views on a central topic of Liepmann's theories, imitation.

Jackson's principle fails

The German–British neuropsychiatrist Wilhelm Mayer-Gross (1935, 1936) analyzed the tasks used for the examination of constructional apraxia in terms of the automatic versus voluntary action dichotomy. He concluded that typical constructional performances like the arrangement of matches, colored mosaics, or bricks in accordance with a given pattern are non-routine because they have not been practiced and are removed from the sphere of daily life. For example, patients are asked to arrange matches in geometrical patterns rather than using them for the habitual purpose of lighting. For most subjects this holds also for drawing, the non-automaticity of which contrasts with the highly practiced routine of writing. Jackson's principle of relative sparing of automatic actions from the effects of brain damage would predict particularly severe impairment of such artificial tasks and relative sparing of everyday routines, but Mayer Gross brought forward observations which did not fit into this schema. For example, an artist who had suffered bilateral parietal infarctions had completely lost the skill of drawing:

> Although his handling of the pencil was quite normal, the destruction of his drawing faculty was almost incredible. Even his placing of the drawing on the sheet of paper demonstrated the severe spatial disturbance. Some lines and some fixed schemata in designing disclosed the professional hand, otherwise his drawings were like a child's. (Mayer-Gross, 1935, p. 1207)

Not only had he lost his highly practiced skill of drawing, he also displayed a reverse dissociation between preserved and disturbed routine and non-routine capabilities:

> In writing he used block letters almost exclusively. Single letters were entirely correct; there were few mistakes in spelling in larger words. But these mistakes increased and made the whole word unrecognizable when he tried to write in cursive script. He could never write his signature in cursive style. (Mayer-Gross, 1936, p. 751)

There was no indication that he used to write in block letters rather than script before the cerebral accidents, and presumably his signature was among his most practiced motor routines. The dissociation between routine and non-routine actions was thus the reverse of what it should be according to Jackson's principle.

Earlier in this chapter we cited Marie's lively description of the difficulties with dressing in "planotopokinesia." Some 20 years later the British neurologist Russell Brain (1941) described "apraxia for dressing" as a distinct manifestation of visual disorientation following right brain damage. The French neuropsychiatrists, Henry Hécaen and Julian de Ajuriaguerra[16] endorsed the proposal to recognize dressing apraxia ("apraxie de l'habillage") as a clinical entity of its own (Hécaen & De Ajuriaguerra, 1945). They admitted that most cases are associated with constructional apraxia but maintained that dressing apraxia can be analyzed relatively independently from other constructional difficulties. Indeed the matching of the complex spatial structure of pieces of dress with the anatomical structure

[16] De Ajuriaguerra was born in Spain and ultimately became a professor in Geneva, Switzerland, but his formation and the major part of his scientific achievements took place in France, and he received French citizenship in 1950.

of the body certainly challenges the "manipulation of the three dimensions of space, and particularly the translation of an object from one spatial dimension into another" which had been identified by Critchley (1953, p. 191) as the core problem in constructional apraxia. A salient difference between dressing apraxia and constructional apraxia lies in the kind of tasks used for diagnosing them. Constructional apraxia is examined by rather artificial and unfamiliar tasks like reproducing abstract spatial patterns (see earlier). In contrast, there is hardly any complex motor action more familiar and more practiced than dressing. Its disturbance thus undermines Jackson's principle. Moreover, Hécaen and Ajuriaguerra noted that some patients ultimately succeeded in getting properly dressed, but had lost the automatic flow of actions:

> They succeed only after trying different movements or by orienting themselves on visual marks. It is interesting to note that they have lost the automatic actions. To dress is certainly a very automatic action for civilized man. Thus it seems difficult to subscribe to the proposal, based on Jackson's doctrine, that the severity of apraxia is inversely correlated to the degree of automatization of the afflicted functions. (Hécaen & De Ajuriaguerra, 1945, p. 132)

Telling right from left

The idea that the body is a multipart object occupying a place in external space and entertaining spatial relationships with other objects was captured in the popular notions of "body schema" or "body image" (Lhermitte & Trelles, 1933; Schilder, 1935). Critchley's formulation that constructional apraxia affects "particularly the translation of an object from one spatial dimension into another" (Critchley, 1953, p. 191) can be applied to imitation of body configurations or gestures. By this logic the object to be transferred is a particular configuration of the human body and the spatial dimensions which must be translated are the different positions of one's own and the examiner' bodies. One aspect for which this translation is particularly error prone is the distinction between the left and the right side of the body.

Indeed difficulties with replicating the laterality of movements were a regular feature in case reports of constructional and dressing apraxia (Marie et al., 1922; Strauss, 1922; Brain, 1941; Stengel, 1944; Hécaen & De Ajuriaguerra, 1945). Some patients already confused the sides when verbally asked to point to right- or left-sided body parts with either the right or the left hand, but difficulties became more conspicuous, and were in some case even restricted to imitation of such actions. In this situation patients regularly imitated as in a mirror even when the instruction unequivocally demanded moving and touching body parts on the nominally same side of the body as the examiner. This deficiency is reminiscent of the errors described by Head in patients with aphasia (Head, 1920). Indeed the "Hand, Eye, and Ear Test" was frequently used to detect confusion of right and left in the patients with constructional and dressing apraxia. There was, however, a crucial difference between these patients and those examined by Head: The patients with constructional or dressing apraxia had no aphasia at all or, at best, mild and recovered language disturbances. Their difficulties with the transfer of laterality from another person's to their own body clearly invalidated Head's contention that the adherence to mirror imitation is due to a deficiency of the "power of verbalization" or, more generally, of symbolic thought. Rather than betraying the government of action by "lower, primitive, inherited psycho-physical mechanism" (Gordon, 1922, p. 298) the errors indicated a mundane deficiency of spatial thinking.[17]

The Austrian–American neurologist Paul Schilder summarized:

> It is, of course, possible that some of Head's patients had difficulties in verbalization. But there is no question that in the great majority of cases these difficulties are based on inability to use the body schema for action. (Schilder, 1935, p. 49).

Constructional apraxia and imitation

Liepmann's model of apraxia included three domains of actions: use of tools and objects, performance of communicative gestures, and imitation of gestures. Dressing is certainly an instance of object use, and dressing apraxia can thus be categorized not only as a manifestation of constructional apraxia but also as an apraxia for use of tools and objects. There is less overlap between constructional apraxia and the performance of communicative gestures, and several case reports of constructional apraxia emphasized the absence of any difficulties with the production of emblems or pantomime (Marie et al., 1922; Strauss, 1922; Lhermitte et al., 1928; Mayer-Gross, 1936; Hécaen & De Ajuriaguerra, 1945). Few case reports noted some spatial inaccuracies of communicative gestures, but they were distinctly less conspicuous than the aberrations in constructional tasks (Lhermitte & Trelles, 1933; Stengel, 1944). The most important overlap between constructional apraxia and Liepmann's apraxias was in the domain of imitation. In his initial description of "optical apraxia" Poppelreuter noted:

> One of the most remarkable failures with optic apraxia is the incorrect imitation of demonstrated body movements, for example of hand- and arm-movements. (Poppelreuter, 1990, p. 202)

Based on a thorough examination of one patient with predominantly right-sided brain damage diagnosed as multiple sclerosis[18] the Viennese neurologist Benno Schlesinger (1928) gave a lucid analysis of disturbed imitation accompanying constructional apraxia. He wrote:

> The similarity between disturbed imitation of finger and hand postures and constructional-apraxia is so striking that there can be no doubts on their common basic disturbance ("Grundstörung"). The disturbance which becomes manifest in the imitation of movements and the postures reached by them, is nothing else than "constructional apraxia on the own body." (p. 672)

---

[17] Modern neuropsychology would classify the disorder as insufficient mental rotation (Goldenberg, 1989; Corballis & Sergent, 1989) and provide a less ideological explanation for the superior performance of boys by considering it a further instance of the better performance of male subjects on mental rotation tasks (Moore & Johnson, 2008; Jansen & Heil, 2010).

[18] Given the very limited diagnostic tools available at the time and the absence of a post-mortem examination the diagnosis is rather insecure. However, the clinical examination yielded unequivocal signs of right sided plus diffuse brain damage.

Schlesinger emphasized that defective imitation was typically confined to "abstract" movements, that is, meaningless gestures but spared "concrete" movements, that is, meaningful and familiar gestures:

> If imitation of concrete spatial configurations is required, the required movements are not produced directly from perception (that is, by parallel movements) but by a detour to their meaning. Rather than being copied in a strict sense, the parallel movements are replaced by movements from memory. (p. 691)

Finger agnosia

Defective imitation was a regular feature in all cases of constructional apraxia where it had been looked for, but in some cases it was confined to finger postures (Marie et al., 1922; Schilder, 1935; Mayer-Gross, 1936) while in others the body part specificity of disturbed imitation included finger and hand (Schlesinger, 1928; Mayer-Gross, 1935; Stengel, 1944) or was not specified (Lhermitte et al., 1928).

In some patients defective imitation of finger postures was associated with defective selection of single fingers on verbal command (Mayer-Gross, 1935; Stengel, 1944). The different manifestations of insufficient location of fingers had been subsumed under the heading of "finger agnosia" (Gerstmann, 1924; Schilder, 1935). The Austrian–British neurologist Erwin Stengel demonstrated the close relationship between finger agnosia and constructional apraxia in an elegant experiment. It was carried out with a woman who had suffered bilateral parietal damage from eclampsia:

> Naming, recognizing and presenting a particular finger were equally impaired, and the same applied to other persons' fingers and toes. She was unable to perform specified movements of her fingers to order or to imitate such movements.
>
> Two sets of matches were laid out, each consisting of five matches arranged either parallel or converging like fingers of the hands; the patient was requested to choose one particular match, e.g. the middle match of the right set, etc. In this test she was equally helpless as when requested to choose a particular finger on her own or another person's hand or on a diagram of a hand. She also failed when she had to choose between the matches of one set only. (Stengel, 1944, p. 754)

Stengel concluded that the configuration of the hand is perceived like that of an external object and that consequently one and the same disturbance can affect both the spatial evaluation of the external multipart object and the own hand:

> The hand belongs to the "dynamic body scheme,"[19] but is at the same time something comparatively independent, acting outside the body, connecting personal and outer space. This conception states clearly the peculiar position of the fingers, which in acting become to a certain extent external objects.

[19] The "dynamic body schema" had been introduced by Paul Schilder (1935) to denote knowledge about the current configuration of one's body which is necessary for planning goal directed movements. More detailed discussions of the validity and function of this purported entity can be found in Gallagher (1986), Goldenberg (2005), and de Vignemont (2010).

> Finger agnosia is the inability to appreciate the position of individual fingers amongst its fellows, and is an instance of the inability to locate correctly a part of a multiplicity of objects forming an organized whole. (p. 759)

Constructions on earthly ground

Constructional apraxia was an offspring of the traditional apraxias. Children grow up and eventually leave their family to find a new home. We have already mentioned the warm welcome of constructional apraxia by the growing family of disorders of spatial thinking. In the last third of the twentieth century constructional apraxia ultimately left the house where it was born. Although some researchers continued to use the epithet "apraxia" for visuo-constructive disorders, their connection to the traditional apraxias of imitation, symbolic gestures, and tool use have ceased to be a topics of research and are rarely mentioned at all (Gainotti, 1985; Carlesimo et al., 1993; Laeng, 2006; Trojano & Conson, 2008).

During the approximately 30 years when constructional apraxia lived in one house with the traditional apraxias, it made important contributions to their development. Arguably, its major merit was to shake the solidity of the hierarchical model of action control. Research on constructional apraxia and spatial thinking undermined the prevailing "holistic" tendency to make the struggle between higher and lower levels of control the central principle of apraxia if not of all psychological manifestations of brain damage. As we have discussed in detail, the observation of dressing apraxia, a variant of constructional apraxia, called into question Jackson's principle of voluntary and automatic control. Analysis of the human body as a multipart object occupying a place in external space reduced right–left confusions from being a manifestation of a "lower, primitive, inherited psycho-physical mechanism not involving the 'higher centres'" (Gordon, 1922, p. 298) to a mundane weakness of mental rotation.

Revisiting the corpus callosum

Unilaterally left-sided apraxia following destruction of the corpus callosum was a core argument for Liepmann's model of apraxia and for the localization of brain functions in general. The observation that the interruption of their connections to other regions can deprive cortical regions from functional competencies was considered as an impressive demonstration of the validity of anatomy as an explanatory concept for psychological symptoms. Unsurprisingly, callosal disconnection lost its popularity when holistic theories and psychological reasoning dominated the field. Liepmann's discussion of the importance of callosal disconnection for the symptoms of the imperial counselor and his subsequent publication of a case of left-sided apraxia caused by a callosal lesion (Liepmann & Maas, 1907) had been followed by a number of confirmatory case reports (Van Vleuten, 1907; Hartmann, 1907; Goldstein, 1908; Maas, 1910; Bonhoeffer, 1914), but the tide soon ebbed away, and when the century advanced similar case reports became rare (Pineas, 1924; Hoff, 1931). McDonald Critchley (1930) recognized left-sided ideo-motor apraxia as a regular symptom of occlusions of the anterior cerebral artery which supplies the corpus callosum, but other authors denied any importance of callosal lesions for apraxia (Lhermitte & Trelles, 1933). Generally, however, callosal disconnection was less disputed than neglected. It could offer no contribution to the dominant discourse on psychological topics such as the autonomy of action or spatial thinking (see earlier).

In the middle of the century callosal disconnection re-entered the stage but apparently only to be definitely expelled. Based on the observation that in patients with brain tumors encroaching upon the corpus callosum the frequency of epileptic seizures decreased with increasing destruction of the corpus callosum, the American neurosurgeon William van Wagenen attempted first partial and then complete surgical sections of the corpus callosum in patients with pharmacologically uncontrollable epilepsy (Matthews et al., 2008). The patients were examined shortly after surgery and some of them also in later follow-ups by the psychiatrist Andrew Akelaitis (1942; Akelaitis et al., 1945). The main upshot of his clinical examinations was an absence of lasting deficits which could unequivocally be referred to the callosal disconnection. This absence led prominent neuroscientists to joke that the corpus callosum must have evolved only "to aid the transmission of epileptic seizures from one to the other side of the body" or, alternatively, that the only function of the corpus callosum "must be mechanical, i.e., to keep the hemispheres from sagging" (Finger, 2000).

Indeed Akelaitis found quite numerous abnormalities of left-hand actions and did not hesitate to apply a diagnosis of "idio-motor apraxia" to some of them. Some of his observations were quite spectacular. For example, he described problems encountered by a young woman after section of the posterior half of the corpus callosum:

> The patient noted that frequently her left hand would do exactly the opposite of what her right hand was doing. For example, she would open a drawer with her right hand and put it shut with her left hand, or put her dress on with her right hand and pull it off with her left hand. (Akelaitis et al., 1942, p. 985)[20]

However, he noted that such difficulties recovered within few weeks after surgery, and that all patients displaying them had evidence of additional brain damage outside the corpus callosum. Since the section of the corpus callosum was permanent, the transience of symptoms proved that left-hand control was not contingent on integrity of the corpus callosum.

Akelaitis proposed alternative mechanisms such as sensory abnormalities, ataxia, or forced grasping of the left hand to explain awkwardness and aberrant actions, and for conflicts between the hands he even alluded to psychodynamic factors. Acceptance of such

[20] In the 1942 paper the term "diagnostic [sic!] dyspraxia" was used for these intermanual conflict. In a later paper devoted exclusively to them the name changed to "diagonistic" apraxia. (Akelaitis, 1945). "Diagonistic" is largely synonymous with the more common term "antagonistic." Perhaps it was preferred for emphasizing that the opposing limbs are on opposite sides of the body (dia = through), although Akelaitis included observations of conflicts that did not oppose right- and left-sided limbs, such as desiring to walk forward or stand up from a sitting position and being unable to do so because of an equal urge to walk backward or remain seated. The meaning of "diagnostic apraxia" is a puzzle. Possibly it was due to typing errors or, conversely, to an overzealous but ignorant editor who wanted to correct what seemed to him to be typing errors.

mechanisms would not rule out the possibility of an additional contribution of callosal disconnection, but the apparent absence of any left-sided motor deficiency in patients with complete section of the corpus callosum was definitely incompatible with Liepmann's diagrams. It seemed that both hemispheres were equally capable of converting ideas into motor action, and unilateral left-sided apraxia must be due to right-sided lesions interfering with basic motor abilities of the left hand (Hécaen & Gimeno-Alava, 1960).

Liepmann's model of apraxia had been a flagship of the associationists' endeavor to divide the brain into functionally distinct centers and their connections. Its shipwreck in the encounter with the clinical reality of callosal disconnection seemed to seal the decline of diagram making. In Chapter 4 we will see that its resurrection commenced where it had perished, that is, in the analysis of the effects of callosal disconnection on apraxia.

A latecomer

In 1968 the first volume of the multivolume *Handbook of Clinical Neurology* was published. Volume 4 included a chapter on apraxia written by two psychiatrists from Geneva, Julian de Ajuriaguerra and René Tissot. They combined Morlaas' concept of "spatial dyskinesia" with the developmental psychology of Jean Piaget. Piaget had postulated that "the child masters the space involved in manipulating objects, then the space centered on his body, and finally objective Euclidean space." Ajuriaguerra and Tissot proposed that in apraxia:

> practically all of these stages of integration of represented space in the child may be followed in reverse order . . . Constructional apraxia corresponds to Euclidean space, ideomotor apraxia to the space centred on the body, and ideational apraxia to the concrete space of manipulation. (De Ajuriaguerra & Tissot, 1969, pp. 62–63)

The continuity of functional regression does not lend itself easily to a differential localization of its stages and indeed de Ajuriaguerra and Tissot were very skeptical about the localizing specificity of any variant of apraxia. They thought that the total mass of lesioned brain tissue was more important for determining the form of apraxia than its location.

De Ajuriaguerra and Tissot embedded their theory in a sharp critique of Liepmann and his followers. They disqualified Liepmann's analysis of the imperial counselor as "according to the associationist conceptions in vogue at the time" and deplored the persistence of "authors such as Kleist, and more recently Geschwind, whose ideas still bear the stamp of the classical doctrines" but concluded: "The doctrines of these so-called 'diagram-makers' of apraxia, even in their most recent form, no longer merit criticism" (p. 58).

Nearly 20 years later a new edition of the Handbook was published. The chapter on apraxia was now written by the leading proponent of the "most recent form of diagram making," Norman Geschwind (Geschwind & Damasio, 1985). It did not even mention its predecessor. The pendulum had swung back and the diagram makers had returned (see Chapter 4).

Chapter 4

Return of the ostracized

From Germany to Boston

After World War II the Liepmann tradition of apraxia seemed to have definitely expired, but in the last third of the century it made a forceful comeback. The return started from Boston, USA, and its most influential proponent was the neurologist Norman Geschwind. Geschwind was a brilliant and charismatic clinician, writer, and teacher (Galaburda, 1985; Kean, 1994). He had been a resident under Derek Denny-Brown (see Chapter 3) and originally acquired a rather antilocalization bias which, however, was shaken when he joined the Boston Veteran Administration Hospital. It had an aphasia unit where Geschwind was confronted with the diversity of clinical features of aphasia. The neurology department was headed by Fred Quadfasel. Quadfasel was of German origin. He was not Jewish but had to emigrate from National Socialist Germany because of his political opposition to the regime (Geschwind, 1963). He had been an assistant to Kurt Goldstein and later to Karl Bonhoeffer, both disciples of Wernicke, and brought with him a large library containing many of the original texts of Wernicke, Liepmann, and other proponents of the localizing approach to brain function. The content of these texts opened Geschwind's mind to a reconsideration of the allegedly irrevocably overcome ideas of German associationism.

The rediscovery of callosal apraxia

In 1962, Edith Kaplan, a psychologist working in the same department as Geschwind, drew his attention to a puzzling observation of unilateral agraphia. The patient was a 41-year-old man who had a left frontal glioblastoma, an infiltrating, fast-growing malignant brain tumor. A complete resection of this kind of tumor is impossible, but surgery was nonetheless performed to diminish its extension. During the operation a large branch of the anterior cerebral artery which irrigates the anterior two-thirds of the corpus callosum was amputated. After the operation there was a right-sided hemiplegia which soon recovered and a tendency for right-hand grasping reactions which remained. Two months after the operation, however, Edith Kaplan noted that the patient's left hand produced an unrecognizable crawl intermingled with some well-written but clearly incorrect words when he was asked to write words and sentences to dictation with the left hand. By contrast, writing with the initially paretic right hand was spatially somewhat distorted but legible and linguistically correct. She alerted Geschwind to this peculiar dissociation, and they set up a testing program for exploring the possibility that the unilateral agraphia was caused by destruction of the callosal connection between both hemispheres. It soon became clear that the disconnection between left-hand activity and speech was not restricted to verbal control of writing. When objects, numbers, or letters were placed in the patient's left hand out of sight, he grossly misnamed them, calling, for example, a ring an eraser and a padlock a book of matches, although the left hand manipulated the misnamed objects quite skillfully and could even demonstrate correct use simultaneously with the incorrect verbal accounts. Thus, given a hammer, the patient's left hand made hammering movements while the patient commented "I would use this to comb my hair with." The defect was not confined to transfer of information from the left hand to speech but interrupted also the transfer of information from one hand to the other. The left hand was capable of selecting from an array an object which it had explored tactually out of sight, whereas the right hand was unable to select that object, to write its name, or to draw a picture of it.[1] Conversely, the left hand was unable to select or demonstrate the use of objects which had been tactually explored out of sight by the right hand.

Execution of these tests implied a compliance of the left hand with verbal instructions demanding, for example, writing to dictation or selection of tactually explored objects. However, when the ability to perform verbal commands with the left hand was tested in more detail, difficulties became manifest. Thus, when asked to point to the examiner with the left index finger, the left hand pointed to the patient's own eye. When asked to show how to brush the teeth, the left hand on one occasion made the motions of lathering the patient's face and on another went through the motions of combing his hair. These errors were restricted to performance on verbal command. When asked to imitate the examiner's movements or to manipulate real objects, both hands performed flawlessly.

Geschwind and Kaplan predicted that the patient's lesion must have destroyed large parts of the corpus callosum because:

> It appears to us that the simplest description of this patient's most striking disturbances is that he behaved as if his two cerebral hemispheres were functioning nearly autonomously. (Geschwind & Kaplan, 1962, p. 683)

The tumor continued to grow and few months later the patient died. Post-mortem examination confirmed atrophy of the anterior two thirds of the corpus callosum due to the amputation of the irrigating branch of the anterior cerebral artery.

In their discussion Geschwind and Kaplan referred to the cases of left-sided apraxia published in the early years of the century by Liepmann, Maas, and others (see Chapter 2), but noted that "our testing showed certain unusual features in the apparently apraxic manifestations" (1962, p. 682). They emphasized that the left hand was apraxic for actions which demanded transfer of information from the left to the right hemisphere, such as performance of actions on verbal command, but could perform all other actions, including

[1] One would expect that the hands were also unable to pantomime the use of objects identified tactually by the other hand, but apparently this was not tested.

imitation and real tool use, without difficulties. Apraxic difficulties could also be induced in the right hand when actions were contingent upon communication between the hemispheres as, for example, right-handed drawing of objects which had been tactually explored by the left hand. Geschwind and Kaplan concluded that the apraxia of their patient was exclusively caused by insufficient transfer of information between the hemispheres, and did not denote an inherent inferiority of right-hemispheric action control.

Dissecting the unity of man

Geschwind's rehabilitation of callosal apraxia received reinforcement from new studies on the effects of surgical section of the corpus callosum, first in animals and then in a new series of patients with intractable epilepsy. Using more refined examination techniques than Akelaitis in the first series of such patients (see Chapter 3), these studies demonstrated that the two hemispheres could indeed be isolated from each other and continue to function independently (Gazzaniga et al., 1967). The proof that interruption of fiber tracts could dissect the brain into independently functioning parts opened the door for speculation about the consequences of disconnecting not only one hemisphere from the other but also one area from another within a hemisphere. In other words, it reinstated the associationist model of centers and their connections which had been the basis of the despised art of diagram making.

In 1921 Henry Head had published his vigorous critique of the diagram makers on 78 pages of *Brain*, the most prestigious journal in neurology (Head, 1921). In 1965 the same journal published a two-part paper of 116 pages by Norman Geschwind titled "Disconnexion syndromes in animal and man" (Geschwind, 1965). The winds had turned: holism had given way to a new era of localization of functions. Geschwind summarized this turn:

> For the past forty years there have been schools of thought which have stressed the importance of thinking of the patient as a whole, of seeing his responses as those of an integrated unitary structure, even in the face of damage. When Edith Kaplan and I were studying our patient, we constantly found that many confusions about the patient in our minds as well as in those of others resulted from failure to do the exact opposite of what the rule to look at the patient as a whole demanded, i.e. from our failure to regard the patient as made of connected parts rather than as an indissoluble whole. (Geschwind, 1965, p. 637)

Geschwind's paper proposed disconnections between anatomically and functionally distinct areas of the brain as an explanation for an amazing multitude of disorders in animals and man. Thirty-two of its 116 pages were devoted to apraxia. Geschwind's and Kaplan's single case still formed the fundament of this topic, but it was augmented by other clinical observations, and the theoretical account of apraxia was substantially revised and expanded. Up until his death in 1984 Geschwind published several additional papers on apraxia (e.g., Geschwind, 1975; Geschwind & Damasio, 1985). Throughout their course, the exclusive concentration on disconnection gave way to a more complete associationist model considering both connections and centers.

Refining the posterior to anterior stream of action control

Geschwind adopted Liepmann's basic idea of a posterior to anterior stream of action control but amended both its exact anatomy and its function (see Figure 4.1). He shifted its anterior end from motor to premotor cortex, and its origin from visual association cortex to "Wernicke's area" in the posterior superior temporal lobe which has traditionally been recognized as a center for language comprehension (Wernicke, 1874). The fiber connection from the posterior to the anterior end of the stream was identified with the arcuate fasciculus which runs below the inferior parietal lobe. Both ends of the streams were starting points of callosal fibers connecting them with homologous areas of the opposite hemisphere.

Functionally, the displacement of the anterior end of the stream to premotor cortex separated it from motor primary cortex and thus suggested the possibility that lesions damaging the anterior end of the stream spare the motor cortex and cause bilateral apraxia without hemiplegia of the right limbs.[2] The displacement of the posterior end of the stream into an area devoted to comprehension of verbal commands constituted a more profound deviation from Liepmann's original conception. It changed the origin of the stream from a multimodal, predominantly visual, mental image of the intended action into a verbal command. Geschwind described the functioning of the revised stream of action control during the examination of movements to verbal command:

> When the subject receives an order to carry out a movement with the right hand, this order is probably transmitted from Wernicke's area through the lower parietal lobe to the left premotor region. The pre-motor region, in turn, probably controls the precentral motor cortex which . . . activates the nerve cells controlling the muscles.
>
> When a command is given to the subject to carry out an action with the left hand, the order must also pass through Wernicke's area in the left hemisphere. Two alternative routes routes might be taken from this point. One goes from Wernicke's area to the left premotor region, from there via the corpus callosum to the premotor region of the right hemisphere, and from there to the right precentral motor cortex which controls the left limbs. The alternative route goes from Wernicke's area to the corresponding region in the right hemisphere and from there to the right premotor and precentral motor regions. This alternative route is probably not the one primarily used, since damage to this pathway [that is, the posterior portion of the corpus callosum] does not lead to apraxia in the left arm. (Geschwind, 1975, p. 198)

Thus far, the diagram claims a leading role for the left hemisphere for controlling movements on verbal commands for both the right and the left limbs but it entails no other asymmetry between both hemispheres' control of their contralateral hands. The right hemisphere, though unable to understand verbal commands, should be capable of imitating movements, to use tools and objects, and to pantomime their use when stimuli are presented visually. This constellation corresponded to Geschwind's and Kaplan's first

[2] If you are a very careful reader you may note that the anterior end of the posterior to anterior stream had already been shifted to premotor cortex by Kleist (see Figure 3.1). However, Kleist supposed that lesions of premotor cortex cause limb-kinetic apraxia of the opposite hand rather than bilateral ideo-kinetic apraxia.

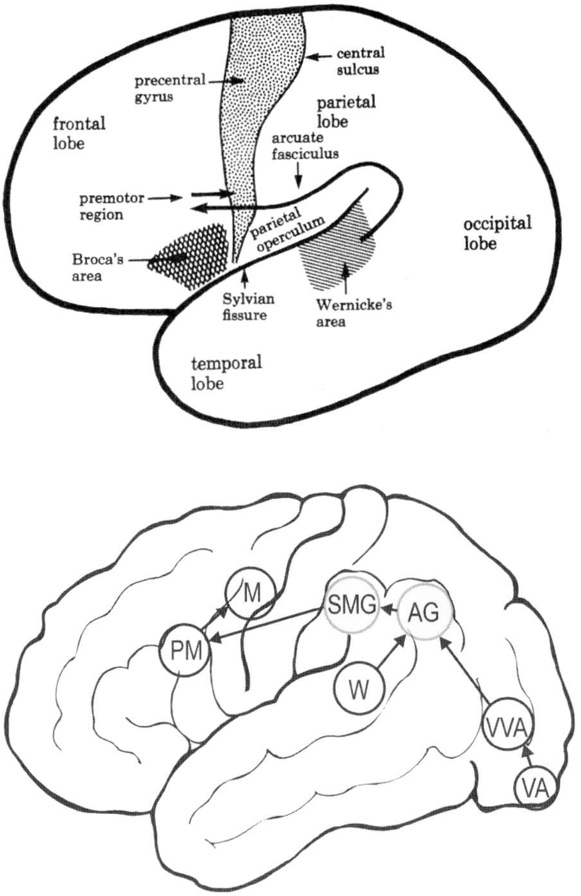

Figure 4.1 Top: Geschwind's (1975) first version of the posterior to anterior stream of action control placed its origin into Wernicke's area which is conceived as a center for language comprehension. In this version apraxia is due to a disconnection between verbal comprehension of commands and their motor execution. Reproduced from Geschwind, N. The apraxias: Neural mechanisms of disorders of learned movements. *American Scientist*, *63*, p. 189, figure 1 © 1975, *The American Scientist* with permission. Bottom: Geschwind's final version of the posterior to anterior stream was elaborated and popularized by Heilman and Rothi (1993). It postulates storage of "time–space motor representations" in the supramarginal or angular gyrus (possible differences between these two portions of inferior parietal lobe were not discussed). The stored engrams can be addressed from verbal commands or, in imitation and tool use, from vision. PM: premotor area; M: motor cortex; SM: supramarginal gyrus; AG: angular gyrus; W: Wernicke's area; VA: primary visual area; VVA: visual association area. Reproduced from Heilman, K. M. and Rothi, L. J. G. Apraxia. In K. M. Heilman and E. Valenstein (Eds.), *Clinical Neuropsychology*, p. 151 (1993) Oxford University Press, by permission of Oxford University Press. (See Plate 4.)

case report. However, after that publication, Geschwind continued to study the literature and found that the preservation of imitation and actual tool use by the apractic hand was exceptional when compared with early reports of callosal disconnection.[3] Moreover, a seminal group study by his Boston colleagues Harold Goodglass and—again—Edith Kaplan (1963; see "A replication of Liepmann's 'mass study'" section) confirmed Liepmann's assertion that patients with left-hemisphere damage and apraxia also fail when they are requested to imitate the gestures which they are unable to produce on verbal command.

A storehouse of learned motor skills

Since left-hemisphere language dominance was not sufficient to account for difficulties with imitation and actual tool use after left brain damage, Geschwind turned his attention to the left-hemisphere superiority for motor control as manifested by right-handedness in the majority of persons. He proposed that the "the hemisphere dominant for handedness is a storehouse of the learning involved in the acquisition of motor skills." He continued:

> Even normal individuals often fail to imitate actions correctly. The protracted learning periods for such motor acts as the proper use of a pen, eating utensils or golf clubs illustrates this point. In other words, the correct imitation of many learned motor skills depends, in fact, on learning and practice. If the right hemisphere is deficient in motor learning, it will imitate poorly. (Geschwind, 1975, p. 191)

In other words, Geschwind postulated that correct imitation of motor acts presupposes that they had been learned and practiced before. Because left-hemisphere lesions destroy the traces of previous learning they cause apraxia for imitation. Since the deficit concerns retrieval of previously learned motor skills, it does not extend to novel and meaningless movements.[4] Consequently, in the last version of his theory, Geschwind explicitly excluded disturbances of the control of "non-learned, non-representational movements" from the realm of apraxia. He declared that they "add to our knowledge of the physiopathology of movement but do not really relate to the understanding of the phenomenon of apraxia" (Geschwind et al., 1985, p. 430).

---

[3] Geschwind referred preferentially to Liepmann and Maas's (1907) report of left-sided apraxia caused by an autopsy proven callosal lesion as a classical example of defective imitation by the left hand. Curiously the cited paper does not mention imitation of gestures at all. The patient's left hand could neither write to dictation nor copy script, and it misused objects, but imitation of gestures was simply not examined. Liepmann and Maas remarked in a footnote: "Unfortunately the patient died before we could complete our examinations in all directions" (1907, p. 216).

[4] Although in principle possible, learning and practicing of meaningless movements is very unlikely to occur in real life. Moreover, the very act of learning will associate them with other knowledge, such as, for example, the reason for, and circumstances of, learning, perhaps even with a name. In other words, the act of learning and practicing will make the action meaningful. Meaninglessness thus remains tightly coupled with novelty. Consequently, authors who investigated imitation of meaningless gestures took their novelty for granted (Kimura & Archibald, 1974; Kolb & Milner, 1981; Goldenberg & Hagmann, 1997).

Geschwind described the storehouse of learned motor skills as a "master control for the kind of representational limb movements impaired in apraxia" and he localized it in the lower left parietal region (Geschwind et al., 1985, p. 429). The similarity to Kleist's postulate that the left parietal lobe stores engrams of single actions (Kleist, 1934; see Chapter 3)[5] is as obvious as is the contradiction to Liepmann's strict refusal of a "praxis center" located in the left parietal lobe (Liepmann, 1908; see Chapter 2). Geschwind had resuscitated this praxis center.

The shift in emphasis from interruption of fiber paths to destruction of cortical centers is highlighted in Geschwind's anatomical interpretation of left inferior parietal lesions. In his monumental survey of disconnection syndromes he reported that "Liepmann repeatedly insisted that the critical lesion in the region of the supramarginal gyrus involved not the cortex but the white matter running beneath the gyrus" (Geschwind, 1965, p. 612; see Chapter 2). In this paper Geschwind dismissed the alternative explanation that memories for movements were stored in the supramarginal gyrus with the argument that lesions located anteriorly of the supramarginal region could cause apraxia. Such lesions can interrupt the fiber tracts leading from the posterior to the anterior end of the stream of action control but do not destroy the putative memories located in supramarginal cortex.

By contrast, in his last paper on apraxia Geschwind stated that "apraxia in patients with lower left parietal lesions indicates that, in most individuals, this region of the brain probably contains the master control for the kind of representational limb movements impaired in apraxia" and distinguished between lesions which impair the master control itself and others which interrupt its activation from verbal or visual commands or block its outflow to premotor cortex and to the other hemisphere (Geschwind & Damasio, 1985). This late version of Geschwind's model of apraxia degraded Wernicke's center to a supplier of verbal input for the parietal praxis center which, in turn, was promoted to being the origin of the posterior to anterior stream of action control. This final version of the posterior to anterior stream of action control was further elaborated and popularized by Geschwind's disciple Kenneth Heilman (Heilman, 1979; Heilman et al., 1982; see figure 4.1).

Levels of action control

For Liepmann, the posterior to anterior stream of action control was the neural substrate for translating mental images of intended actions into motor commands. These mental images could depict familiar and frequently practiced actions but were not restricted to them. On the contrary, highly practiced motor routines were assumed to be stored as "limb kinetic memories" directly in the motor cortex and thus be excepted from the conversion along the posterior to anterior stream. The posterior to anterior stream was a general mechanism for conversion of mental images into motor commands which should be able to accommodate novel actions. We have argued that for Liepmann the conversion of mental images into

[5] Geschwind never mentioned this aspect of Kleist's contributions to apraxia. Apparently he arrived at the postulate of a "praxis center" without knowledge of its historical predecessors. The reinvention of the praxis center testifies of its appeal which, as we will see, continues to influence theories of apraxia until today.

motor commands was equivalent to "the government of the limbs by the mind" and led from the psychological to the physiological side of action control (Liepmann, 1913). Arguably, the ability to create mental images of novel actions and to realize their motor execution is a prime example of the subjugation of motor control under high-level mental processes.

Geschwind's premise that the praxis center and its connections support only the production of previously learned movements changed the purpose of the posterior to anterior stream of action control from a mechanism for converting mental images into motor commands to a path for the transport of motor skills from their storehouse to the place of execution. It deprived apraxia of its significance for understanding the relation between the mental and the motor side of action control, because it did not consider the possible role of mental images preceding and dominating the employment of motor skill. Whereas Liepmann attempted to understand the relationship between a superior, mental, and an inferior, motor, level of action control, Geschwind's model acknowledged only the motor level. The denial of two levels of action control diminished the interest into the duality of ideational or ideo-motor apraxia. Geschwind noted that Liepmann had used the term ideo-motor to refer to the failure of a single movement with an object, and ideational apraxia for the failure to produce a sequence of movements, but he did not search for an anatomical basis of their division except noting that ideational apraxia is often seen in patients with advanced Alzheimer's disease (Geschwind & Damasio, 1985). Usually he used the term apraxia without specification of its type.

The resurrection of body part specificity

Body part specificity of apractic errors had been precious to Liepmann as a trace imprinted by the anatomy of motor control on the government of the limbs by the mind. He thought that the distribution of symptoms reflected the somatotopic organization of motor cortex (see Chapter 2). Geschwind proposed an alternative version of body part specificity. It was also based on the anatomy of motor control and distinguished between efferences originating from the motor cortex and from other brain areas.[6]

Geschwind observed that patients who were unable to follow even very simple commands with the limbs could carry out much more complex movements with the whole body. One particularly impressive patient, whom he described repeatedly:

> could carry out a command such as, "Stand up, turn around twice and then sit down again" although he had been unable to perform such simple commands as "Make a fist."
>
> One of the most dramatic manifestations of this discrepancy was seen when the patient was asked to assume the position of a boxer.[7] He immediately assumed the boxing stance, leading correctly with the left fist. When asked to punch he looked perplexedly at his fist. Several different terms were then used—"punch," "jab," "uppercut," but none of these succeeded in eliciting a response. (Geschwind, 1965, pp. 621–622)

---

[6] Otto Sittig had already proposed dissociations between disturbed hand, and preserved axial, movements but had referred them to the different complexity of distal and proximal movements (see Chapter 3).

[7] Geschwind's patients were ex-servicemen which makes it plausible that the patient had experience with boxing.

Geschwind identified the anatomical basis of the dissociation between axial and limb movements with the distinction between pyramidal and non-pyramidal motor systems. The majority of pyramidal efferences originate from the primary motor cortex and cross to the opposite side of the spinal cord where they control movements of the opposite limbs. Their integrity is particularly important for the swift execution of finely tuned individual finger movements. In contrast, non-pyramidal efferences have their origin in widespread regions outside the primary motor cortex. Their efferent fibers end mostly in the brainstem where they connect with cerebellar and spinal afferences to form a system controlling bilateral whole-body movements like walking or turning.[8] Geschwind assumed that a substantial portion of non-pyramidal efferences have their origin in Wernicke's area. When a lesion anterior to Wernicke's area interrupts the transmission of verbal commands to the motor cortex and its pyramidal efferences, non-pyramidal efferences from Wernicke's area can still command the bilateral coordination of axial movements for whole body movements like walking, turning, or assuming a boxer's stance. As a further consequence of the sparing of non-pyramidal efferences not only to the trunk but also to proximal portions of the limbs, apraxia of limb movements will be most severe for their most distal portions, that is, for shaping the hand and moving individual fingers.

Geschwind soon noted that this theory was not sufficient to explain all instances of preservation of axial movements in severe apraxia. He observed aphasic patients with clinical and even post-mortem evidence for destruction of Wernicke's area who could nonetheless execute axial whole-body movements on verbal command. He described one of them:

> He showed no evidence of comprehension of simple questions and statements and made no response to simplest commands for movement of the limbs or face.
>
> In remarkable contrast to these failures, he responded promptly and correctly to such three-part axial commands as "Roll over, stand up, and then turn around." (Geschwind, 1975, p. 194)

Since the left-hemisphere center for language comprehension had been destroyed, the intact performance of axial movements must have been accomplished by the right hemisphere. Apparently, non-pyramidal efferences from the right hemisphere were capable of controlling bilateral axial movements. The bilaterality of right-hemisphere motor control was less surprising than its exertion on verbal command. Geschwind concluded:

> We were therefore drawn to a surprising conclusion: the human right hemisphere appears to have a special capacity to comprehend axial commands, although it may lack comprehension of other aspects of spoken speech. The reasons are not clear why the right hemisphere might have a special ability to understand axial commands or, stated more broadly, to innervate non pyramidal motor systems in response to verbal command. Certain speculative possibilities are raised; perhaps the capacity to carry out axial commands is a phylogenetically older capacity that was present in both hemispheres at some earlier stage of evolution before the full development of cerebral dominance. (Geschwind, 1975, p. 194)

---

8 The relation between pyramidal and non-pyramidal efferences is more complicated than this account suggests. For example, there is a substantial portion of pyramidal fibers which do not cross to the other side of the spinal cord and hence control ipsilateral muscles. However, since this chapter is devoted to the history of apraxia I am following faithfully Geschwind's account of the laterality of motor systems.

The idea that evolution had implanted in the human brain a special mechanism for carrying out axial movements on verbal command is not very convincing. It rather reminds of Geschwind's own warning that for thinking in terms of disconnexions "perhaps the greatest danger is that of 'working backwards' and of inventing pathways to correspond to every difference in behaviour" (Geschwind, 1965, p. 636).

A replication of Liepmann's "mass study"

In parallel with Geschwind's development of a comprehensive theory of disconnection, his Boston colleagues Harold Goodglass and Edith Kaplan undertook a replication of Liepmann's seminal first "mass study" of apraxia (Liepmann, 1908; see Chapter 2). Unlike Liepmann who had classified patients according to the laterality of hemiplegia, Goodglass and Kaplan (1963) compared aphasic patients to brain damaged patients without aphasia. Their study was aimed at distinguishing whether apraxia can best be explained as a disorder of motor execution as conceived by Liepmann or as an expression of general asymbolia:

> The principal questions at issue are (1) whether with age and post-morbid intellectual level controlled, there is a difference between the aphasics and controls in ability to use gesture and pantomime, and (2) whether such a difference, if it is found, should be attributed to a central "communication disorder" in aphasia. Defining a defect in gesture as part of an aphasic communication disorder requires that it be correlated with the severity of aphasia. Furthermore, it should be distinguished from an apraxia by the absence of any related difficulty in purposeful movement *per se*, as in imitation of the examiner or in object manipulation. (Goodglass & Kaplan, 1963, p. 705)

In this study the production and comprehension of gestures by 20 patients with aphasia was compared to those of 19 patients with brain damage in different locations but without aphasia. The gestures included "natural expressive gestures" like showing "how you would hold your nose when you smell something terrible," "conventional gestures" like saluting or showing "thumbs down," "simple pantomimes" describing the physical properties of objects such as the contour of a drawing pin, and "actions without objects" like demonstrating "how you would stir sugar in your coffee." Production of gestures was required by verbal command but in addition the capacity for imitation was probed for gestures which had been executed poorly.

The aphasic patients scored lower than the non-aphasic controls on all tests of gesture and pantomime. In both groups the accuracy of gestures and pantomimes correlated with general intellectual efficiency as measured by the Wechsler Intelligence Scale. Gestural performance of aphasic patients correlated also with the severity of aphasia which in turn was correlated with intellectual efficiency. However, the authors argued that the presence of a relationship between intellectual efficiency and the gesture and pantomime scores in the controls indicates that "intellectual efficiency is the primary determinant and hence one may conclude that increasing severity of aphasia has little influence on gestural ability, beyond the effects of the accompanying drop in intellectual efficiency" (Goodglass & Kaplan, 1963, p. 711).

In both groups the proportion of well-formed gestures rose significantly when they were tested on imitation rather than on verbal command, but the rate of improvement was higher in the non-aphasic group, indicating at least a relative deficit of imitation in aphasic patients beyond their problems with performance on verbal command.

Finally, Goodglass and Kaplan analyzed the locations of brain damage in the non-aphasic control group and found that patients with bilateral or left-sided lesions tended to score more poorly on the gestural tests than those with unilateral right-sided lesions. They considered this finding as a replication of Liepmann's observation that left-hemisphere lesion can cause apraxia also in the absence of aphasia.

The results of this replication were certainly not as clear-cut as those reported by Liepmann in his original "mass study." In particular, the pervasive relationship between gestural competency and general intellectual efficiency makes it unlikely that defective motor execution was the only reason for the degradation of gesture and pantomime. In the final conclusions of their paper Goodglass and Kaplan noted this relationship but nonetheless concluded:

> Aphasics have a gestural deficiency which is best understood as an apraxic disorder consequent to a left hemisphere lesion; the concept of a general communication disorder is not supported.
>
> The disturbance of gestural ability now appears to be adequately subsumed under the heading of idiokinetic apraxia, as defined by Liepmann. (Goodglass & Kaplan, 1963, p. 719)

Body parts as objects

The different types of gestures included in the study were not equally difficult. Pantomiming the use of objects ("actions without objects") elicited more errors than performance of conventional gestures in both aphasics and controls. Goodglass and Kaplan analyzed not only the number but also the nature of errors and found that particularly for pantomiming object use their distribution differed between aphasics and controls. Aphasics produced more "body part as object" (BPO) errors, where the configuration of the hand does not reproduce the pretended grasp of the object but the shape of the object itself. For example, when asked to show how one is sawing, the edge of the flat hand touches the table and is moved forward and backwards as if it were the blade of the saw, and when asked to show how one combs their hair, the fingers actually touch and arrange the hair rather than pretending to hold the comb in appropriate distance from the head.

The interest in this particular type of error was presumably brought into the study by Edith Kaplan who, before moving to Boston, had collaborated with Heinz Werner, a developmental psychologist who had emigrated from Austria. They had studied the development of expressive gestures in children (Werner, 1952) and had found that body part as object demonstrations are a regular developmental step preceding the differentiation between hand grip and pretended object. Werner was a proponent of organismic and Gestalt psychology and thus of the "holistic" thinking. In this theoretical framework, BPO errors were manifestations of increasing but yet incomplete competency for conveying symbolic information (Cermak et al., 1980). In other words, the aphasic patients' BPO errors reintroduced the concept of asymbolia which Goodglass and Kaplan claimed to have invalidated. Indeed their discussion of this particular error sounds suspiciously similar to the reasoning of Henry Head, Kurt Goldstein, and other authors emphasizing the loss of autonomy and abstract attitude in aphasia (see Chapter 3):

> When one observes the impaired patient (or young child) in response to the instruction to carry out an action with a pretended object, there is frequently an effort to find some actual object to take the place of the absent one. With something actually in hand to manipulate, the task no longer involves a pretended object, but an actual one. In a personal communication, Professor Heinz Werner suggested that the subject behaves as though he really had to "stir his coffee," "comb his hair," etc. and uses his fingers out of necessity. Thus, BPO may permit the aphasics to evade the difficult task of reproducing a movement sequence outside of the concrete context which ordinarily elicits it. (Goodglass & Kaplan, 1963, p. 718)

Norman Geschwind took up the challenge of reintegrating BPO into his associationist account of apraxia. He interpreted them as a manifestation of the body part specificity of apraxia. He reasoned that the non-pyramidal systems which are preserved in apraxia can direct whole body and proximal limb movements but are capable of only crude approximations of discrete movements in individual limbs, especially the hand or fingers. On this account BPO are nothing more than a consequence of reduced individual variability of finger configuration and subsequent coarsening of hand shaping.

It is not difficult to find counter-examples for this proposal. For example, a typical BPO error for demonstrating cutting with scissors is to open and close the angle between the extended index and middle fingers while holding the other fingers bent. Real use and hence correct pantomime would afford moving the thumb against the block of the other four fingers. As one can easily convince oneself by trying both versions, demands on individual finger movements are higher in the BPO version than in the correct pantomime. Geschwind's attempt to expel asymbolia and abstract attitude from the explanation of BPO was not convincing.

Chapter 5

High and low levels of action control

The renaissance of Liepmann's concepts of apraxia ends our historical review. The second part of this book will be concerned with current empirical evidence for theories of apraxia rather than with their historical development. Before we leave history I will sum up the main conclusions.

The excursion into history has revealed a basic dichotomy shining through many theoretical accounts of apraxia. It opposes a higher mental to a lower motor level of action control. In some accounts this dichotomy was explicitly spelled out and formed the core of the theory. Liepmann's classification of ideational and ideo-kinetic apraxia is the most prominent example of this way of thinking. Other accounts did not explicitly postulate such a dichotomy but defended the supremacy of one level and contested the importance of the other. An early example of this kind of argument is provided by Finkelnburg who attributed gestural expression to a pervasive deficiency of "symbolic cognition" and declined any importance to differences between the motor acts of gesturing, speaking, or any other variants of symbolic expression. Conversely, Munk's concept of mind-palsy was developed in animal experiments and consequently took into consideration only mechanisms of motor control which are similar in dog and man.

Arguably, the distinction between a higher and a lower or, respectively, a mental and a motor level of action ultimately refers to the distinction between mind and body.

Table 5.1 lists different aspects of this basic dichotomy. Since they all have been discussed extensively in the foregoing chapter I will describe them only briefly and without detailed citation of the references.

Body part specificity of errors

Body part specificity of apraxic errors was attributed to the somatotopy of motor cortex by Liepmann and Foix, and to the anatomy of pyramidal and extrapyramidal motor efferences by Geschwind. For both of them, body part specificity was a mark imprinted upon apraxia by anatomy and a manifestation of the influence of low-level motor mechanisms on the distribution of apraxia. This interpretation of body part specificity was not unanimously accepted. Like Geschwind, Sittig postulated an increase of severity of apraxia from proximal to distal body parts, but attributed this body part specificity to general principles of brain function rather than to the anatomy of motor control. He reasoned that distal movements are more diverse and more complicated than proximal ones and hence put higher demands on voluntary control which, according to Jackson's principle, should

Table 5.1 Examples of the comparison of high versus low level of action control

	High/mental	**Low/motor**
Body part specificity of symptoms	Due to different complexity of movements	Reflects somatotopic layout of motor cortex
Autonomy of action	Autonomous generation of action plan	Actions are determined by environmental stimuli
Cerebral representation of intended actions	Multimodal	Modality specific motor memories (motor engrams)
Cerebral localization	Whole cortex	Localized centers
Anatomy and psychology	Anatomy can constrain but not replace psychological mechanisms	Anatomy is congruent with psychological mechanisms
Constructional apraxia	Translation from one spatial dimension to another	Association of visual percepts with motor engrams
Left hemisphere dominance	Related to language	Related to handedness
Actions predominantly affected by apraxia	Novel actions	Familiar and well-practiced actions

be predominantly affected by brain lesions. Another possibility for separating body part specificity from the anatomy of motor control derived from the analysis of imitation in constructional apraxia. Errors were observed mainly for movements and postures of hand and finger, that is, again, for distal body parts, but were referred to the spatial complexity of finger postures and a general inability to locate single elements within a spatial compound rather than to peculiarities of motor control of finger and hand.

Autonomy of action

The autonomy of human action was a central topic for the holistic approach to human action. Proponents of holism like Head, Goldstein, or Grünbaum, distinguished actions which are automatically elicited by environmental stimuli from voluntary actions that are planned and executed independently from, or even in contradiction to, environmental exhortations. The classification of these two modes of behavior as corresponding to a higher and a lower level of action control is evident. Arguably, the postulated loss of autonomy following brain damage is equivalent to Liepmann's formulation that apraxia abolishes "the government of the limbs by the mind."

Modality of the mental representation of actions

Here, the low level account is constituted by Kleist's and Geschwind's assumption that voluntary movements arise from motor-specific engrams storing kinetic features of learned movements and the high-level position by Liepmann's proposal that the mental images preceding motor execution are multimodal with a preponderance of visual information. The incorporation of multimodal images into the realm of high-level mental processes was emphasized by the observation that they are accessible to introspective consciousness, whereas unimodal motor images are excluded from introspective analysis. Consequently, Liepmann regarded unimodal motor images, that is, motor engrams, as low-level physiological rather than high-level psychological concepts.

Cerebral localization

Generally, accounts which emphasize higher-level mental function tended to be associated with skepticism regarding the importance of cerebral localization of functions, whereas localization was foundational for theories grounded in the physiology of motor control. The association of high-level accounts with a refusal of narrow localization was, however, not mandatory. A notable exception was Pierre Marie who regarded both aphasia and apraxia as expression of a general loss of intelligence. Although the concept of intelligence refers to high-level cognitive functions, Marie localized its cerebral substrate narrowly in Wernicke's area.

Anatomy and psychology

Theories that acknowledge the localization of functions come in two variants. Associationist diagrams explained psychological functions directly by the structure and function of cortical areas and their connections. They constitute a radically reductionist approach to mental function. A less radical concept of localization is exemplified by Morlaas' thesis. He assigned different manifestations of apraxia to different locations of lesions, but did not postulate congruence between the spatial layout of regions and the functional relationships between their functions. On the contrary, Morlaas considered the possibility that spatial proximity between lesions could conceal the functional independence of the afflicted functions. In the dichotomy of low- and high-level accounts, the associationist reduction of psychology to anatomy favors the supremacy of the lower level, whereas the liberation of psychological processes from strict congruence with their anatomical substrate provides space for high-level mental processes.

Left-hemisphere dominance

In a right-handed person apraxia is mainly caused by left hemisphere lesions. This laterality coincides with left-hemisphere dominance for language and with motor control of the dominant right hand. Liepmann and Geschwind considered the association with handedness crucial. This association is based on the anatomy of motor control and can thus be classified as acting on a low level. By contrast, Steinthal, Finkelnburg, and Head emphasized the affinity of apraxia to aphasia and hence to language, which is among the highest achievements of human mind. They thus defended a high-level explanation for the left lateralization of lesions causing apraxia.

Although Liepmann placed the main emphasis on handedness he also conceded significance to the relationship between apraxia and language, but rather than regarding apraxia as a manifestation of the loss of high-level aptitudes in aphasia, he reduced language to the motor act of speaking and proposed that aphasia is due to apraxia of the articulators.

Constructional apraxia

Kleist thought that constructional apraxia is due to the interruption of fiber paths connecting visual with motor areas. Being based on the anatomy of modality-specific engrams this account can be classified as low level. By contrast, the descriptions of constructional apraxia by Critchley, Paterson, and others emphasized the translation of spatial relationships from one frame of reference to another. They subsumed constructional apraxia in the disorders of spatial thinking and credited minor importance to the motor act of reproducing spatial relationships. They thus defended a high-level, psychological approach to spatial errors in constructional tasks.

Novelty of action

The opposition between voluntary and automatic actions which was central to Jackson, Goldstein, and the adherents of holistic theories placed novel actions on a higher level than routine actions, because novel actions put higher demands on conscious planning and on creativity. Accordingly, apraxia was held to affect predominantly novel and unusual actions while sparing highly practiced routine acts. By contrast, Kleist and Geschwind postulated that apraxia is due to the loss of motor engrams of familiar actions. Geschwind's formulation that apraxia affects "learned" actions paraphrases the familiarity of affected actions, because learning is associated with an increase of familiarity of the learned actions. At least from the point of view of the holistic theories, the alleged loss of motor engrams interferes with a lower level of action control than the inability to produce novel motor actions.

Introducing modern evidence

In the following chapters of this book I will review modern empirical evidence concerning manifestations of apraxia and related phenomena of motor control like handedness or intermanual conflicts. Throughout this survey the opposition between high and low levels of motor control will be a central thread. The criteria listed in Table 5.1 will serve as a guideline for identifying and classifying its appearances. As in the historical part, I will look for the high- versus low-level dichotomy on both sides of scientific reports, one being empirical observations and results, and the other the methods used for acquiring the empirical data and their theoretical interpretation (Latour, 1993). The opposition between high and low levels of control may oppose different elements of the empirical evidence, but it may also oppose different methodical approaches for exploring and interpreting the same piece of empirical evidence.

Names of the mind

In the historical chapters I have followed the habitual nomenclature of their time and used the expressions "mind," "mental," "psychic," and "psychological" for characterizing the higher pole of the high- versus low-level dichotomy. In the modern literature the prevalent designations for this level are "cognition" and "cognitive." Although the names have changed, the basic meaning has remained the same. All of these designations indicate explanations of human behavior that refer to mental processes like thinking, knowing, remembering, or problem solving rather than explaining behavior directly by the physiology and anatomy of underlying neural processes. In the context of this book, the neural processes at issue are predominantly the physiology and anatomy of motor control.

Chapter 6

Imitation: A direct route from vision to action?

We start our survey of the evidence with imitation of gestures. Imitation of gestures was introduced into the clinical examination of apraxia by Liepmann (see Chapter 2). To Liepmann, disturbed imitation was important because imitation is essentially a nonverbal test. Once the general instruction is understood, the command to imitate a particular gesture is given without words by demonstration of that gesture. Since disturbed imitation cannot be attributed to deficient verbal comprehension it underlines the independence of apraxia from aphasia. To be sure that performance is not influenced by paresis or other elemental motor deficits patients are asked to imitate with the hand ipsilateral to their lesion. In accordance with the natural tendency to use the hand on the same side of space as the demonstration rather than the nominally same hand (see Chapter 3), the examiner demonstrates "like a mirror," using the right hand when the patient uses the left and vice versa.

Healthy persons imitate meaningless gestures like those shown in Figure 6.1 swiftly and virtually errorless. By contrast, some patients encounter massive difficulties. Their hand approaches the face but ends up in a position that deviates grossly from the demonstrated target posture. The path of the hand may consist of swift and secure movements leading to the wrong position or, more frequently, of hesitating and searching movement which sometimes ends up in the correct target position but more frequently misses it (Hermsdörfer et al., 1996).

Imitation and the posterior to anterior stream of action control

The importance given by Liepmann to disturbed imitation was not exhausted by the demonstration of the independency of apraxia from aphasia. Remember that in his model of the posterior to anterior stream of action control mental images of intended actions are transformed into motor commands, and that disturbances can affect either the generation of the mental image or its translation into motor command. Liepmann took for granted that the demonstration of the gesture by the examiner secured the patient's correct mental image of the gesture. Consequently, errors in imitation testified that "the guidance of the left hand by mental images of the shape of the movement is disturbed" (Liepmann, 1908).

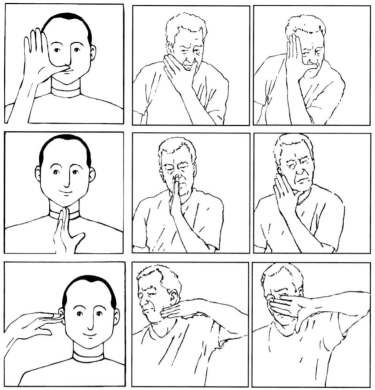

Figure 6.1 Imitation of meaningless hand postures by a patient with a left parietal lesion: the left image shows the model, the middle image a stage in the searching movements, and the right image the final position.

The assumption that defective imitation indicates defective execution of correctly conceived gestures still prevails in modern literature. For example, the Italian neurologist Ennio de Renzi wrote:

> It must be recognized, that it is not always easy to decide whether the patient has the representation of the gesture clear in his/her mind, . . . and this is one of the reasons why imitation tests are often preferable to verbal commands in testing ideomotor apraxia. Since the examiner provides the model of the action and the patient must simply copy it, errors can only be due to an executive deficit. (De Renzi, 1990, p. 246)

Liepmann had proposed that problems with the translation of mental images into motor acts would come to the fore most conspicuously when movement are made wholly from memory rather than resulting from interactions with external objects. This definition applies not only to imitation of meaningless hand postures but also to the production of communicative gestures. The conversion of mental images into motor commands constitutes a common final path for all gestures regardless of whether the mental image preceding them is generated from the examiner's demonstration for imitation, from knowledge about the use of tools for pantomime of tool use, or from knowledge about the conventional shape of emblematic gestures. In the theoretical framework of the posterior to anterior stream of motor control, imitation is supposed to probe the integrity of the final portion of the path regardless of the nature of its origin. This leads to the prediction that patients who fail imitation should also fail the production of communicative gestures on command.

Figure 6.2 shows a diagram illustrating this prediction for imitation and generation from memory of pantomime of tool use (Roy & Square, 1985).

Clinical evidence contradicts this prediction. There are patients who have severe problems with the imitation of gestures but can produce pantomimes of tool use and

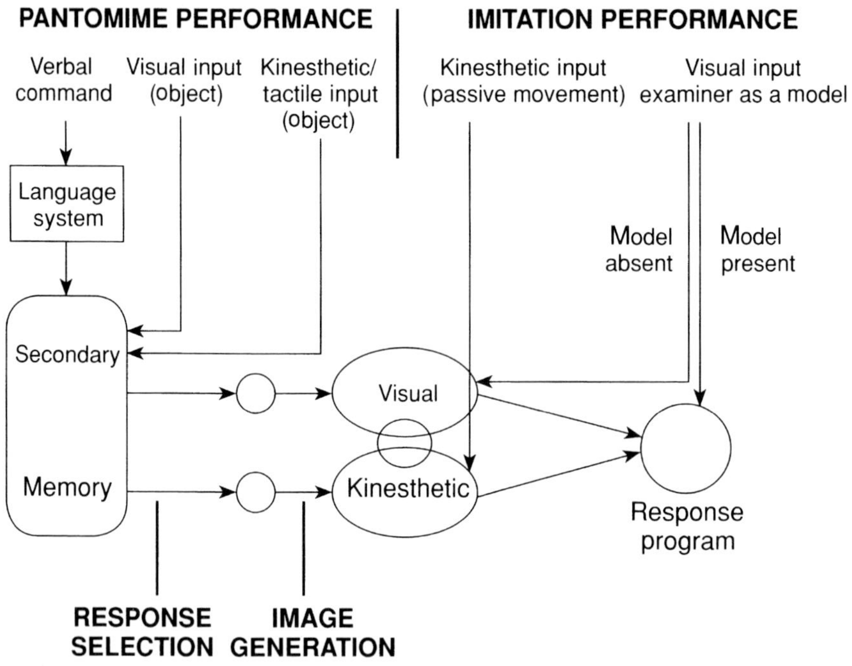

Figure 6.2 A model illustrating the putative relationship between pantomime of tool use and imitation of gestures (Roy & Hall, 1992). It distinguishes two phases of gesture production. In the first phase a mental image of the pantomime is created from long-term memory, and in the second phase the image is converted into motor response programs. Production of the pantomime in response to a verbal, visual, or kinesthetic command taps both phases whereas imitation requires only the second phase. The two phases are arranged sequentially. Pantomimes conceived in the first phase must pass through the second phase for motor execution. Consequently, breakdown of the second phase disturbs not only imitation but also the production of pantomimes that are retrieved from long-term memory. This is an abstract model of functions that does not specify the anatomical location of its components. However, the sequence of a first phase where a mental image of the gesture is created, and a second phase where the image is converted into motor acts, is easily recognizable as a descendant of Liepmann's version of the posterior to anterior stream of motor control (see Chapter 2, Figure 2.4). Adapted from Roy, E. A. and Hall, C. Limb apraxia: A process approach. In L. Proteau and D. Elliott (Eds.), *Vision and Motor Control*, p. 270, © 1992, The Authors, with kind permission.

emblematic gestures flawlessly. This condition has been termed "visuo-imitative apraxia" (Mehler, 1987; Goldenberg & Hagmann, 1997; Cubelli et al., 2000; Peigneux et al., 2000; Bartolo et al., 2001). The dissociation between defective imitation and preserved production on command can be quite impressive. For example, the request to imitate the hand posture of touching the temple with the tip of the middle finger of the horizontally extended flat hand may lead to searching movements that finally result in a touch of the forehead with the thumb of the vertically aligned hand, while the request to show a military salute is promptly answered by the same gesture that the patient was unable to produce in imitation.

Two routes for imitation

The gestures shown in Figure 6.1 are meaningless. Thus, the dissociation between their defective imitation and the preserved production of gestures on verbal command is at the same time dissociation between defective production of meaningless, and preserved production of meaningful, communicative gestures. This ambiguity can be resolved by asking patients to imitate meaningful gestures. Indeed, the imitation of meaningful gestures can be perfectly preserved in patients with visuo-imitative apraxia (Goldenberg & Hagmann, 1997; Peigneux et al., 2000; Bartolo et al., 2001). Apparently the problem in visuo-imitative apraxia is not a general defect of imitation but a specific defect of imitation of meaningless gestures.[1]

Figure 6.3 shows a model which can account for visuo-imitative apraxia (Rothi et al., 1997). It has its roots in Geschwind's (Geschwind 1975; Geschwind & Damasio, 1985) reinterpretation of the posterior to anterior stream of action control. Geschwind had postulated that defective imitation is due to destruction of a storehouse of learned motor skills. Because meaningless gestures are generally novel, Geschwind explicitly excluded imitation of meaningless gestures from the realm of apraxia (see Chapter 4). Rothi's model proposes two significant amendments to Geschwind's schema. First, the "storehouse of learned motor skills" is conceived as an "action lexicon" storing the shape of gestures, and this lexicon is duplicated resulting in an action input and an action output lexicon. Both are connected to a central semantic memory storing knowledge related to the meaning of the gestures. The action input lexicon mediates understanding of the meaning of perceived gestures and the action output lexicon their production for expression of meaning. Imitation of familiar meaningful gestures is accomplished by transfer of the gesture from the

[1] The apparently selective deficit of imitation of meaningless gestures does not exclude the possibility that patients with visuo-imitative apraxia are generally unable to perform meaningless gestures, regardless of whether they are presented for imitation or for performance on verbal command. However, production of meaningless gestures on verbal command is difficult to assess. Since these gestures have no names, the verbal command must consist of a description of the spatial features of the gesture. Comprehension of such a command is not trivial for patients with left brain damage who have some degree of aphasia and restrictions of verbal working memory. In any case it would be difficult to decide whether errors are due to insufficient production of gestures or to insufficient comprehension of the instruction.

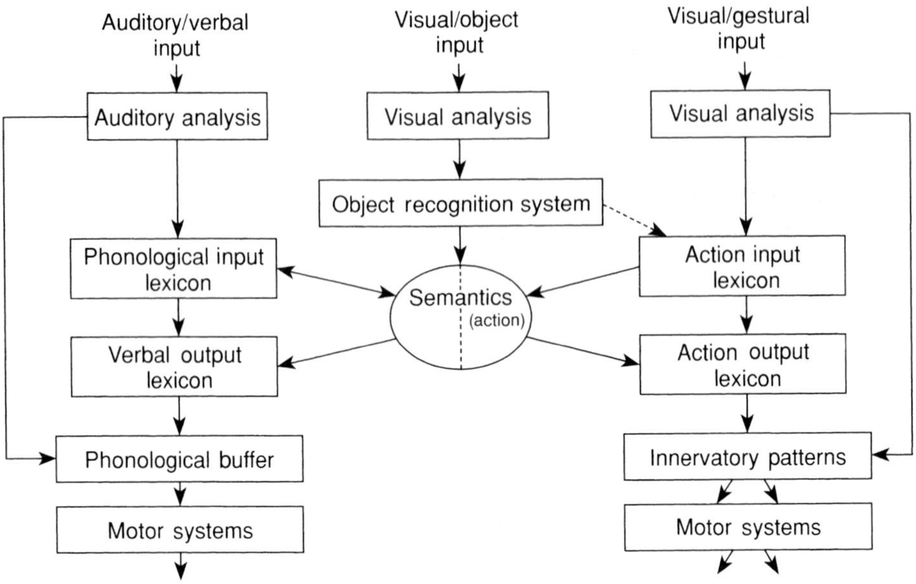

Figure 6.3 Another functional model that can account for dissociations between production of pantomime of tool use on command and imitation of gestures (Rothi et al., 1991). The model emphasizes the parallels between the processing of language and gestures. The direct path from visual analysis to innervatory patterns can accommodate imitation of both familiar meaningful and novel meaningless gestures. The alternative ways from input to output lexica or via semantic memory are reserved to familiar and meaningful gestures. Interruption of the direct route thus causes a selective disturbance of imitation of novel and meaningless gestures. Reproduced from Rothi, L. J. G., Ochipa, C., and Heilman, K. M. A cognitive neuropsychological model of limb praxis. *Cognitive Neuropsychology*, *8*, p. 456 © 1991, Taylor and Francis, with permission.

input to the output lexicon. The transfer can pass via the direct connection between the lexica or take the detour via their meaning stored in the central semantic memory.

The second amendment is the addition of a direct route leading from visual analysis of gestures to the innervatory patterns of their motor replication and bypassing storage of the shape and meaning of familiar gesture in lexicons and semantic memory. This route can accommodate imitation of meaningless gestures. Its interruption would interfere with imitation of meaningless gestures but spare the imitation of meaningful gestures via the lexicons, and thus bring forward visuo-imitative apraxia.

Imitation and mirror neurons

Thus far, we can conclude that the route from visual perception to motor replication of gestures can be direct insofar as it bypasses recognition of the meaning of the gesture. It is another question whether the route is constituted by a direct connection from vision to motor control or includes interpolated stages where the visual information is translated into a format compatible with the direction of motor actions. The idea that the connection from vision to motor execution of gestures is direct also in the sense that it includes no interpolated stages has become very popular in recent years. The popularity was nourished by the detection of "mirror neurons" in monkey premotor cortex (Di Pellegrino et al., 1992; Rizzolatti et al., 2002; Rizzolatti & Sinigaglia, 2008). These neurons are similarly active when the monkey sees another monkey or a human perform an action and when it performs the same actions. The conclusion that they provide a substrate mirroring observed actions by their motor replication is tempting but not straightforward. Indeed, the monkeys in whom mirror neurons had been detected do not imitate motor actions (Subiaul et al., 2004). Furthermore, whereas the putative human direct route accommodates novel and meaningless gestures, mirror neurons in monkey react only to biologically meaningful and familiar actions (Ferrari et al., 2005). Nonetheless, the attractiveness of mirror neurons has encouraged the development of theories as to how imitation could be built upon a direct link from vision to motor execution of gestures.

One such account posits that the basis for imitation is laid by children's observations of their own movements. The co-occurrence of the motor action and its visual perception increases the strength of associations between neurons mediating the visual perception of an action and neurons directing its motor execution (Keysers & Perrett, 2004; Brass & Heyes, 2005). Because the view of oneself performing an action is similar to that of another person doing the same, the association between visual perception and motor execution of actions generalizes to the perception of other person's actions. Seeing the action reactivates the association between vision and motor control and elicits motor execution of the perceived action, that is, imitation. The motor neurons that become activated by vision of the action and direct its motor replication become "mirror neurons."

The association between perception and execution of actions lends itself to being activated automatically. Vision of the action elicits activation of mirror neurons by simple association regardless of whether subjects are intending to imitate the action or not. Indeed, automatic activation of motor cortex by mere observation of actions has been brought forward as evidence for the existence of mirror neurons in human (e.g., Fadiga et al., 1995; Buccino et al., 2001; Aziz-Zadeh et al., 2002; Watkins et al., 2003; Clark et al., 2004; Ehrsson et al., 2006). This automatic motor activation was somatotopic. Observation of a movement activated precisely those parts of the motor cortex which control the moving body part. The parallel to the historical theories postulating an influence of the somatotopic layout of motor cortex on body part specificity of apraxia is striking. We will come back to body part specificity of imitation disturbances in Chapter 7.

Strategic choices

Rothi's model (see Figure 6.3) predicts selective impairment of imitation of meaningless gestures when the direct route is interrupted but not necessarily the converse dissociation of selective impairment of imitation of meaningful gestures when the lexical route is disturbed, because failure of the lexical route could be compensated by the direct route treating the meaningful gestures as if they were meaningless and mediating their imitation by connecting their visual analysis to their motor execution. There are, however, a few reports of patients who could imitate meaningless gestures but failed the imitation of meaningful gestures (Bartolo et al., 2001; Tessari et al., 2007). A possible explanation of this unexpected dissociation is the exertion of strategic control on the use of either the direct or the indirect route. Particularly when meaningful and meaningless gestures are presented for imitation in a mixed sequence, subjects prefer to treat both kinds of gestures as meaningless and copy their shape via the direct route without paying attention to the meaning and familiarity of the meaningful gestures. This strategic choice is advantageous in that it takes away the need to select the appropriate strategy for each gesture individually, but it veils the possibility of selective disturbance or selective preservation of only the lexical route. When, however, meaningful and meaningless gestures are presented for imitation in separate blocks, subjects are inclined to select the appropriate route for each block and to adhere to their choice through the whole block even when single items give rise to difficulties. This adherence to the strategic choice prevents compensation of insufficient imitation via the lexical route by application of the direct route and may thus reveal selective deficits of imitating meaningful gestures (Tessari & Rumiati, 2004; Tessari et al., 2007).

The conclusion that subjects can choose whether or not they employ the direct route for imitation of meaningful gestures cast doubts on its automatic activation by mere vision of gestures.

The goals of imitation

Further evidence that the route from perception to replication of gestures can be modulated by strategic choices was provided by developmental studies (Bekkering et al., 2000; Gattis et al., 2002; Bekkering et al., 2005). They revived the historical "Hand, Eyes, and Ear" Test (Head, 1920; Gordon, 1922; see Chapter 3). Children were seated opposite the experimenter who demonstrated touching of either the left or the right ear with either the left or the right hand. The children were instructed to imitate the experimenter's actions like in a mirror. Children always reached to the correct ear but frequently replaced contralateral by ipsilateral reaching, that is, they reached for the right ear with the right hand although the experimenter had touched the spatially opposite left ear with her right hand, and vice versa. When, however, the examiner touched both of her ears simultaneously the children imitated correctly not only when each hand reached for its ipsilateral ear, but also when the hands were crossed for reaching the contralateral ears (see Figure 6.4). The authors speculated that the children had established a hierarchy of goals for the imitation, and that the laterality of the targets of reaching, that is, the ears, were on top of this hierarchy. The laterality of the instruments of reaching, that is, the hands, were lower valued and not protected from being neglected. Thus the unfamiliar and motorically somewhat cumbersome reach of the contralateral hand could be replaced by the more comfortable and faster reaching of the ipsilateral hand (see Schofield (1976) for evidence that reaching across the midline is difficult for children). In the bimanual condition the target of reaching remained constant, as both ears were touched in all trials. Consequently, attention could be withdrawn from the laterality of the touched ears and directed to the position of the arms. The choice of the

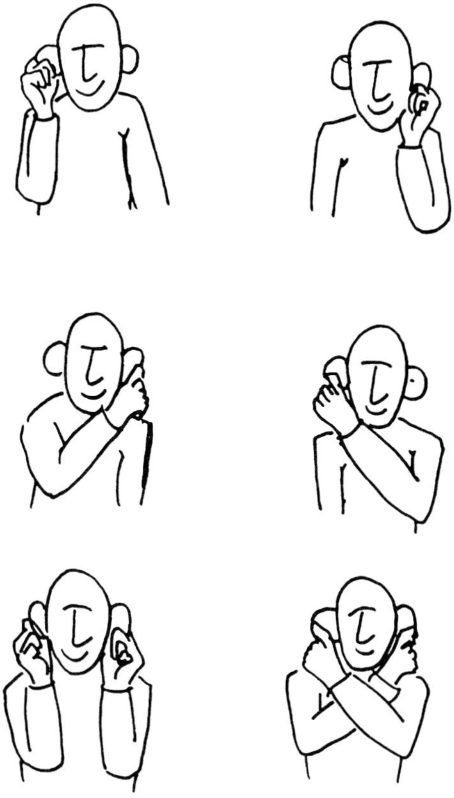

Figure 6.4 The gestures examined by Bekkering et al. (2000). In the unimanual condition (top and middle row) children tend to replace contralateral reaching (middle row) by ipsilateral reaching to the indicated ear (top row). When reaching with both hands to both ears (bottom row) they faithfully copy the lateralities of the reaching hands. Reproduced from Bekkering, H., Wohlschläger, A., and Gattis, M. Imitation of gestures in children is goal-directed. *Quarterly Journal of Experimental Psychology, 53A*, p. 156, © 2001, Taylor and Francis, with permission.

hand now ascended to the top of the goal hierarchy and the children imitated faithfully not only ipsilateral, but also contralateral reaching.

In a further experiment the children were asked to imitate reaching to a spot on the table located either on their right or the left side with either the right or the left hand. There were two conditions: in one the target positions were marked by black dots whereas in the other there was no visible mark and the target of pointing was indicated by the examiner's demonstration. Children virtually never failed to touch the correct side of the table, but in the dot condition they frequently used the hand ipsilateral to the dot although the experimenter had demonstrated pointing with the contralateral hand. This error occurred only very rarely when there were no visible dots. The authors speculated that in the dot condition the children had assigned the highest position in the goal hierarchy to reaching the correct dots and neglected the alternations between crossed and uncrossed pointing. When, however, there were no visible dots, the type of movement became the dominant goal and crossing or uncrossing of the hand was replicated correctly. The authors concluded that their results speak:

> against the notion that imitation involves a direct mapping of a non-composed action pattern. Imitation involves more than a direct mapping between perceptual input and motoric output. Observed behaviours are coded as constituent goals and those goals are the units from which subsequent action patterns are composed. (Gattis et al., 2002, p. 201)

In a similar line of research, Franz and colleagues (2007) manipulated the habitual preference of normal subjects for imitation like in a mirror over imitation with the nominally same hand. The preference reversed in favor of imitation with the nominally same hand when salient markers were affixed to the hand used by the experimenter for demonstration and to the nominally same hand of the subject. Apparently the similarity between demonstrated and imitated gesture can be given different specifications. Contextual cues can induce a change of the dominant specification. The malleability of the mapping from perception to execution of actions is difficult to reconcile with the automatic activation of a direct route from vision to motor control.

How direct is the direct route?

The direct routes in Rothi's model and in the "mirror neuron" account share the seemingly self-evident assumption that the motor act of imitation is the same as the motor act of the demonstration. If the model touches the temple with extended fingers, the imitating person also touches their temple with extended fingers. However, imitation of gestures can be seen differently. It can be classified as one particular instance of the transposition of a body configuration from one body to another.[2] In imitation the configuration is transposed to the own body of the person performing the transposition, but this correspondence can be torn apart. For example, the person can be asked to replicate the demonstrated body configuration on a manikin instead of their own body. The manipulation of the manikin is a motor act too, but its features are substantially different from those of the movements and body configurations that have been demonstrated for replication. In order to approach the extended fingers of the manikin to its temple, the person manipulating the manikin must neither touch their own nor the manikin's temple, and must clench their hand around the hand or the wrist of the manikin rather than extending it.

I have conducted a clinical study based on this paradigm (Goldenberg, 1995). Imitation of hand postures was tested in two conditions. First, the examiner sat opposite the subject and demonstrated the postures and the subject was asked to repeat them. Then, the examiner sat beside a life-sized wooden manikin (without lower body) whose arm and hand could be moved like those of a human. He demonstrated the hand postures again, and the subject was asked to replicate the posture with the manikin's hand. There were three groups of subjects: patients with left brain damage and aphasia, patients with right brain damage, and healthy controls. Patients imitated with the hand ipsilateral to the lesion and manipulated the same hand of the manikin. Half of the controls used the left and half the right hand, but results did not differ between them.

The results were quite straightforward. Healthy controls and patients with right brain damage imitated the gestures with nearly no errors. By contrast, out of 35 patients with

[2] Note the similarity of this definition to the historical accounts of constructional apraxia as affecting the translation of an object from one spatial dimension into another (Critchley, 1953) and to Schlesinger's (1928) proposal that the disturbance which becomes manifest in the imitation of movements and the postures reached by them, is nothing else than "constructional apraxia on the own body" (see Chapter 3).

left brain damage, 15 made more errors than controls and were classified as apraxic. The results on the manikin replicated those of imitation: while normal controls, patients with right brain damage, and non-apraxic patients with left brain damage made only a few errors, the apraxic patients scored dramatically worse.

Manipulating the distance between model and replication

Transposition of body configuration from one body to another can be tested without any substantial demands on motor action by asking subjects to match photographs of gestures performed by different persons and seen under different angles of view. In a single case study, Alan Sunderland (2007) examined matching of hand postures in a patient with a severe disturbance of imitation caused by a left parietal lesion. The patient had no difficulties in selecting the same postures from photographs showing the postures with identical or mirror-reversed orientation, but committed many errors when asked to match photographs to cartoons showing the same gestures. Sunderland concluded that the patient could exploit visual similarity for matching gestures but failed when the match had to be mediated by a more abstract conceptual representation of the gestures.

The importance of the perceptual distance between demonstration and replication of gestures was demonstrated in a series of experiments probing the imitation of three- to five-step sequences of combined hand and finger postures (e.g., touch table with index—touch table with back of flat hand—touch table with thumb—touch table with fist) (Jason, 1983a, 1983b). Patients with left brain damage, about one-half of which committed errors on clinical testing of imitation, needed more trials than patients with right brain damage to learn such a sequence and performed more slowly and with more errors even after successful learning. When, however, the examiner was seated beside the patient, demonstrated the sequence with the same hand as the patient, and maintained each position until the patient had copied it, imitation of the sequence became errorless. Moreover, when the examiner gradually accelerated the pace of the demonstration, left brain damaged patient could follow as fast and as errorless as the right brain damaged patients. The procedure of simultaneous imitation had minimized the perceptual distance between demonstration and replication, and had thus rendered intermediate cognitive processing superfluous. The observation that patients who have apraxia for imitation on clinical testing perform as well as right brain damaged patients without apraxia on this variant of imitation strongly suggests that their problems concern interpolated processing stages that mediate equivalence between perceptually distant motor actions.

High and low routes to imitation

Before we leave this discussion of imitation we should reconsider its implications for the high- versus low-level dichotomy. Liepmann's proposal that defective imitation testifies the inability to direct the limbs according to mental images addresses this dichotomy and identifies defective imitation with insufficient control of the low level of motor control by the high level of mental images or, in his words, “the governance of the limbs by the mind” (Liepmann, 1913). By contrast, a direct route connecting perception to motor execution of gestures bears unmistakable hallmarks of belonging entirely to the low level of motor physiology: it functions automatically, bypasses semantic knowledge about the meaning of gestures, and is body part specific. Analysis of the empirical evidence, however, casts doubts on the reality and ubiquity of these features. The malleability of the mapping from vision to execution of gestures rimes poorly with an automatic replication of the perceived motor act. Its susceptibility to interpretations of the goals of an experiment and to cues highlighting the correspondence between the nominal laterality of the model and the subject’s hands, strongly suggest the intervention of higher-order cognitive processes in the functioning of the direct route. Finally, the observation that apraxic patients who fail imitation on their own body have similar problems when trying to replicate the body configuration on a manikin implies that imitation involves spatial representations beyond the “innervatory pattern” (Rothi et al., 1991) of motor actions. We will discuss the possible nature of these representations in Chapter 7 where we also return to the topic of body part specificity of disturbed imitation. At this stage we can summarize that an explication based exclusively on low-level neuronal mechanisms and neglecting the intervention of high-level cognitive processes cannot give a satisfactory account for imitation of gestures.

Chapter 7

Body part specificity

In the historical part of this book we have repeatedly emphasized that body part specificity of apraxia was attributed to the anatomy of cerebral motor regions and their efferent connections. Body part specificity was seen as the mark stamped on apraxia by the physiology and anatomy of motor control. In this approach, the mechanisms of body part specificity were rooted in the hidden anatomy of neural motor control rather than in the visible structure of body parts.

However, you do not need to study the brain to divide the body into parts. Distinctions between upper and lower limbs, trunk, neck, and head, and, within the head, ears, eyes, mouth, and nose are perceptually and functionally salient. Their universal recognition is documented by different names for different body parts in all languages, although more fine-grained distinctions as, for example, between leg and feet are subject to cultural variations (van Staden & Majid, 2006; Enfield et al., 2006). Body parts are distinguished by their position relative to other body parts as well as by their local structure and by biomechanical constraints on their mobility. It appears conceivable that the different sensitivity of different body parts to apraxia has its basis in such differences between the body parts themselves rather than in the layout of the cerebral structures directing their movements.

A salient division of body parts affected by apraxia opposes movements of mouth and face to movements of the limbs. My research and this book are devoted nearly exclusively to limb apraxia, but I will here interpose a short summary of basic findings concerning apraxia of mouth and face and their relationship to limb apraxia.

Apraxia of mouth and face

Apraxia of mouth and face had been recognized since the very beginning of the scientific history of apraxia. Indeed, Jackson's "Remarks on Non-Protrusion of the Tongue in some Cases of Aphasia" (Jackson, 1878/1932b) is one of the earliest descriptions of phenomena which later had been subsumed under the conceptual umbrella of apraxia. Facial apraxia was also diagnosed in Liepmann's imperial counselor. Whereas his limb apraxia was unilateral, face apraxia was bilateral. Liepmann gave a lively description of his futile attempts to stretch out the tongue:

> Asked to show his tongue he throws the head backwards, opens widely the eyes and the mouth and produces snatching movements with the jaws. (Liepmann, 1900, p. 23)

Like Jackson, Liepmann observed dissociation between the failure to make oral and facial movements on command and preservation of natural movements like chewing or swallowing. He interpreted these preserved actions as further examples of "short cut" actions which do not depend on connection between the motor region and other cortical areas (see Chapter 2) thus drawing a parallel with the preserved manual skills of the imperial counselor.

Apraxia of face and mouth continued to be mentioned in case reports of more extensive apraxia (e.g., Van Vleuten, 1907; Hartmann, 1907) but did not evoke discussions of specific mechanisms underlying it. Apparently it was considered as just one manifestation of general apraxia, obeying the same principles and mechanisms as apraxia of other body parts. This belief was shaken by a seminal paper by the British neurologist Peter Nathan (1947). He observed that there are patients with apraxia of the mouth who have no limb apraxia but that all of them have difficulties with articulation of words. Most of the patients with mouth apraxia had left-hemisphere lesions but there were also cases with right-sided lesions.

In the last third of the twentieth century a number of group studies confirmed the absence of a close link between apraxia of the mouth and the limbs (Alajouanine & Lhermitte, 1960; De Renzi et al., 1966; Tognola & Vignolo, 1980; Raade et al., 1991) but a regular association of mouth apraxia with dysarthria. Studies which used computed tomography for determining the site of responsible lesions localized them in the lower part of the precentral gyrus, that is, close to the face and mouth area of the motor cortex. By contrast, parietal regions, generally thought to play a prominent role for limb apraxia, were not involved (Tognola & Vignolo, 1980; Kimura, 1982; Raade et al., 1991). A recent couple of studies confirmed and refined Nathan's observation of mouth apraxia in patients with right-hemisphere damage. They documented an interaction between the body part executing the gestures and their sensitivity to right and left brain damage (Bizzozero et al., 2000; Della Sala et al., 2006b): whereas oral movements like sticking out the tongue or puffing out one cheek were predominantly affected by left brain damage, movements of the upper face like blinking with one eye were equally disturbed by right or left brain damage.

Two studies (De Renzi et al., 1966; Bizzozero et al., 2000) determined a rank order of difficulty of the gestures. Protrusion of the tongue, failure of which had been emphasized in Jackson's original description, turned out to be among the easiest items. Interestingly the most difficult items included gestures demanding asymmetric and unusual movements like "puff out your left cheek" (Bizzozero et al., 2000). By contrast the meaning of the gesture did not seem to play a major role. While pretending to give a kiss was among the easiest items, a "Bronx cheer" (sticking out the tongue between the lips and blowing to make a sound reminiscent of flatulence) was among the most difficult.

Both of these studies tested the imitation of gestures. On scrutiny, imitation of oral gestures is not necessarily equivalent to imitation of manual gestures. Whereas the model for imitation of manual gestures is constituted by the sight of the body part performing the gesture, demonstration of oral gestures may consist of a visible consequence of the target gesture rather than its direct sight, as for example when patients are asked to bite the inside of one cheek, which was one of the most difficult items in Bizzozero et al. (2000). For some oral gestures the model consists of the sound produced by mouth movements rather than the sight of the movement, as, for example, when patients are asked to click their tongue, imitating a horse galloping, which turned out to be the most difficult gesture in the study by De Renzi et al. (1966).

A distant relative

The short survey of mouth and face apraxia raises doubts on their communality with limb apraxia. Statistical correlations between their severities are weak. Factors which are decisive for the classification of limb apraxia, such as the meaningfulness of gestures or their interactions with tools and objects, do not play a major role for apraxia of mouth and face. Relationships to aphasia have been postulated for both, but whereas the communality was sought at the highest level of symbol formation and abstract attitude for limb apraxia, it concerns the motor act of articulation for oral apraxia. Finally, evocation of gestures by imitation poses problems for oral gestures which are absent for gestures of the limbs.

If the different variants of limb apraxia were conceived as a family, oral and face apraxia might be compared to distant relatives who happen to live in the neighborhood but lead a life on their own. We will not invite them to our further explorations of the structure and peculiarities of this family, but will concentrate entirely on apraxia of the limbs.

Hand, finger, foot, and axial movements

My own research on the body part specificity of imitation concentrated on meaningless gestures involving three categories of body parts: hand postures, finger postures, and feet postures. Their imitation was tested in blocks rather than in an intermingled sequence of different categories (Tessari et al., 2007). Patients imitated with the limbs ipsilateral to their lesions and demonstration was made like "in a mirror," that is, the examiner demonstrated with the right hand when the patients used their left hand and vice versa. Scoring evaluated the final position of the acting body part regardless of whether it was reached with a straight movement or after hesitations and self-corrections.

Generally, our studies included patients who had suffered a first unilateral stroke in one hemisphere. If not mentioned otherwise, patients with left brain damage had aphasia, and those with right brain damage hemineglect[1] and/or visuo-constructional difficulties.

Hand postures

Healthy subjects imitate the hand postures shown in Figure 7.1 swiftly and with a virtually errorless performance (Goldenberg, 1996). The same applies for most patients with right brain damage. Only right brain damaged patients with very severe hemineglect have some difficulties. By contrast, imitation can be very difficult for patients with left brain damage. As a group, they score significantly worse than either controls or right brain damaged

1 Patients with hemineglect fail to pay attention to the side of space opposite to a lesioned hemisphere. It is more common and persistent after right brain lesions, and it is frequently associated with a general narrowing of the focus of attention.

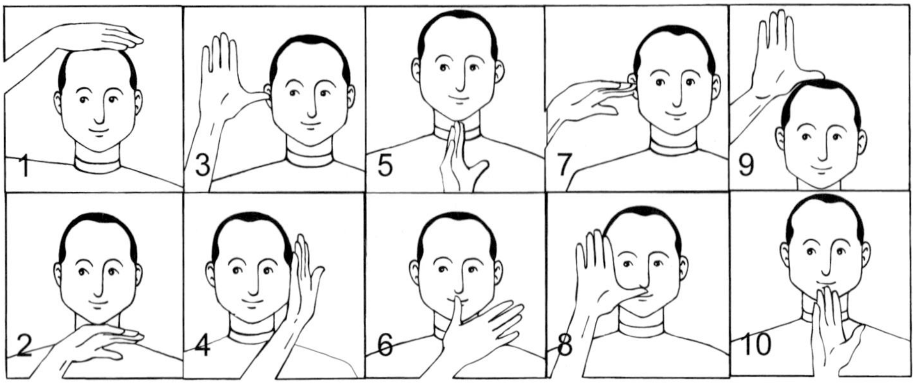

Figure 7.1 Ten hand postures used for testing imitation of meaningless gestures. Postures are arranged according to their difficulty for patients with left brain damage. Error rates increase from left-sided to right-sided columns and within each column from top to bottom. The numbers correspond with the increasing difficulty. Adapted from *Neuropsychologia*, *39* (13), Georg Goldenberg, Kerstin Laimgruber, and Joachim Hermsdörfer, Imitation of gestures by disconnected hemispheres, p. 1436, Copyright (2001), with permission from Elsevier.

patients (Goldenberg, 1995, 1996, 1999; Goldenberg & Strauss, 2002). However, as is frequently the case with group comparisons, their low mean scores are in fact a composite of patients who have no particular problems and others whose inability to copy the postures is quite dramatic. One patient with a severe problem has been shown in Figure 6.1. This patient had a lesion restricted to the parietal lobe.

The crucial role of integrity of the left parietal lobe for the imitation of hand postures was confirmed by a lesion subtraction study (Goldenberg & Karnath, 2006): lesions of left brain damaged patients visible on magnetic resonance imaging (MRI) were transcribed to corresponding slices of a standard brain, and with the help of a dedicated programme (MRIcron; Rorden & Karnath, 2004; Rorden et al., 2007) the lesions of patients whose scores on imitation of hand postures fell within the normal range were subtracted from those of patients who scored in the pathological range. Such subtraction reveals the location of lesions which distinguish patients with impaired imitation from those with normal imitation of hand postures. This crucial location turned out to be the inferior parietal lobe (Figure 7.2).

The selective impairment of imitation of hand posture following left parietal lesions was replicated in a further lesion mapping study using the same hand postures by Dovern et al. (2011), while two further studies by other groups (Bekkering et al., 2005; Della Sala et al., 2006a) confirmed that imitation of hand postures is severely impaired in left brain damaged patients but spared in patients with right brain damage.

Finger postures

The finger postures shown in Figure 7.3 look more complicated than the hand postures, and indeed the mean scores of controls for copying them are somewhat lower than

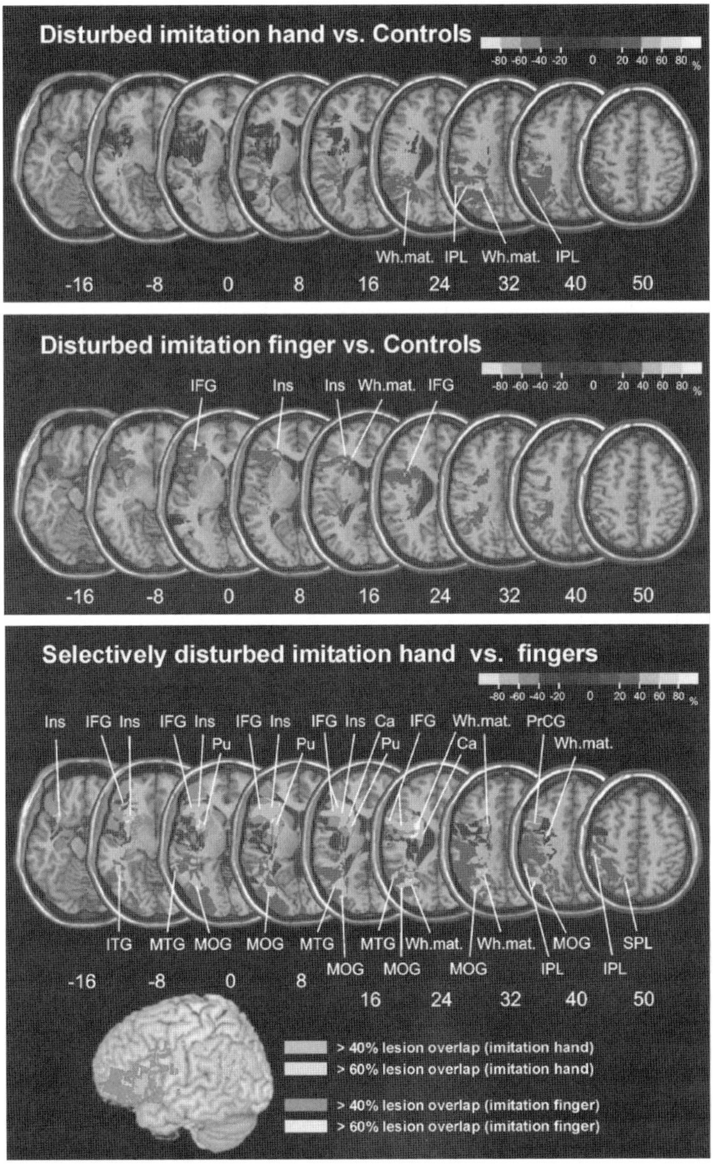

Figure 7.2 Lesion subtraction delimiting the crucial lesions for defective imitation of hand or finger postures in patients with left brain damage and aphasia. The colors indicate the difference between the frequencies of lesions in patients with and without the target symptom. The upper two figures show differences between patients with defective imitation of either hand or finger postures and patients with intact imitation of the same kind of postures regardless of whether imitation of the alternative body part is also impaired. The bottom figure compares only patients with selective deficits of either hand or finger imitation. The red to yellow part of the color scale indicates higher frequencies of lesions in patients with disturbed imitation of hand postures, and the blue part higher frequencies in patients with disturbed imitation of finger postures. Ca: capsula interna; IFG: inferior frontal lobe; Ins: insula; IPL: inferior parietal lobe; ITG: inferior temporal gyrus; MOG: middle occipital gyrus; MTG: middle temporal gyurs; Pu: putamen; SPL: superior parietal lobe; Wh. matt: white matter. Adapted from Goldenberg G. and Karnath, H. O. The neural basis of imitation is body-part specific. *Journal of Neuroscience*, *26*, p. 6284 © 2006, The Society of Neuroscience, with permission. (See Plate 5.)

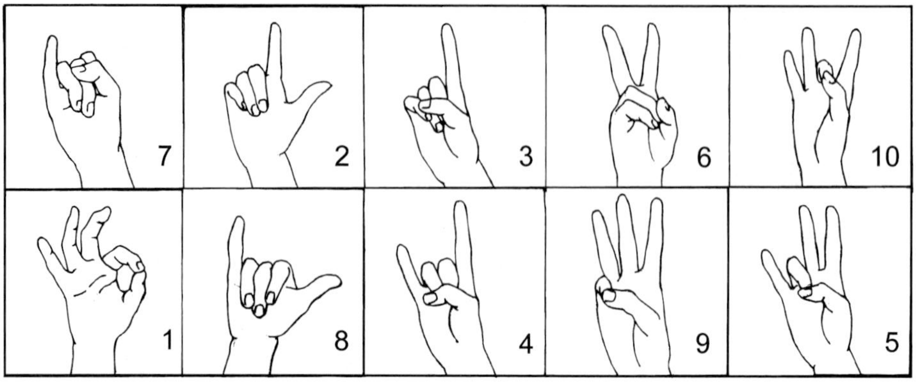

Figure 7.3 Ten finger postures used for testing imitation of meaningless gestures. Postures are arranged according to their difficulty for patients with left brain damage as in Figure 7.1, whereas the numbers indicate the ranking of difficulty for patients with right brain damage. Higher numbers indicate higher error rates. For example, the leftmost upper posture is the easiest one for left brain damaged patients, but occupies the seventh rank in the rank order of increasing difficulty for patients with right brain damage. Adapted from *Neuropsychologia*, *39* (13), Georg Goldenberg, Kerstin Laimgruber, and Joachim Hermsdörfer, Imitation of gestures by disconnected hemispheres, p. 1436, Copyright (2001), with permission from Elsevier.

for copying hand postures (De Renzi et al., 1980; Goldenberg, 1996). A more exciting difference to hand postures concerns the sensitivity to left brain and right brain damage. In contrast to hand postures, difficulties with imitation of finger postures are not restricted to patients with left brain damage. Imitation of finger postures is about equally affected by right and by left brain damage (Goldenberg, 1995, 1996, 1999; Goldenberg & Strauss, 2002)

The vulnerability of finger postures to right brain damage had already been observed and published in earlier group studies (Kimura & Archibald, 1974; De Renzi et al., 1980), but the two studies replicating the specific vulnerability of hand postures to left brain damage failed to replicate the susceptibility of finger postures to right brain damage (Bekkering et al., 2005; Della Sala et al., 2006a). A closer look at their method sections revealed an important difference concerning the selection of patients: whereas we included only right brain damaged patients with hemineglect and/or visuo-constructional difficulties, these studies excluded patients with hemineglect. We will come back to the influence of hemineglect on imitation later in this chapter.

In groups of left brain damaged patients the mean scores tend to be somewhat higher for finger than for hand postures (Goldenberg, 1995, 1996, 1999; Goldenberg & Strauss, 2002; Bekkering et al., 2005; Della Sala et al., 2006a), but this mild global difference conceals complete dissociations between single patients. There are left brain damaged patients whose defective imitation of hand postures contrasts with perfect imitation of finger postures and others who show the reverse dissociation. Lesion subtraction revealed an anatomical basis of these dissociations. Whereas defective imitation of hand postures is bound to left parietal lesions, defective imitation of finger postures is predominantly a symptom of precentral and inferior frontal lesions (Haaland et al., 2000; Goldenberg & Karnath, 2006; Dovern et al., 2011; see Figure 7.2).

Foot postures

Although deficient imitation of leg movements had already been mentioned in Liepmann's report of the imperial counselor, apraxia of the legs and feet has rarely been included in modern research on apraxia. There are only three studies examining the imitation of leg and feet gestures in patients with left brain damage. Two of them probed movements like "kick forward" or "trace a cross on the floor using your foot" in patients with left brain damage (Lehmkuhl et al., 1983; Ambrosoni et al., 2006), whereas the third one tested imitation of static foot postures (Goldenberg & Strauss, 2002; see Figure 7.4). The three studies agreed that defective imitation of leg gestures is usually associated with defective imitation of hand gestures, and that there are no instances of unequivocal dissociation between these two variants of limb apraxia. Ambrosoni et al. (2006) analyzed the lesions and found them to be larger in patients with deficient imitation of leg movements than in those who had problems only with imitation of arm and hand gestures.

Our study (Goldenberg & Strauss, 2002) was the only one also including patients with right brain damage. They scored significantly worse than controls but their impairment was less severe than that of left brain damaged patients.

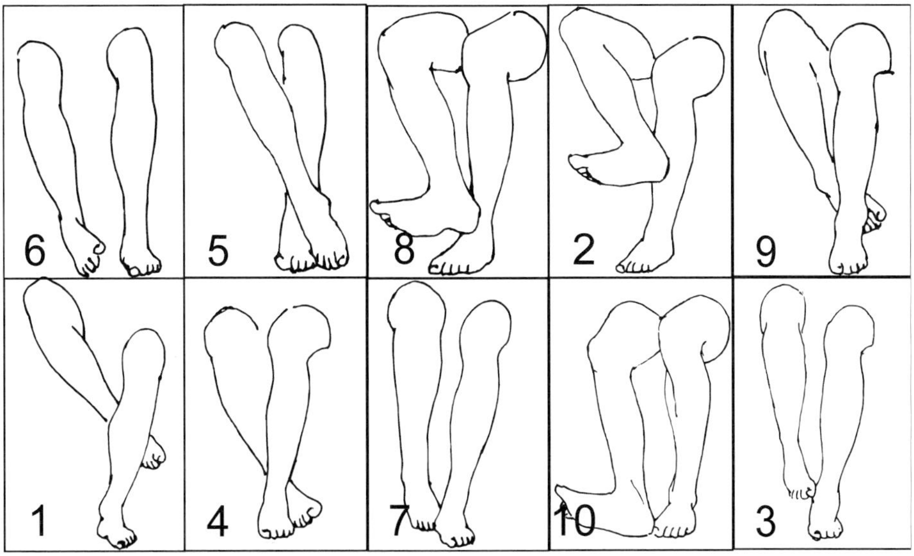

Figure 7.4 Ten foot postures used for testing imitation of meaningless gestures. The arrangement of the images and their numbering follow the same system as in Figure 7.3.

Axial movements

In the last chapter of the historical part we encountered Geschwind's patient who could on command assume the position of a boxer leading with his left fist but was unable to execute commands with that fist or to use either leg correctly in response to such commands as "Kick" or "Show me how you would stamp out a cigarette." The preservation of the boxer's stance was presented as an example for sparing of "axial" movements. Other examples of preserved axial movements included "dance steps, bowing, kneeling, marching, or standing at attention" which are all associated with distinct movements of the legs (Geschwind, 1975, p. 192). Apparently the preservation of axial movements was assumed to include leg movements on condition that they formed part of synergistic whole body actions.

The ambiguity of the distinction between individual leg movements and the involvement of the legs in whole body synergies made it difficult to probe the reality of Geschwind's observation in methodically sound group studies. For sake of clarity, group studies aiming at verification of Geschwind's claim excluded leg movements and limited the range of gestures to movements of trunk, neck, and eyes like: "lift both shoulders," "turn your head to the left," "look to the left," or "close your eyes firmly"[2] (Alexander et al., 1992; Poeck et al., 1982; Hanlon et al., 1998). This restriction changed the nature of the required actions from complex whole body synergies to simple local movements.

The results of these studies were controversial. A first study did not find significant differences between imitation of axial and of limb movements in aphasic patients but was later criticized for using too lenient statistical criteria (Poeck et al., 1982; Howes, 1988). Two other studies confirmed a lower error rate for axial than for limb movements (Alexander et al., 1992; Hanlon et al., 1998) but it remains questionable whether the lower error rate of axial movements is due to differences between the neural substrates of axial and limb movements. Alternatively it might simply indicate that the range of possible axial movements is much smaller than the range of possible limb movements, and that consequently axial movements provide fewer opportunities for errors than limb movements.[3] The difference between limb and axial movement may thus have its cause in the anatomy of the executing body parts rather than in the anatomy of their neuronal control.

Sources of body part specificity

So far, our review demonstrated the reality of body part specificity of disturbed imitation but left open their cause. We will first discuss possible explanations based on the anatomy of cerebral motor regions and their efferent connections.

[2] Note that closing of the eyes could also be classified as an examination of face apraxia (see Chapter 6).

[3] The higher complexity of arm and hand movements had already been brought forward by Sittig (1928; Maas & Sittig, 1929) as a cause for sparing of axial movements from apraxia (see Chapter 3).

Motor dominance of the left hemisphere

The neural organization of motor control is, in principle, symmetric. The motor cortex of the right hemisphere controls the left limbs, and vice versa. By contrast, the neural organization of apraxia is asymmetric, since unilateral lesions cause bilateral disturbances of motor actions. Liepmann resolved the exception by postulating a general dominance of the left hemisphere for motor control of both sides. As he put it:

> The right sided hand centre which in most cases has learned all higher achievements only after the left one, remains lifelong to some degree dependent on the left hemisphere. (Liepmann, 1908, p. 35)

This proposal can account for bilateral apraxia caused by left brain damage, but it fails when confronted with the variability of lateralization: as we have seen, exclusive bilateral control by the left hemisphere is confined to hand postures. Bilateral deficits of imitation of finger and foot postures can be due to lesions in either hemisphere. This bilaterality creates a conflict between two definitions of motor dominance. If motor dominance means that only lesions of the dominant hemisphere cause deficits, neither hemisphere is dominant for the control of finger and foot gestures. If, however, motor dominance means that lesions of the dominant hemisphere cause bilateral motor deficits, both hemispheres are dominant. Obviously, the concept of motor dominance fails to explain body part specific effects of unilateral brain lesions.

Somatotopy of motor cortex

Another possible source of body part specificity is the somatotopy of motor cortex. In primary motor and adjacent premotor cortex the neurons sending commands to body parts are arranged in a sequence that more or less replicates their neighborhood relations in the real body. The lowest part, adjacent to Broca's area controls the mouth, the tongue and the articulatory muscles. Upwards, it is followed by the fingers, the arm, the trunk, and finally the leg (Grünbaum & Sherrington, 1901; see Figure 7.5). According to this sequence, one might expect that the effects of lesions depend on their position along the inferior to superior extension of the brain, so that lesions of inferior portion cause apraxia of the mouth, lesions of the middle part apraxia of fingers and arms, and lesions of the upper part apraxia of the legs. This expectation is fulfilled for the mouth (see beginning of this chapter) but not for the other body parts. Our lesion study (Goldenberg & Karnath, 2006) demonstrated that dissociations between imitation of finger and hand postures depend on the location of lesions in frontal or parietal regions rather than in the lower or upper parts of the central region (Figure 7.2).

Proximal versus distal motor control

Greater frequency and greater severity of apraxia of distal body parts has been suggested by Sittig (1928) and by Geschwind (1975), but they based their suggestions on different aspects of the anatomy of cerebral motor control. Sittig reasoned that the greater extension of cerebral motor areas devoted to distal body parts makes them more vulnerable to the

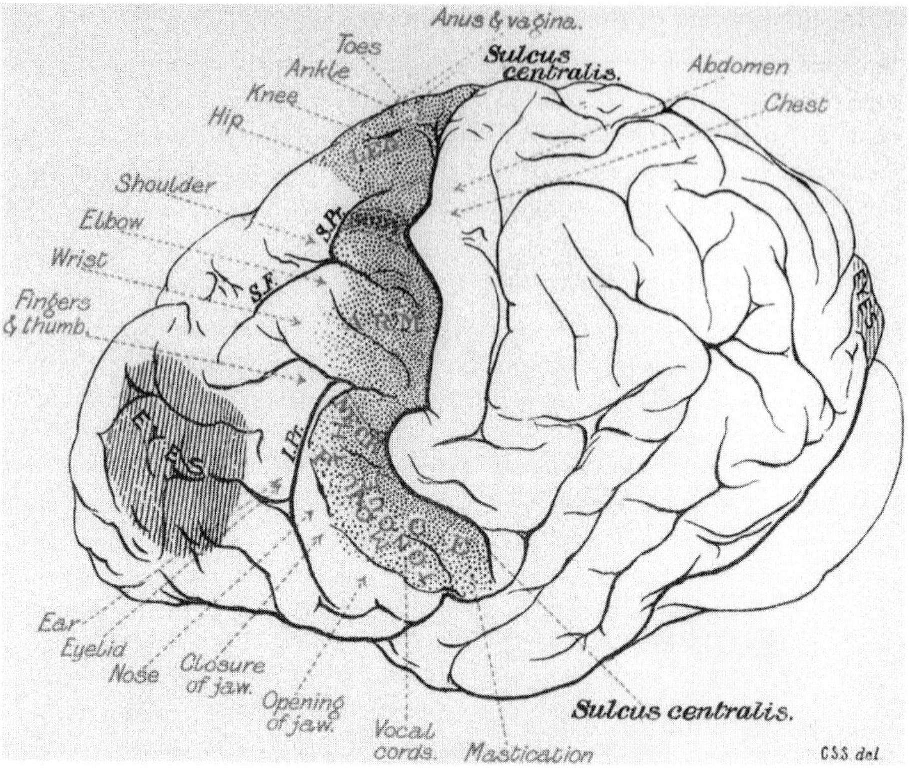

Figure 7.5 This early depiction of the somatotopy of motor cortex was derived from electrical stimulation and partial excisions of the cerebral cortex of a chimpanzee. It does not substantially differ from the somatotopy of human motor cortex. From dorsal (top) to ventral (bottom) there is a sequence of motor representations of leg, arm, wrist, and fingers. Reproduced from Grünbaum, A. S. F. and Sherrington, C. S. Observation on the physiology of the cerebral cortexs of some of the higher apes. *Proceedings of the Royal Society of London*, *69*, 206–209, plate 4 © 1901, The Royal Society. (See Plate 6.)

effects of brain damage. Geschwind deduced the preferential affection of distal body parts from their exclusive control by crossed pyramidal nerve fibers (see Chapters 3 and 4).

The predicted sparing of proximal body parts has indeed been confirmed for movements of the trunk and the head (Hanlon et al., 1998), but we already discussed that this dissociation might simply indicate that the range of possible axial movements is much smaller than the range of possible limb movements, and that consequently axial movements provide fewer opportunities for errors than limb movements.

Finger postures are more distal than hand postures. When the distal versus proximal dichotomy is applied to finger and hand postures, the empirical support dwindles. Our studies found double dissociations between deficient imitation of finger and of whole hand postures but no general advantage of hand over finger postures. Approximately equal frequency of defective imitation of finger and whole hand movements in patients with left brain damage was also reported in a previous group study using other finger and hand gestures (De Renzi et al., 1980).

Patients with right brain damage do have significantly more difficulties with finger than with whole hand postures, but they also encounter difficulties with leg postures, although the muscles moving the leg are not farther away from the trunk, and hence not more distal, than those moving the whole hand. Moreover, neither Sittig's nor Geschwind's proposals provided any clue as to why the principle of predominant affection of distal body parts should apply only to patients with right brain damage.

Matching gestures

Further evidence against the dependence of body part specificity on the anatomy of motor control was provided by an experiment exploiting the idea that imitation is the translation of body postures from one human body to another. We asked healthy controls and patients with either left or right brain damage pages to match photographs of gestures produced by different persons and seen under different angles of view (Goldenberg, 1999, see Figure 7.6). After matching, imitation of the same gestures was tested.

In this sample, patients with left brain damage had fewer difficulties with the imitation of finger than of hand postures while the right brain damaged patients' difficulties were

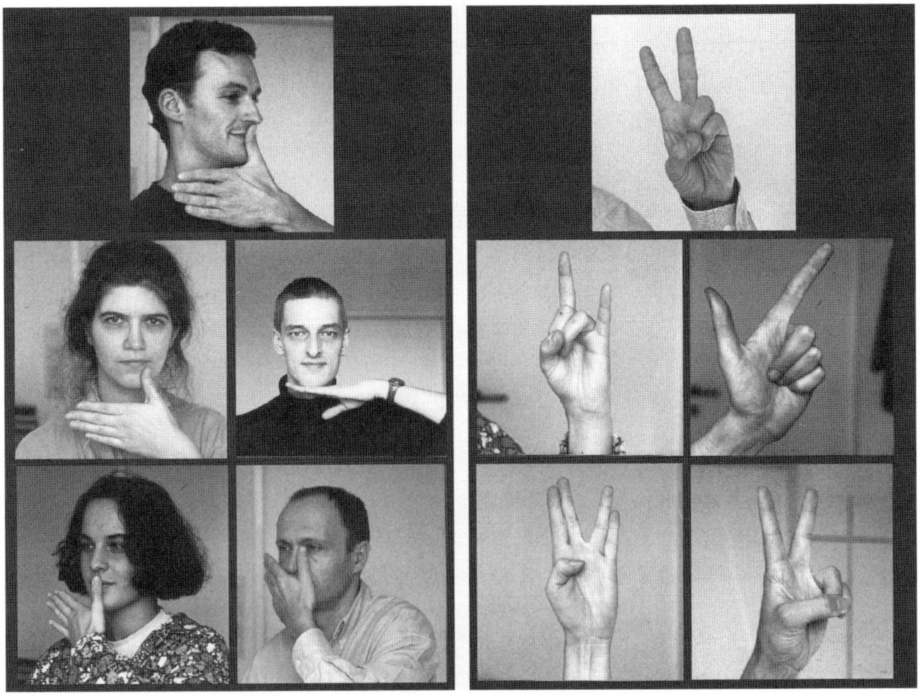

Figure 7.6 Pages from the test of matching gestures: subjects were asked to select from the array of four gestures the one that matches the target shown on top.

restricted to finger postures. The matching test replicated this body part specificity: left brain damaged patients made more errors with matching of hand than finger postures while right brain damage patients showed the reverse pattern. Since the motor act of pointing to a picture was the same for selection of hand and finger postures, their differential sensitivity to left and right brain damage cannot be due to the anatomy of motor control. The sources of body part specificity of defective imitation must be looked for in factors beyond the anatomy of motor control.

Body part coding

Do you need some distraction, and is there another person around? Then I suggest a little experiment: demonstrate the ten hand postures shown in Figure 7.1 and ask the other person to imitate them. In all probability, imitation will be fast and virtually free of errors. Exceptions to error-free performance become conspicuous only when the experimental subject is your little daughter or son (or any other child) below the age of seven, because it is only about this age that children reach adults' level of competence for imitating the postures (Aouka et al., 2003; Weidinger et al., in preparation).

The ease of imitating these hand postures is not trivial. They are essentially novel. This does not mean that you have never before happened to make one or the other of them, but in all probability you performed them substantially less often than, say, the gesture of scratching your nose, and you never practiced them in order to improve their performance. Some of them share elements with more common and natural gestures. Rather than facilitating their execution, this partial similarity may become a source of disturbing interference (Petreska et al., 2010). For example, the three most difficult postures of our collection (see Figure 7.1) evoke touching the mouth (gesture 10), the hair (9), and the face (8), but they deviate from natural touch in that the palm of the hand looks away from face and head rather than touching them. By contrast, the easiest gesture (1) replicates natural touch of the hairs (or the bald head). The order of difficulties refers to patients with left brain damage. Healthy subjects are nearly errorless when imitating even the counterintuitive difficult gestures.

In order to understand the imitation of meaningless gestures we must seek a mechanism that enables imitation of novel gestures without practice and even in the face of interference by partially similar, more natural, gestures. The mechanism should be independent of the motor execution of gestures and apply to all instances of the translation of gestures from one human body to another. The nature of that mechanism should make it plausible that it matures only at an age when children are already competent language users. Finally this mechanism should provide a basis for body part specificity of imitation disturbances. I have proposed that this mechanism is body part coding (Goldenberg, 1995; Goldenberg & Strauss, 2002; Goldenberg & Karnath, 2006; Goldenberg, 2009).

The proposal maintains that the association between perception and replication of meaningless gestures is mediated by body part coding. Body part coding reduces the gestures to simple spatial relationships between defined body parts. For example, gesture 2 of Figure 7.1 could be described as "back of hand touches underside of chin," gesture 4 as "back of hand touches contralateral cheek," gesture 6 as "thumb crosses middle of mouth, back of hand looks away from head," gesture 8: "thumb touches underside of nose, palm of hand looks away from head," and gesture 10: "middle finger crosses center of mouth, palm looks away from head." These examples are not meant to suggest that subjects verbalize the gestures before they imitate them. We will come back to the role of language for development of body part coding in the next section.

Body part coding solves the "correspondence problem" (Brass & Heyes, 2005) between perception and execution of gestures because it creates descriptions which apply independently of whether the gesture is perceived or executed and independently of the different perspectives and modalities of perceiving one's own and other bodies. Furthermore, body part coding reduces the load on working memory where the gesture must be held from demonstration until completion of replication, because it reduces the multiple visual features of the demonstration to simple relationships between a limited number of elements.

A non-trivial prerequisite of body part coding is the segmentation of the continuity of the human body into defined body parts (de Vignemont et al., 2006, 2009). This requires knowledge about features and boundaries of body parts that pertain to all instances of human bodies regardless of individual variations in size or shape and regardless of changes in body configuration brought about by movements of limbs and whole body. The continuous transitions from one body part to another are transformed into sharply defined boundaries, while variability within the defined borders of a part is neglected. This kind of perceptual processing has been termed "categorical" (Kosslyn et al., 1990; Laeng et al., 2003) or "topological" (de Vignemont et al., 2006; Wang et al., 2007; He, 2008). Authors who speculate about the cerebral basis of categorical or, respectively, topological perception agree that it is bound to left hemisphere function (Laeng et al., 2003; Jager & Postma, 2003; Wang et al., 2007; He, 2008).

If there are several persons around you, you may carry out a further experiment illustrating the application of categorical segmentation to body part coding and imitation. Put an index finger on the bridge of your nose so that the tip of the finger is approximately halfway between tip and root of the nose, and ask your subjects to imitate this posture. Ask them to maintain the position of the finger and inspect them carefully. You will probably find that none of them deviated from the bridge of the nose to its flanks but that the position of the fingertip varies from the tip of the nose to its root. The variance of the position extends across the whole length of the nose which is several centimeters. By contrast, the distance between the bridge and the flanks of the nose is only a few millimeters. Nonetheless the boundary between bridge and flanks is respected while the position along the axis from tip to root is neglected. The interpretation of this inequality is that the border between bridge and flanks of the nose is significant for categorical classification, whereas the distances to tip and root of the nose are not. All positions along the extension from tip to root belong to the same category, that is, bridge of the nose. Subjects coded and replicated the gesture as "tip of index touches bridge of nose."

Body part coding and language

We have already mentioned that imitation of hand and finger postures reaches adult levels only around seven to eight years (Aouka et al., 2003, Weidinger et al., in preparation). At that age children are competent users of language and begin to master paralinguistic skills like reading, writing, and calculation. Interestingly naming of body parts reaches adult levels at about the same age (Poeck & Orgass, 1964). The coincidence evokes a suspicion that the acquisition of categorical knowledge about body part is identical with the learning of their name and that body part coding for imitation of gestures is accomplished by verbalization of the demonstrated gesture.[4] There is, to my knowledge, neither experimental proof nor disproof of this idea. My own experience from asking subjects for their strategies does not endorse a major role of covert verbalization of the body part code of demonstrated gestures. It seems, however, plausible that learning the names of body parts facilitates acquisition of knowledge about their conceptually significant features and boundaries. Hearing and producing the same name for a body part regardless of whether it is on the own or another person's body and regardless of whether it is seen, felt, or moved, augments coherence between features reliably associated with that name and cancels out features which are accidently associated with single instances of perceiving or moving that body part (Lupyan et al., 2007). Learning the names of body parts thus promotes recognition of their permanent features and significant boundaries. Once this knowledge has been acquired, it can probably be used for body part coding without a need for verbal labeling.

Body part coding and the left inferior parietal lobe

Thus far I have argued that body part coding is a general mechanism for imitation of novel gestures. This leaves open the question as to how it can explain differences between the neural substrates of imitating gestures made by different body parts. A possible explanation starts from the assumption that the difficulty of body part coding increases with increasing number and diversity of body parts involved in the gesture. Both are exceptionally high for hand postures and exceptionally low for finger postures (see Figures 7.1 and 7.3). Positions of the hand relative to parts of head and face demand access to knowledge about the determining features and boundaries of a multitude of very different body parts like chin, lips, bridge and flanks of the nose, cheek, ears, palm, and back of hands. By contrast, finger postures are, with a possible exception for the thumb, constituted by a set of uniform elements which differ only in their serial position. Thus body part coding of finger postures can be reduced to numbering extended and flexed fingers according to their serial position from index to small fingers. If this reasoning is correct, the neural substrate of body part coding should be located in a region whose damage can cause a selective deficit

[4] In a way, this hypothesis would be a variant of Head's ideas concerning the "power of verbalization" necessary for correct imitation in spite of diverging laterality of the examiner's and the patient's acting hand (see Chapter 3).

of imitation of hand postures coupled with preserved imitation of finger postures. This definition applies to the left inferior parietal lobe.

Autotopagnosia

A crucial role of the left inferior parietal lobe for body part coding is supported by case reports of the rare but impressive syndrome of autotopagnosia (Pick, 1922; De Renzi & Scotti, 1970; Poncet et al., 1971; Sirigu et al., 1991b; Denes et al., 2000; Buxbaum & Coslett, 2001). Patients with autotopagnosia become insecure and commit errors when asked to point to body parts on themselves, on another person, or on a model of the human body. Most frequently they search for body parts in their vicinity, e.g., for the wrist on the forearm, but they may also confound them with body parts of similar functional properties, e.g., the elbow with the knee. Both types of errors combine when they point to the nearest body part with a similar function, e.g., the elbow for the wrist.

Errors occur not only when the body parts are designated by verbal command but also when they are shown on pictures or when the examiner demonstrates correct pointing to a body part and the patient tries to imitate. By contrast, patients are able to name the same body parts when they are pointed at either on their own body or on a model, and they can select a named body part when given an array of drawings of isolated body parts. Nor is there a general inability to point to distinct locations on their own body: they reach them accurately when asked to indicate the typical location of accessories (e.g., a wrist watch) or the location of objects which had been temporarily fixed to a body part (Semenza, 1988; Sirigu et al., 1991b; Denes et al., 2000).

A possible explanation for this pattern of preserved and disturbed abilities could be that patients have global knowledge about shapes and locations of body parts but lack knowledge of their defining features. Their knowledge suffices for recognizing and naming body parts when they are presented in isolation or are set off from other body parts by the examiner's pointing, but not for defining its boundaries when the body part appears integrated in the continuous structure of the body. They are unable to segment the body into its parts.

Segmentation of the continuity of the body into defined body parts is the core prerequisite of body part coding. Imitation of gestures differs from pointing at single body parts by the need to apply body part coding to combinations of multiple body parts rather than to the localization of only one body part. This makes imitation more difficult than pointing to single parts and leads to the prediction that patients who fail the easier task of pointing to body parts will invariably also fail the more difficult imitation of gestures. Indeed, when imitation of gestures has been examined in patients with autotopagnosia it was regularly found to be defective (De Renzi & Scotti, 1970; Poncet et al., 1971; Assal & Butters, 1973; Ogden, 1985; Denes et al., 2000; Buxbaum & Coslett, 2001; Felician et al., 2003).

Right brain damage and the focus of attention

Enhanced demands on body part coding can explain the heightened sensitivity of imitating hand postures to left parietal brain lesions. This is, however, unlikely to be the only mechanism contributing to the body part specificity of disturbed imitation. Another possible mechanism could consist of different demands on the allocation of attention to the spatial layout of the demonstrated gesture. For analyzing this aspect of imitation we will return to the imitation of finger postures.

We have already mentioned that studies excluding patients with left hemineglect found imitation of finger postures by patients with right brain damage preserved, whereas our studies which included only right brain damaged patients who had either hemineglect or visuo-constructional difficulties revealed impairment. The suspicion that the conflicting results were due to the presence or absence of hemineglect was borne out by a further study examining imitation of hand and finger postures in right brain damaged patients who were not preselected for either absence or presence of hemineglect.

The results were straightforward: there was a tight relationship between the severity of hemineglect and the number of errors in imitation of finger postures, and in patients with very severe hemineglect there was also some impairment of imitating hand postures (Goldenberg et al., 2009; see Figure 7.7). An obvious explanation for this correlation could be that patients with severe hemineglect failed to attend to the fingers on the left side of the demonstrated gesture. Since the right brain damaged patients used their ipsilesional right hand for imitation, the examiner demonstrated the posture with their left hand. From the

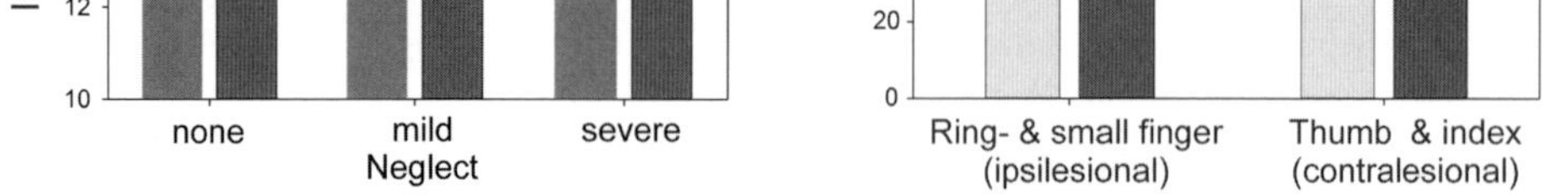

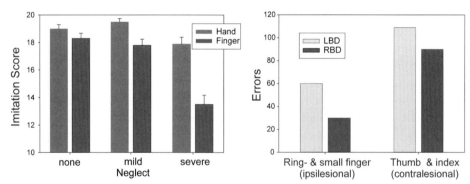

Figure 7.7 Left: Correlation between severity of hemineglect and accuracy of imitation in patients with right brain damage. Right: Distribution of errors in left and right brain damaged patients. All patients used the hand ipsilateral to the lesioned hemisphere. Since the examiner demonstrated the posture "like in a mirror" with the other hand, the thumb and the index finger appeared on the contralesional side and was hence vulnerable to hemineglect. We classified the laterality of the fingers that were in incorrect positions for 100 consecutive errors each of consecutive patients with right or left brain damage. Both groups of patients made more errors with thumb and index than with ring finger and small finger, but the difference was significantly higher in patients with right brain damage. Reprinted from *Neuropsychologia*, *47* (13), Georg Goldenberg, Udo Münsinger, and Hans-Otto Karnath, p. 2952, Copyright (2009), with permission from Elsevier. (See Plate 7.)

patient's perspective the thumb and the index fingers of the examiner's hand were located on the left side and were hence susceptible to hemineglect. Indeed, analysis of the distribution of errors revealed more incorrect configurations of thumb and index than of ring finger and small finger. The same bias of error distribution was also detected in left brain damaged patients who saw the demonstration of thumb and index finger on the right side of the examiner's hand, but the asymmetry of error distribution was stronger in the patients with right-sided lesions (see Figure 7.7).

However, neglect of the left side of the demonstrating hand cannot be the whole story, because one-third of the errors of the patients with right brain damage concerned the ring and the small fingers which, from their perspective, were located on the right side of the examiner's demonstrating hand. A possible cause for non-lateralized errors could be a general narrowing of the focus of attention. Such narrowing has been postulated to be a regular companion of the lateral displacement of attention in spatial hemineglect (Heilman & Van Den Abell, 1980; Halligan & Marshall, 1994; Husain & Rorden, 2003).

Inspection of the gestures (see Figures 7.1 and 7.3) gives clues as to why the effects of narrowing the focus of attention are more severe for finger than for hand postures. Configuration of any of the five fingers can make a difference between otherwise identical finger postures. Correct imitation requires attention to each of the five fingers and hence deployment of attention across the whole extension of five spatially distinct but otherwise uniform elements. By contrast, the defining features of hand postures are concentrated in the small region where the hand contacts the face or head and consist of combinations of the hand with perceptually salient and unique body parts like chin, lips, midline and tip of the nose, cheek, or ears. A narrow focus of attention suffices for appreciation of such spatially concentrated and perceptually salient features but not for analysis of the relationship between five spatially distributed but perceptually uniform elements.

Finger agnosia

Similar to the correspondence between defective imitation of hand postures and autotopagnosia, defective imitation of finger postures has a counterpart concerning the identification of single fingers that has been named "finger agnosia" (Gerstmann, 1924; Schilder, 1935). Patients with finger agnosia confound fingers when asked to designate single fingers of either the own or the examiner's hand on verbal command, as well as when asked to show on a diagram which of their fingers had been touched or to move a finger demonstrated on a diagram (Benton, 1961; Kinsbourne & Warrington, 1962; Poeck, 1969; Gainotti et al., 1972; Mayer et al., 1999; Anema et al., 2008). Since the selection of single fingers is already disturbed, imitation of complex finger postures is invariably defective. Like defective imitation of finger configurations, finger agnosia is found with approximately equal frequency in patients with left or right brain damage (Kinsbourne & Warrington, 1962; Poeck & Orgass, 1969; Sauguet et al., 1971; Gainotti et al., 1972).

The term finger agnosia was introduced by the Viennese–American neurologist Joseph Gerstmann who considered it as a minor form of autotopagnosia (1924, 1942).[5] This classification is not tenable, because there are patients with finger agnosia who can point to proximal body parts and hence have no autotopagnosia (Gerstmann, 1924; Roeltgen et al., 1983; Mayer et al., 1999; Anema et al., 2008), as well as patients with autotopagnosia who can localize single fingers and hence have no finger agnosia (De Renzi & Scotti, 1970; Poncet et al., 1971; Assal & Butters, 1973).

In Chapter 3 we mentioned that finger agnosia had been conceived as a manifestation of a general "inability to locate correctly a part of a multiplicity of objects forming an organized whole" (Stengel, 1944). This inability was supposed to affect the fingers as much as external objects, because "their peculiar position outside the body, connecting personal and outer space makes them to a certain extent external objects." Recent studies suggest that the position between personal and outer space is less important for the emergence of finger agnosia than their uniformity. These studies demonstrated that patients with finger agnosia have similar difficulties with the selection of toes as with the selection of fingers (Tucha et al., 1997; Mayer et al., 1999; Moro et al., 2008). Toes share with fingers the structure of five uniform elements distinguished only by their serial position, but can hardly be said to connect personal and outer space more than other body parts.

Body part specificity and the anatomy of motor control

We have identified two main mechanisms that make complementary contributions to body part specificity of disturbed imitation and are bound to opposing laterality of responsible lesions: Body part coding is bound to left parietal lesions and affects hand postures more than finger postures, whereas narrowing of the focus of attention is bound to right hemisphere lesions and affects finger postures more than hand postures. These conclusions, however, exhaust neither all possible variants of imitation that can be examined, nor all possible mechanisms that may contribute to failures of imitation. For example, we have not analyzed the interplay of left and right brain lesions in determining the success of imitation of leg postures (see Figure 7.4), and we have not tried to account for defective imitation of finger postures by patients with left inferior frontal and precentral lesions. We will come back to the influence of left inferior frontal lesions on imitation of finger postures in the chapter on pantomime of tool use (Chapter 10) but rather than trying to make up an exhaustive list of factors influencing other variants of imitation, I want to draw a couple of general conclusion that come forward quite clearly.

[5] Later, Gerstmann proposed that finger agnosia is regularly associated with disturbances of writing, calculation, and right–left confusions, and that this combination is indicative of a left parietal lesions. The assumption that the "Gerstmann syndrome" is based on a common basic deficit has been challenged by studies demonstrating that its single components are more likely to be related to symptoms not included in the syndrome than to the other components of the syndrome (Benton, 1961; Poeck & Orgass, 1966). Nonetheless the syndrome continues to be a topic of research (Tucha et al., 1997; Mayer et al., 1999; Rusconi et al., 2010).

Body part specificity of errors is a robust finding, but, contrary to the suggestions of Liepmann and Geschwind, it does not reflect the anatomy of motor control and hence cannot be taken as proof for the dependence of apraxia on low-level mechanisms of motor control. It rather derives from the interaction of general cognitive aptitudes, like categorical perception or spatial deployment of attention, with structural properties of body parts.

Body part coding and the levels of motor control

Body part coding is based on segmentation of the body into its parts. Imitation is achieved by segmenting the demonstrated gestures into the constituent body parts and their spatial relationships and subsequent combination of these elements. The sequence of segmentation and combination makes body part coding a "generative system" where a multitude of formations can be produced from combination of a limited number of elements (Abler, 1989; Corballis, 1991). The most important generative system is language (Chomsky, 1957). The generative potential of body postures is much lower than that of language but it suffices for creation and replication of a multitude of novel gestures. In Chapter 6 we submitted that comprehension and production of novel actions have been recognized as evidence for the intervention of higher-level action control. According to this line of thought, body part coding qualifies as a constituent of high-level motor control. It is noteworthy that it is the only component of imitation that appears to be strictly bound to the integrity of the left parietal lobe.

Chapter 8

Use of single tools

Misuse of tools was the topic of the first printed appearance of the term "apraxia." Chajm Steinthal (1871; see Chapter 1) used the term for the description of an aphasic composer who grasped the pen upside down, took hold of a spoon and fork as if he had never used them before, and gripped his violin so awkwardly that it was impossible to play on it. All of these errors concern the use of single familiar tools. In the further historical course, authors who adhered to the dichotomy of ideo-kinetic and ideational apraxia were nearly unanimous in classifying misuse of tools and objects as a manifestation of the ideational variant, meaning that these patients' impressive errors were due to a loss of knowledge about the proper use of tools rather than to faulty motor execution of correctly conceived actions.[1] This apparent unanimity can easily conceal that there were indeed two contrasting interpretations of the "ideational" deficit. One, proposed by Pick and supported by Liepmann, maintained that ideational apraxia is "a mental insufficiency which manifests itself in the domain of action but has its roots in deficits which are not specific for action" (Liepmann, 1929), while the other one, brought forward by Morlaas (1928) and resuscitated for modern neuropsychology by de Renzi and Lucchelli (1988) postulated that knowing "how to use and to construct objects is a specialized function, isolated and independent from other specialized functions."

It is noteworthy that the opposing interpretations were illustrated by different kinds of observations. Pick described difficulties and errors of demented patients in the completion of everyday chores and emphasized that many errors were bound to the coordination and sequencing of multiple steps of everyday actions like dressing, cleaning, or preparing a pipe for smoking. By contrast, Morlaas' examples concentrated on the misuse of single tools and objects in the clinical examination of aphasic, but not demented, patients who were presented with a tool and asked to demonstrate its use. For example, a patient was presented with a pen and asked to write but failed because she held the pen upside down (see Chapter 3).

I will argue that the apparent conflict between two interpretations of one syndrome can be resolved by acknowledging that they describe in fact two different disturbances which may co-occur and interact in individual patients but are based on different mechanisms

[1] Exceptions to this view were made by Zangwill (1960) and Poeck (1982) who believed that both variants of apraxia may interfere with use of tools and objects but can be distinguished by an analysis of the nature of errors.

and bound to different locations of responsible lesions. Therefore, there will be two chapters devoted to misuse of tools and objects. This one will concentrate on misuse of single tools and objects while Chapter 9 will discuss difficulties with multistep actions involving multiple tools and objects.

The taxonomy of disturbed tool and object use

The application of the term "ideational apraxia" to two different syndromes is confusing and has motivated proposals for alternative designations. One of them suggests calling difficulties with single tools and objects "conceptual apraxia" and those with multistep actions "ideational apraxia" (Heilman & Rothi, 1993; Raymer & Ochipa, 1997). It has not found many supporters, because it is difficult to unequivocally define the difference between an "idea" and a "concept" and to find reasons why one of them should be more suitable for use of single tools and objects, and the other for multistep actions. A more influential taxonomic development identified "ideational apraxia" with defective use of single tools and objects as described by Morlaas and De Renzi, but proposed a new entity "action disorganization syndrome" for problems with everyday multistep actions involving multiple tools and objects (Schwartz et al., 1995; Humphreys & Forde, 1998). The domain of actions affected by the action disorganization syndrome was further specified as "naturalistic action by which we mean movement in the service of commonplace, practical goals like food preparation and consumption" (Schwartz & Buxbaum, 1997, p. 269). This additional qualification implicates an opposition between the mainly laboratory-based diagnosis of "ideational apraxia" and the coping with tools and objects in everyday life.

Following my suggestion to designate variants of apraxia according to the affected domains of action rather than their place in a putative hierarchy of "ideational" and "ideomotor" apraxia, I will use the attribute "single tools and objects" for the domains of Morlaas' and De Renzi's apraxia of tool use, and "multistep actions with multiple objects" or "naturalistic action" for that of Pick and Liepmann.

Knowing how to use a tool

We will discuss the lateralization and localization of lesions interfering with single tool use later in this chapter, but in order to give a realistic impression of afflicted patients we anticipate that in patients with circumscribed lesions, misuse of single familiar tools and objects is invariably bound to extensive left-sided lesions (De Renzi et al., 1968; Goldenberg & Hagmann, 1998b). Aphasia is a regular and right-sided hemiparesis, a frequent companion of their apraxia.

Misuse of everyday tools and objects is an impressive manifestation of apraxia (Figure 8.1). Patients try to cut paper with closed scissors, to eat soup with a fork, or to write with the wrong end of the pencil. They bite on the toothbrush, press the knife into the loaf without moving it to and fro, press the hammer upon the nail without hitting, and close the paper punch on top of the sheet without inserting the sheet. Patients with right-sided hemiparesis must use the tools one-handed with their less skillful left hand, but the

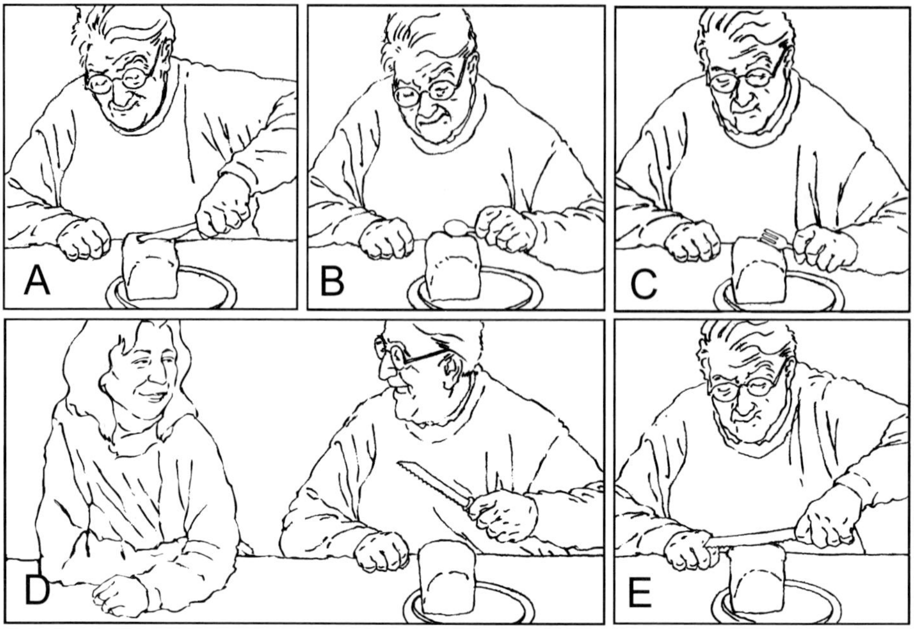

Figure 8.1 Attempts of a patient with right-sided hemiplegia, global aphasia, and apraxia to cut a slice of bread: in addition to the bread knife, a spoon, a fork, and a butter knife were laid out as distracters. All of these tools were easily visible and in a comfortable grasping distance for the patient. A: The patient first takes the butter knife and presses it upon the loaf but quickly realizes that this does not work. B and C: He tries the spoon and the fork. D: Eventually his gaze falls on the bread knife. He recognizes it as the correct tool and raises it triumphantly. E: He presses the knife upon the loaf but omits the slicing movement.

deviation of their errors from regular use obviously transgresses the natural inferiority of left-hand skill.

The independence of errors from inferior deftness of the left hand becomes unequivocally evident when clinical testing involves not only use but also selection of tool and recipient. Usually, patients are given the tool and its matching recipient and are asked to use them together. For example, they are handed a hammer and a block with a half-inserted nail and are asked to pound in the nail. When, however, they are given the tool and a selection of possible recipients or, conversely, a recipient and several tools, it may turn out that their failure concerns not only the proper handling of the tool but also the matching of the tool with its appropriate recipient. They may try to use a spoon for cutting or scissors for severing a nail.

Steinthal's formulation that patients behave as if they had never used the tools before is a pertinent but not exhaustive description of their difficulties. Healthy persons who have never in their lives seen spoons would nonetheless not try to use them for cutting bread, because it is obvious to them that for cutting you need a sharp-edged blade which a spoon does not have. This observation raises a suspicion that experience with the tool

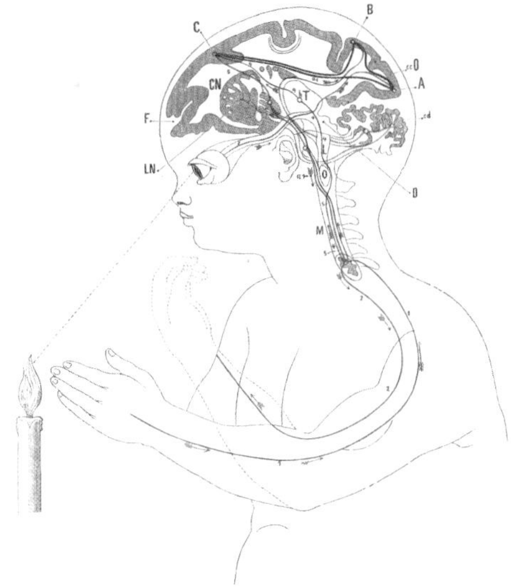

Plate 1 An associationist schema illustrating the motor reaction of the hand to the sight of a candle and the sensation of heat. The blue lines indicate centripetal, the red lines centrifugal, and the black lines association tracts. In this schema, neural processing beyond the incoming of sensation and outgoing of motor commands is limited to uninterrupted connections from the cortical end points of the sensation tracts (A and B) to the origin of the motor command (C). A: a point within the visual center; B: a point within the center for cutaneous sensations; C: a point within the territory of innervation sensations; ccO: occipital cortex; F: frontal cortex; 1: tract leading sensations from hand; 2: tract of movement of arm; 4C: tract for sensations of innervation; 5: centrifugal tract originating from C. Reproduced from Meynert, T. *Klinische Vorlesungen über Psychiatrie auf wissenschaftlichen Grundlagen für Studirende und Aerzte, Juristen und Psychologen*, p. 147 © 1889, Wilhelm Braumüller. (See Figure 1.1.)

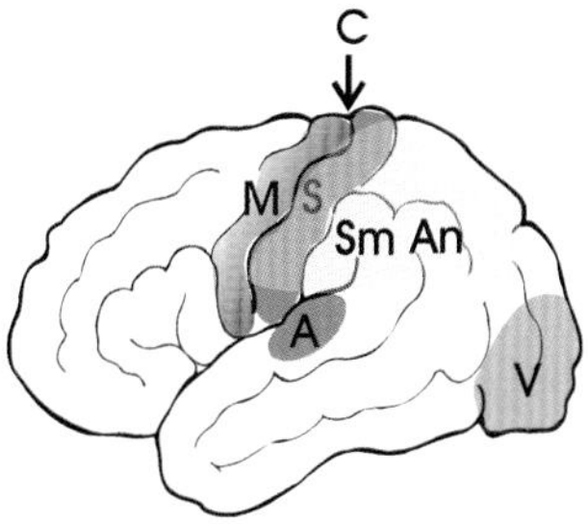

Plate 2 A schematic side view of the brain illustrating the anatomical considerations that underlay the discussions about the neural substrate of mind-palsy. According to the associationist model of brain function, memory images are stored close to the location where the original sensations have been received or the original motor commands have been sent out. Motor memories are thus stored in front of the central sulcus, and sensory memories behind it. The postulate that voluntary actions start with a mental image of the sensation of the completed movement and that this sensation is automatically transferred into motor action thus necessitating a stream of association from postcentral parietal to precentral motor areas constitutes a rudimentary form of a posterior to anterior stream of action control (see Chapter 2). A: acoustic cortex; C: central sulcus; M: motor cortex; S: somatosensory cortex; Sm: supramarginal gyrus; An: angular gyrus; V: visual cortex. Blue regions receive sensory afferences from the periphery, whereas the red region sends motor efferences to the periphery. Green denotes the extension of the parietal lobe. (See Figure 1.3.)

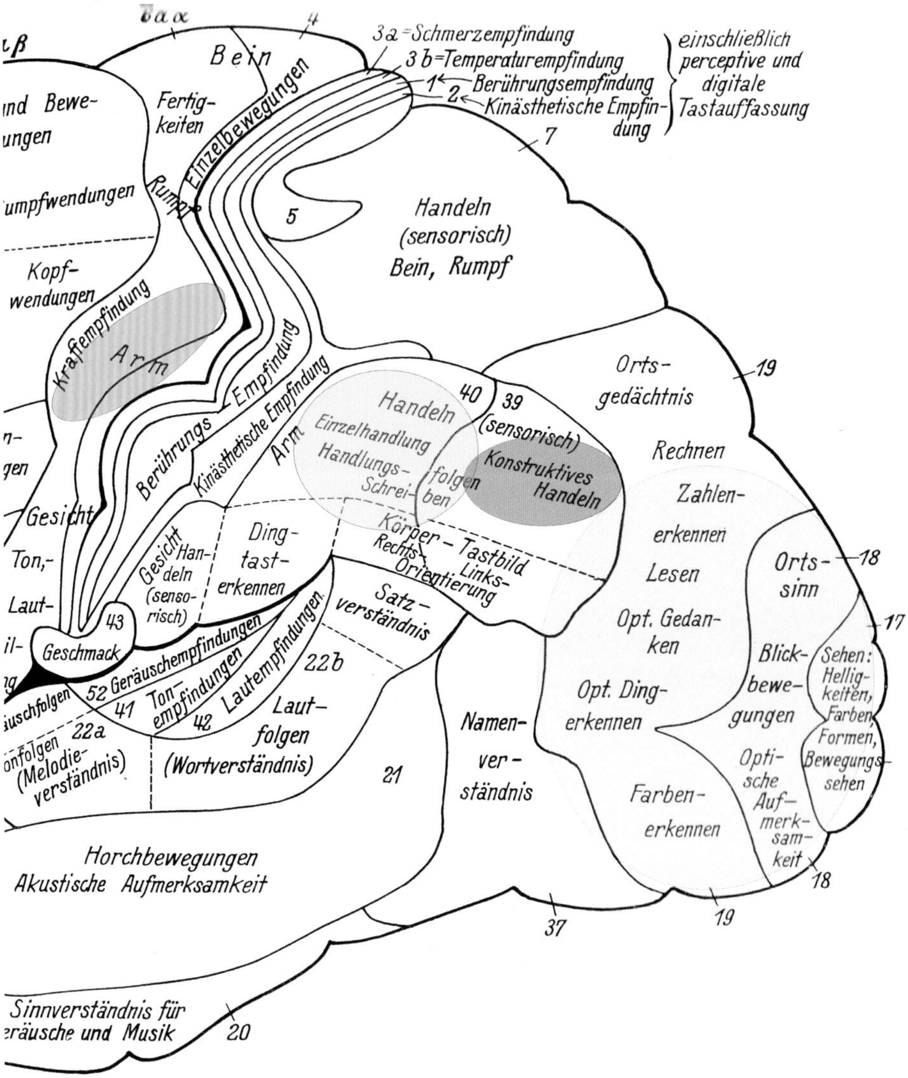

Plate 3 A section of Karl Kleist's famous (for holists rather infamous) brain chart showing the putative assignment of functions to Brodman areas of the cerebral cortex. The inscriptions describe functions of intact areas rather than symptoms of their damage, but in the text the clinical symptoms of their damage are elaborated. The colored field indicate the location of lesions causing limb-kinetic apraxia (orange; Brodman area 6a), ideokinetic apraxia (yellow; Brodman area 40), and constructional apraxia (green; Brodman area 39). Area 6a: *Rumpf*: trunk; *Arm*: arm (obviously including hand); *Gesicht*: face. Area 40: *Handeln*: action; *Einzelhandlung:* single action; *Handlungsfolgen:* action sequences; *Schreiben:* writing. Area 39: *Konstruktives Handeln*: constructional action. Ideational apraxia results from damage extending across the whole inferior parietal lobe. These lesions combine the disturbance of action sequencing with defective kinesthetic–optic coupling which is conceived as being at the core of constructional action. The section of Kleist's map is reproduced with kind permission from Springer Science + Business Media: *Zeitschrift für die gesamte Neurologie und Psychiatrie*, Bericht über die Gehirnpathologie in ihrer Bedeutung für Neurologie und Psychiatrie, *158*, 1937, p. 163, K. Kleist. (See Figure 3.1)

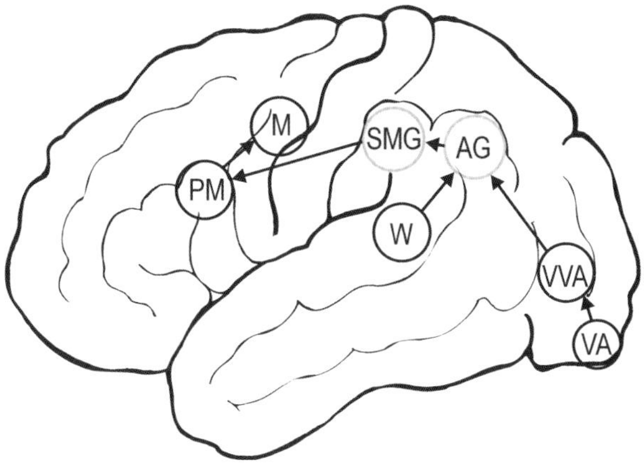

Plate 4 Bottom: Geschwind's final version of the posterior to anterior stream was elaborated and popularized by Heilman and Rothi (1993). It postulates storage of "time–space motor representations" in the supramarginal or angular gyrus (possible differences between these two portions of inferior parietal lobe were not discussed). The stored engrams can be addressed from verbal commands or, in imitation and tool use, from vision. PM: premotor area; M: motor cortex; SM: supramarginal gyrus; AG: angular gyrus; W: Wernicke's area; VA: primary visual area; VVA: visual association area. Reproduced from Heilman, K. M. and Rothi, L. J. G. Apraxia. In K. M. Heilman and E. Valenstein (Eds.), *Clinical Neuropsychology*, p. 151 (1993) Oxford University Press, by permission of Oxford University Press. (See Figure 4.1, bottom.)

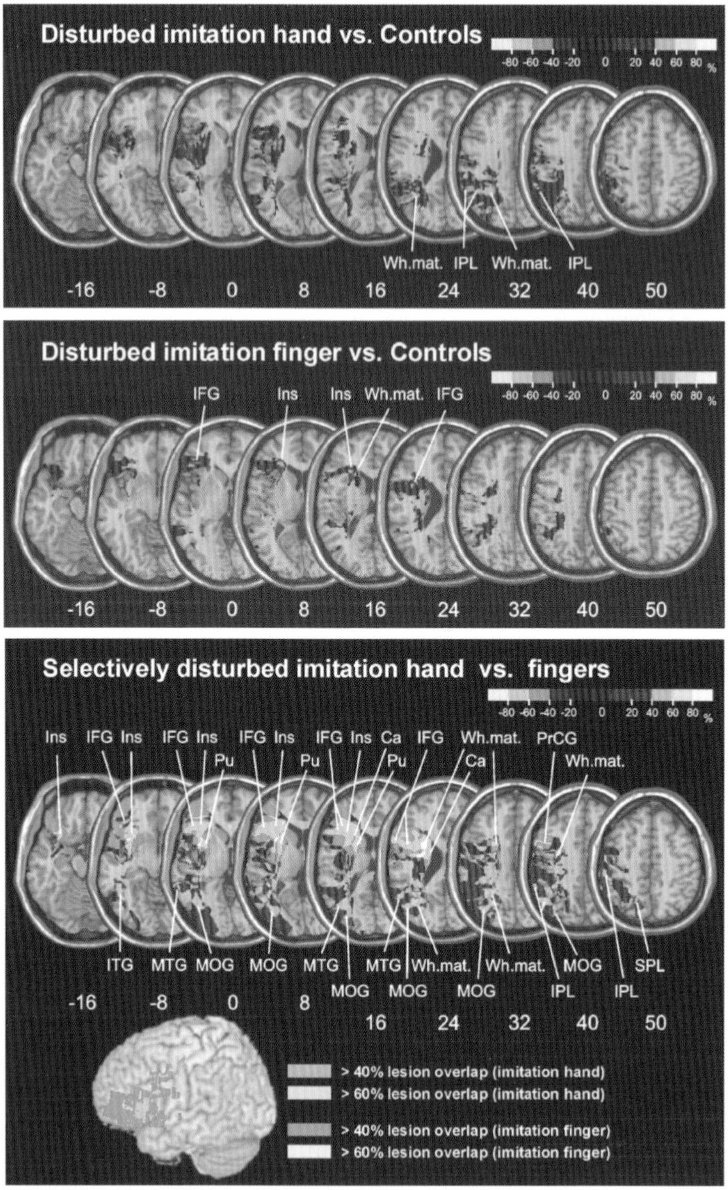

Plate 5 Lesion subtraction delimiting the crucial lesions for defective imitation of hand or finger postures in patients with left brain damage and aphasia. The colors indicate the difference between the frequencies of lesions in patients with and without the target symptom. The upper two figures show differences between patients with defective imitation of either hand or finger postures and patients with intact imitation of the same kind of postures regardless of whether imitation of the alternative body part is also impaired. The bottom figure compares only patients with selective deficits of either hand or finger imitation. The red to yellow part of the color scale indicates higher frequencies of lesions in patients with disturbed imitation of hand postures, and the blue part higher frequencies in patients with disturbed imitation of finger postures. Ca: capsula interna; IFG: inferior frontal lobe; Ins: insula; IPL: inferior parietal lobe; ITG: inferior temporal gyrus; MOG: middle occipital gyrus; MTG: middle temporal gyurs; Pu: putamen; SPL: superior parietal lobe; Wh. matt: white matter. Adapted from Goldenberg G. and Karnath, H. O. The neural basis of imitation is body-part specific. *Journal of Neuroscience*, *26*, p. 6284 © 2006, The Society of Neuroscience, with permission. (See Figure 7.2.)

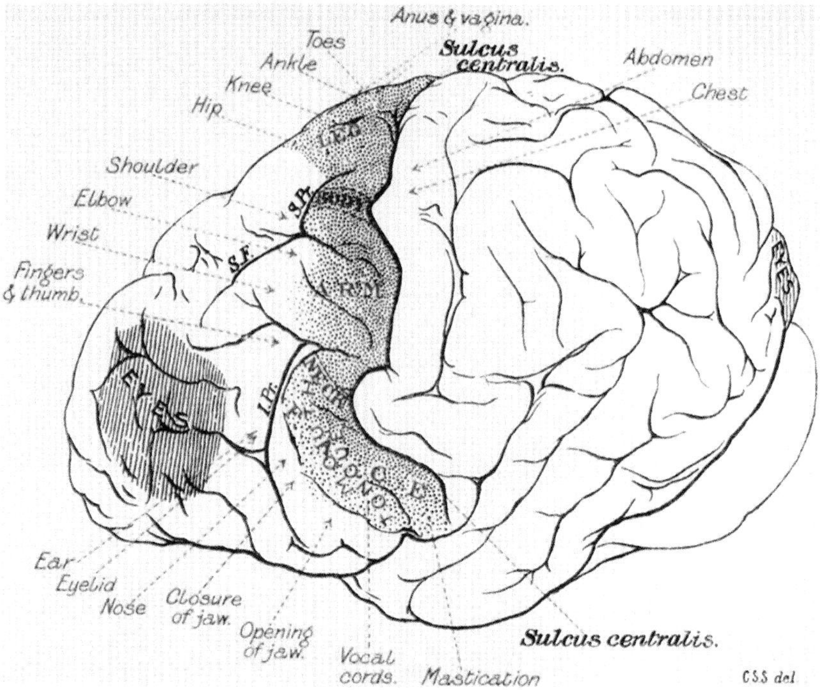

Plate 6 This early depiction of the somatotopy of motor cortex was derived from electrical stimulation and partial excisions of the cerebral cortex of a chimpanzee. It does not substantially differ from the somatotopy of human motor cortex. From dorsal (top) to ventral (bottom) there is a sequence of motor representations of leg, arm, wrist, and fingers. Reproduced from Grünbaum, A. S. F. and Sherrington, C. S. Observation on the physiology of the cerebral cortexs of some of the higher apes. *Proceedings of the Royal Society of London*, *69*, 206–209, plate 4 © 1901, The Royal Society. (See Figure 7.5.)

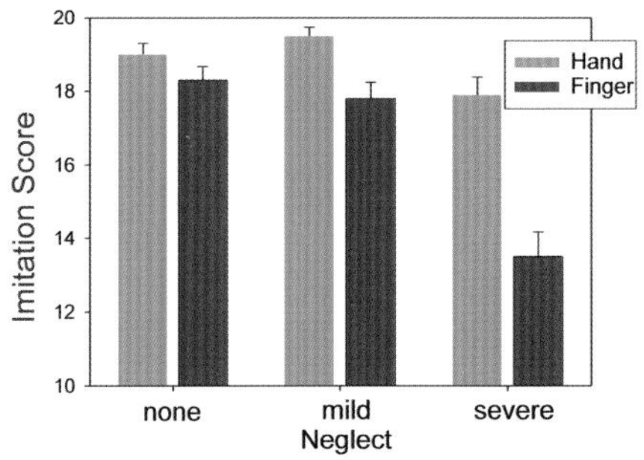

Plate 7 Left: Correlation between severity of hemineglect and accuracy of imitation in patients with right brain damage. Right: Distribution of errors in left and right brain damaged patients. All patients used the hand ipsilateral to the lesioned hemisphere. Since the examiner demonstrated the posture "like in a mirror" with the other hand, the thumb and the index finger appeared on the contralesional side and was hence vulnerable to hemineglect. We classified the laterality of the fingers that were in incorrect positions for 100 consecutive errors each of consecutive patients with right or left brain damage. Both groups of patients made more errors with thumb and index than with ring finger and small finger, but the difference was significantly higher in patients with right brain damage. Reprinted from *Neuropsychologia, 47* (13), Georg Goldenberg, Udo Münsinger, and Hans-Otto Karnath, p. 2952, Copyright (2009), with permission from Elsevier. (See Figure 7.7.)

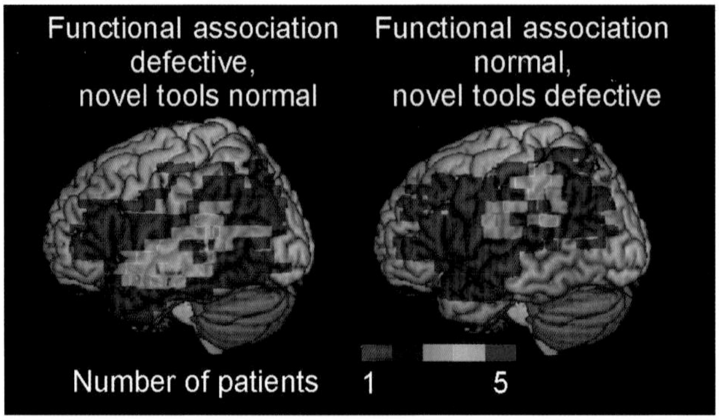

Plate 8 Left: Lesion overlap of five patients with intact mechanical problem solving but defective retrieval of functional knowledge. Right: Lesion overlap of five patients with the reverse dissociation. Adapted from Goldenberg, G. and Spatt, J. The neural basis of tool use. *Brain*, *132*, p. 1650, by permission of Oxford University Press. (See Figure 8.6.)

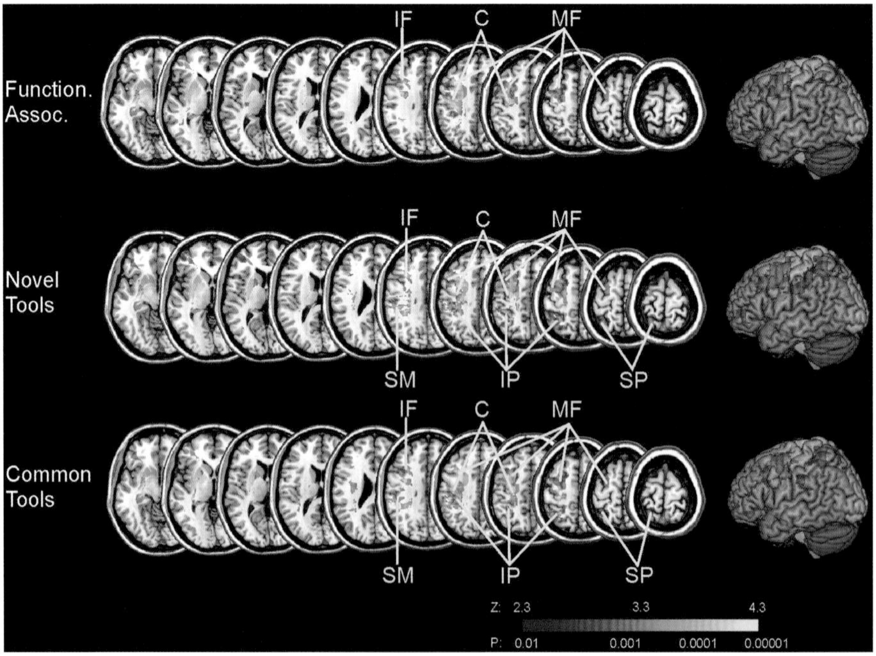

Plate 9 Micro study of lesions responsible for defective retrieval of functional knowledge ("functional associations"), defective mechanical problem solving ("novel tools"), and defective use of common tools ("common tools"). IF: inferior frontal; MF: middle frontal; C: central; SM: supramarginal; IP: inferior parietal; SP: superior parietal. The color scale indicates the strength of the influence of lesions in the colored region on test results. Note that parietal lesions disturb mechanical problem and use of common tools but not retrieval of functional knowledge. Adapted from Goldenberg, G. and Spatt, J. The neural basis of tool use. *Brain, 132*, p. 1649, by permission of Oxford University Press. (See Figure 8.7.)

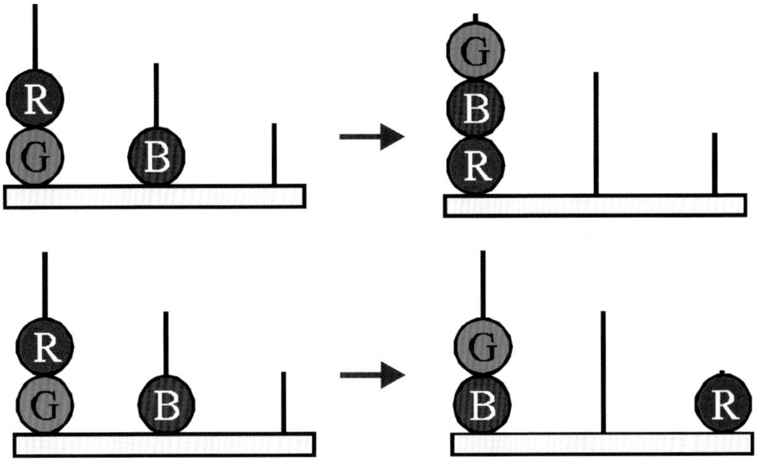

Plate 10 Two five-move problems of the Tower of London (data from Shallice, T. (1982). Specific impairments of planning. *Philosophical Transactions of the Royal Society of London, B, 298*, 199–209). The intuitive beginning by moving the red bead to the empty stick leads into the correct sequence for the first example but into a dead end for the second. Avoidance of the trap necessitates planning ahead of the subsequent moves. (See Figure 9.2.)

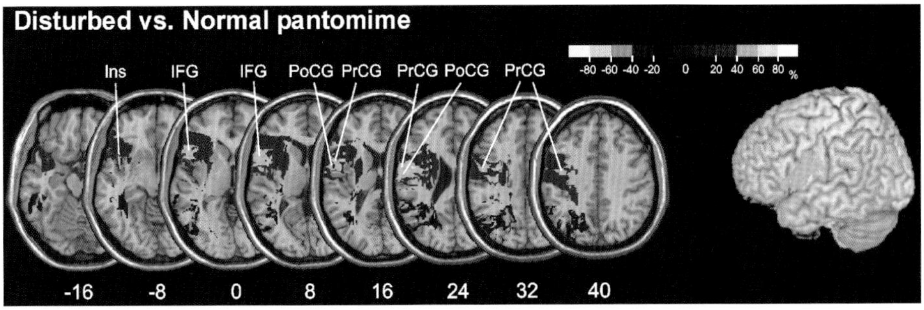

Plate 11 Subtraction of lesions of patients with intact pantomime from those of patients with disturbed pantomime: all patients had left brain damage and aphasia. The two groups did not significantly differ with respect to severity of language comprehension deficits or to size of lesion. The colors indicate the difference between the frequencies of lesions in both groups. IFG: inferior frontal gyrus; Ins: insula; PoCG: postcentral gyrus; PrCG: precentral gyrus. Lesions in inferior frontal and central regions are more frequent in patients with disturbed pantomime. By contrast, parietal regions lesions are even slightly more frequent in patients with intact pantomime. Reproduced from Goldenberg, G., Hermsdörfer, J., Glindemann, R., Rorden, C., and Karnath, H. O. Pantomime of tool use depends on integrity of left inferior frontal cortex. *Cerebral Cortex, 17*, p. 2773, Copyright (2007) by permission of Oxford University Press. (See Figure 10.4.)

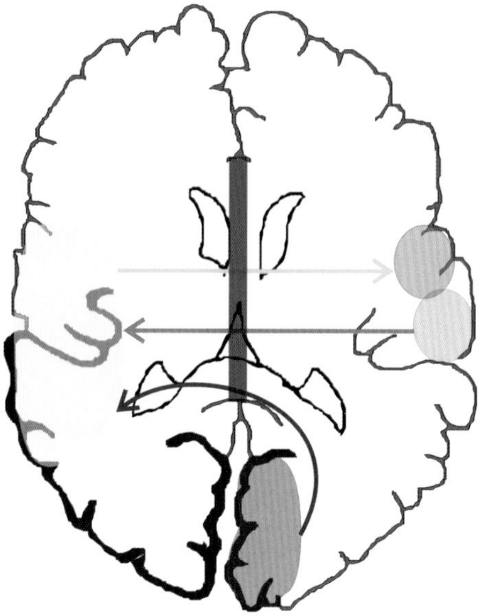

Plate 12 Section of the corpus callosum interrupts the link between left hemisphere linguistic competence and right hemisphere functions. Yellow: left-hemisphere language area. Green: verbal motor disconnection disables movements of the left hand to verbal command. Blue: disconnection between right somatosensory cortex and left hemisphere language areas leads to tactile anomia. Patients palpate objects put into the left hand skillfully and may even be able to demonstrate their use but produce aberrant responses when asked to name them. Red: section of the posterior portion of the corpus callosum causes visuo-verbal disconnection. Patients are unable to name objects and to read letters and words in their left visual hemifield. Beyond these clinical manifestations callosal disconnection can be experimentally exploited for examining the capabilities of isolated hemispheres. For this purpose disconnection between left and right visual cortex is particularly important, because it allows restriction not only of tactile but also of visual input to only one hemisphere. (See Figure 14.2.)

is not the only source of knowledge about its proper use. There must be another source which also enables detection of possible uses for unfamiliar tools. Patients who try to use a fork for eating soup and a spoon for cutting bread must have lost access to both sources. Indeed, even three sources of knowledge about appropriate tool use have been proposed: functional knowledge, manipulation knowledge, and mechanical reasoning (Goldenberg & Hagmann, 1998b; Boronat et al., 2005; Frey, 2007; Canessa et al., 2008; Goldenberg & Spatt, 2009; Osiurak et al., 2011). We will discuss them in turn.

Retrieval of functional knowledge from semantic memory

Knowledge about the use of tools has been termed "functional knowledge" (Sirigu et al., 1991a; Hodges et al., 1999; Rumiati et al., 2001; Bozeat et al., 2002; Canessa et al., 2008). It associates types of tools with their purpose, their recipient, and the action of their use. For example, a screwdriver serves for connecting or disconnecting parts, the recipient of its action is a screw, and the action rotation.

Functional knowledge can exist only for familiar tools and objects, because acquisition and storage of knowledge about an object makes it familiar. If there are several possible uses of a tool, functional knowledge is likely to weight them by their relative frequency and familiarity. Consequently, the prototypical use predominates. For example, a screwdriver is registered as being useful for screwing and unscrewing rather than for stabbing.

Functional knowledge is organized according to types of tools. Knowledge pertaining to one type of tool generalizes across different variants of that tool, but neither to other types of tools nor to general properties of solid objects and the laws of physics governing their interaction. The knowledge that a tool is useful for screwing applies to all sorts of screwdrivers but tells nothing about the proper use of hammers, nor does it specify general laws of physics underlying the use of screwdrivers.

Modality specificity of functional knowledge

Functional knowledge is generally recognized as being part of semantic memory. There is controversy about whether functional knowledge is fully integrated into a single semantic network or constitutes a distinct compartment (Hodges et al., 2000; Bozeat et al., 2002; Boronat et al., 2005; Canessa et al., 2008).[2] The positions in this controversy are associated with conflicting views on the modality specificity of stored knowledge. Proponents of the unified network account postulate that entries in semantic knowledge do not retain the modality of their acquisition. Regardless of whether they had been acquired by verbal instructions or by sensory or motor experience, they become integrated into a single amodal

[2] The structure of semantic memory has been one of the most debated topics in cognitive neuropsychology at the end of the twentieth century and continues to be a central issue in contemporary research. Any attempt to give an exhausting and balanced account of the accumulated empirical evidence and theoretical proposals concerning semantic memory would be far beyond the scope of this book. My account of semantic memory is simplified and selective. It should serve only for sketching the background of different views on the nature of knowledge about the use of tools.

network. The knowledge stored in this network may refer to sensory experiences or motor acts but does not itself consist of modality specific memory traces. The postulated unity of the semantic network gives rise to the expectation that degradation or loss of semantic memory would affect knowledge independently from the mode of its acquisition. Consequently, degradation of functional knowledge should always be associated with degradation of knowledge unrelated to its use (Hodges et al., 2000; Coccia et al., 2004; Silveri & Ciccarelli, 2009). For example, a person who no longer knows whether screwdrivers are used with screws or with nails should also be unable to decide whether they are more likely to be stored in the bathroom or in the garage. Moreover, since activation of knowledge about objects is a necessary prerequisite for naming them (Hodges et al., 1996), they should also be unable to name the screwdriver.

Proponents of the multiple compartment position believe that the network of semantic memory connects modality-specific entries which originate directly from sensory experience or motor actions. For example, knowledge about tools would be constituted by connections between visual entries depicting their shape, motor programs prescribing their proper use, and linguistic representations of their names (Damasio, 1989).[3] Under the plausible assumption that these modality-specific representations are stored in different regions of the brain, lesions might cause a selective loss of only one aspect of knowledge about the object. For our discussion, the most important variant of such modality-specific ignorance would be the loss or degradation of the motor programs for their use. This component of functional knowledge has been called "manipulation knowledge" (Sirigu et al., 1991a; Buxbaum & Saffran, 2002; Boronat et al., 2005). Its reliance on motor representations distinguishes it from other components of functional knowledge and of course also from parts of semantic knowledge which are not related to function. Consequently, patients suffering selective damage to manipulation knowledge should still be able to name tools and to indicate their purpose and the typical recipients of their actions, but unable to manipulate them efficiently for fulfilling their purposes (Sirigu et al., 1995).[4]

Manipulation knowledge

The postulate of modality-specific motor representations subserving the use of familiar tools and objects is easily recognizable as a descendant of Kleist's kinetic engrams. "Manipulation knowledge" is only one of several names that have been given to modern descendants of this old concept. Some authors still use the original label "engram" (Heilman & Rothi, 1993; Buxbaum, 2001; Lewis, 2006) while others designate them as "action knowledge" (Canessa et al., 2008), "movement memories" (Rothi et al., 1991), or "cerebral store of manual postures" (Sirigu et al., 1995). Some authors use more than one of these names

---

3 The idea that semantic memory consists of modality-specific remnants of prior experiences is easily recognizable as a resuscitation of Meynert's and Wernicke's associationist model of mental representations (see Chapter 1).

4 Note the similarity of this prediction to Meynert's "motor asymbolia" (see Chapter 1).

interchangeable (Rothi et al., 1991; Buxbaum, 2001), and still others prefer more descriptive terms like "information about hand and finger movements" (Kellenbach et al., 2003) or "representations of gestures for skilled object manipulation" (Boronat et al., 2005).

On first sight it seems obvious that, like general functional knowledge, manipulation knowledge is organized according to types of tools or, respectively, actions. Engrams of hammering direct all variants of hammering but are useless for screwing. For example, Laurel Buxbaum, (2001) wrote:

> The gesture engram is thought to contain the features of gestures which are invariant and critical in distinguishing a given gesture from others. For a hammering movement, for example, a broad oscillation from the elbow joint is critical, as is a clenched hand posture, and these and other similar gestural features are construed as forming the 'core' of the gesture representation. In other words, the schema for 'hammering' specifies a range of values for the features (or parameters) "elbow joint angle," "shoulder joint angle," "grip aperture" etc. (p. 452)

In the further course of the argument, Buxbaum admits that the actual execution of hammering requires adaptation of its invariant features to the "precise plan and location of the gesture with respect to the environment" but delegates this adaptation to a distinct functional system which combines the stored core features of the movement with changing environmental conditions, as, for example, the vertical or horizontal orientation of the nail. These adaptation results in a wide diversity of hammering actions, but the notion of invariant critical features would not make sense if they would not be present in all of them. Analysis of the features listed by Buxbaum raises doubts on this contention.

Buxbaum's list of invariant and critical features of hammering starts with "a broad oscillation from the elbow joint." Rather than oscillating, that is, repetitively swinging back and forth, hammering can be restricted to a single stroke. For example, Maxwell's silver hammer presumably came down only once for completing its murderous purpose. In a healthier context, tendon reflexes are elicited by single strokes of the reflex hammer. Nor is hammering invariably bound to flexion and extension of the elbow. Indeed, any combination of fixation or movement of the joints of the upper extremity is possible. Light hammers, as, for example, the earlier mentioned reflex hammer, may be driven only by movement in the wrist, while all other joints remain static. Movement of the elbow may be combined with synergistic movement of the wrist, but may also be isolated. The latter possibility is advantageous for hammering with a heavy hammer and with high demands on fine-grained control of the direction and force of the strokes, as, for example, for driving a chisel for sculpting or carving. Grasping the hammer close to its head and immobilizing the wrist permits tight control of the heavy hammer head and protects the wrist from strain after long working. For large hammers, used, for example, for driving-in posts, the stroke is mainly driven by movement in the shoulder and may be augmented by extension and flexion of the whole trunk.

Variability of the clenched hand posture is less extensive but exists. A firm grip is essential for transferring acceleration from the body to the tool, but its width can vary. While the handle of a manufactured hammer is grasped with a narrow cylindrical grip, stones which presumably constitute the oldest type of hammer used by man and even non-human primates are clenched with a wide spherical grip. A modern but unusual type of hammer gained public interest in the early sixties of the last century. In a plenary session of the United Nations General Assembly, the Russian leader Khrushchev underlined his indignation by hammering on the desk with a shoe. Since shoes have no handles he had to form his hand to a wide grip accommodating the width of the shoe. The more habitual version of hammering for emphasizing speech consists of hitting the table with the fist. Although this can be classified as an instance of a "clenched hand posture" it differs from all other variants by the absence of a hand-held tool.

In sum, there are no invariant features of muscular and joint actions for hammering. Joint and muscle actions vary depending on the structural properties of the hammer and on the purpose of its use. There is thus no firm fundament for the storage of manipulation knowledge that specifies invariant features of muscular and joint actions associated with the use of hammers.

Manipulation and structure of tools

Confusion between the motor acts of manipulation and the structure of the manipulated object is a common problem of experimental tests used for differentiating the neural basis of manipulation knowledge from that of general functional knowledge (Kellenbach et al., 2003; Boronat et al., 2005; Negri et al., 2007a; Canessa et al., 2008; Pelgrims et al., 2011). These tests ask for matching objects according either to the similarity between their functions or to the similarity between the manual actions of their use. For example, a piano shares functional properties with a violin but manual actions with a type-writer. However, the different motor actions are contingent upon different structural properties of the object. In this example, the typewriter and the piano share the feature of having multiple keys which can be pushed down independently from each other and from the whole object. The commonality of their manipulation reflects this commonality of their structure. Both devices are operated by downward strokes of selected fingers. Beyond this correspondence to their structural commonality, the motor acts of their manipulations are quite different. For the typewriter, the position of the hand remains static while one finger after the other moves to its target key.[5] In contrast, for playing the piano the whole arm moves for transporting the hand to the high and the low tones. Strokes may be made by the whole forearm and keys may be hit by several fingers simultaneously.

Do we need manipulation knowledge?

The conclusion that use of familiar tools does not depend on the retrieval of stored gesture engrams does not disprove the existence of any dedicated knowledge about motor actions

---

[5] This description applies to skilled typewriting. Unskilled writers may use individual selections of only a few fingers or may even use only one finger of a hand that is held in a fixed bent position while the whole hand moves to the appropriate key and moves downwards to hit the finger on the key. The only constant feature of these variants of typing is that single keys are hit one after the other. This feature is determined by the function of the keyboard.

associated with using tools. Such knowledge could be necessary for special uses of tools like the use of a hammer for sculpting, or for acquisition of specialized patterns of motor coordination like skilled typewriting. In these cases the motor acts of use form part of expert knowledge that must be learned in addition to general functional knowledge about that tool. Such specialized knowledge is not usually probed in the clinical examination for apraxia because the large individual variance of expertise makes the evaluation of its integrity difficult.

A main reason for rejecting a more general role of manipulation knowledge is parsimony. As I will expose in the next section, for conventional single tools the role of manipulation knowledge can also be replaced by combining general functional knowledge with mechanical problem solving.

Inference of function from structure

Functional knowledge associates types of tools with their purpose, their recipient, and their typical action. Identification of a tool activates associated functional knowledge. The sight of a hammer activates the knowledge that it can be used for fixing nails and that its use consists of powerful strokes. Now, look at the tools displayed in Figure 8.2. You probably agree that one is a hammer and the other a screwdriver, but you immediately recognize that the functional knowledge activated by their identification does not apply to these particular exemplars. The source of this immediate insight is a direct inference of possible functions from structure (Sirigu et al., 1991a; Vaina & Jaulent, 1991; Ochipa et al., 1992; Goldenberg & Hagmann, 1998b; Hodges et al., 2000; Spatt et al., 2002; Osiurak et al., 2009; Goldenberg & Spatt, 2009).

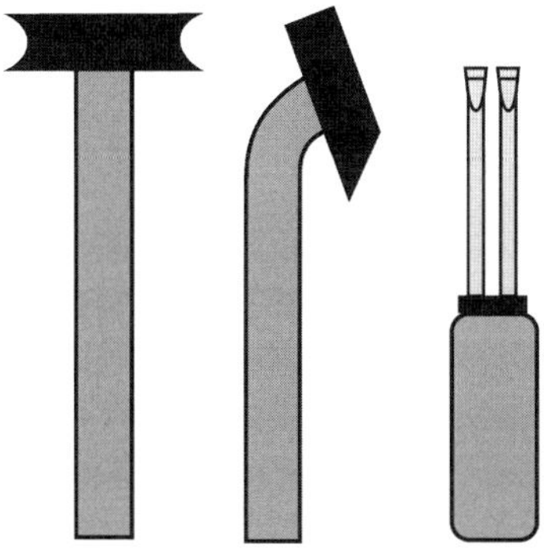

Figure 8.2 The tools shown in this figure are identifiable as two hammers and a screwdriver, but it is evident that functional knowledge about the use of hammers and screwdrivers does not apply to them. The recognition that they are useless must have a different source than retrieval of functional knowledge. Arguably, this alternative source is the direct inference of possible function from structure. Adapted from Goldenberg, G. *Neuropsychologie—Grundlagen, Klinik, Rehabilitation 4. Auflage*, p. 137, Copyright (2007), with permission of Elsevier.

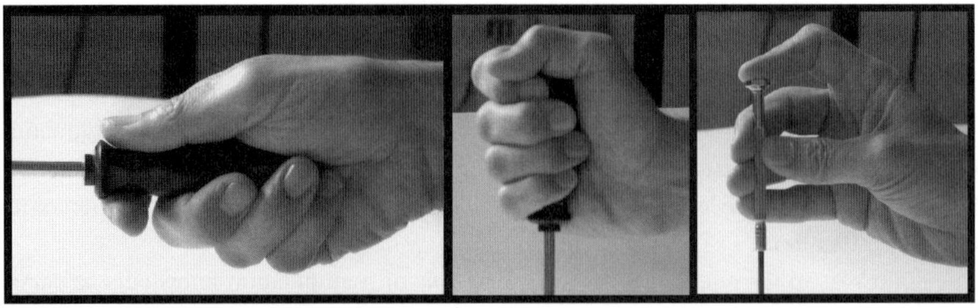

Figure 8.3 Three variants of using a screwdriver illustrate that there are no fixed associations between tools and the manual actions of their use. Left: The most common way of applying a screwdriver is holding it with a lateral grip in prolongation of the forearm and rotating the forearm in the elbow. This manner of screwing becomes awkward or even impossible when biomechanical constraints prohibit alignment of the axis of the forearm with that of the screw. Middle: This variant allows screwing when biomechanical constraints make orthogonal directions of forearm and screw more feasible than congruence of their axes. The screwdriver is held with a narrow cylindrical grip. There are two possible variants of muscular actions associated with this grip: rotation of the screwdriver can be produced by extension and flexion in the wrist. Alternatively, the wrist can be fixated, and the rotation produced by abduction and adduction of the upper arm. The latter variant is advantageous for powerful screwing, because the forearm provides a levering effect that augments the power of the upper arm movements. Right: This clockmaker type of a screwdriver is held with a precision grip. It enables independent control of orientation of the axis, rotation, and pressure. Rotation is produced by flexion and extension of thumb, middle, and ring finger, whereas the direction of the screwdriver axis and the pressure of insertion of the screwdriver blade into the slot of the screw are controlled by the index. Reprinted from *Neuropsychologia*, *47* (6), Georg Goldenberg, Apraxia and the parietal lobes, pp. 1149–59, Copyright (2009), with permission from Elsevier.

The practical value of direct inferences of function from structure is not limited to the rather artificial task of discriminating usable from unusable variants of common tools. It permits the detection of alternative ways for achieving the goals of tool actions, when either the typical tool is absent or mechanical constraints hinder its prototypical manipulation. For example, most persons will easily find out that a coin can replace a screwdriver. Normal subjects can also find out how to use unfamiliar tools, like those shown in Figure 8.3, and at least some of them are capable of inventing novel tools to cope with tasks for which no common tools are available. Finally, mechanical problem solving may be needed for optimizing the adaptation of body movements and manual postures to changing conditions of routine use of familiar tools.

Mechanical problem solving

The ability to detect ways of using unfamiliar tools and objects has already been emphasized in Morlaas' discussion of "agnosia of utilization" (1928; see Chapter 3). He illustrated it by the example of a car driver with "some mechanical understanding" who, when confronted with an unfamiliar type of machine, would by applied reasoning succeed in establishing the plan of the mechanism. Loss of this ability was central to his concept of agnosia of utilization.

In the modern literature the ability to infer functions from structure has been considered as a central component of "mechanical problem solving" (Goldenberg & Hagmann, 1998b), "mechanical reasoning" (Hegarty, 2004), or "technical reasoning" (Osiurak et al., 2009). Although there are subtle differences between these concepts we will use the terms interchangeably with a preference for "mechanical problem solving."

Mechanical problem solving presupposes knowledge about general principles of physics and mechanics. Such knowledge has been acquired by lifelong experience with moving and acting in a three-dimensional world occupied by solid objects (Zago & Lacquanti, 2005). It has been termed "intuitive physics" (McCloskey, 1983) or "folk physics" (Povinelli, 2000). Arguably intuitive physics fulfills criteria for being classified as part of semantic memory (Tulving, 1985), but it is clearly a different kind of knowledge than functional knowledge about individual types of tools and objects. It relates to general rules governing mechanical interactions rather than to functional properties of individual objects. For example, it specifies that objects do not attract each other.[6] This makes the location of contact decisive for the transfer of momentum from one object to another. The active object must contact the side of the recipient object opposite to the direction of its intended movement. In other words, without interpolated devices like hooks, handles, or glue, an object can push but not pull another object.

Mechanical problem solving applies such general rules to concrete constellations of tools and objects. Its elements are not the prototypical functions of entire tools, but the functional compatibilities of their parts (Vaina & Jaulent, 1991). Tools and objects are segmented into functionally significant parts and properties, and combination of these parts and properties with parts and properties of other tools and objects are used for construction of mechanical chains. Since familiar and unfamiliar objects are composed of the same repertoire of functionally significant parts and properties, and since prototypical and familiar applications of tools and objects obey the same physical regularities, mechanical problem solving can accommodate novel tools and objects and detect alternative ways of using familiar tools and objects.

For example, screws have slits on their head which provide a plane opposite to the direction of intended rotation and thus enable the transfer of rotation from the screwdriver to the screw. On the side of the screwdriver, the functionally decisive part is the blade and its functionally decisive property is rigidity. The shape and thickness of the blade must match the width and the form of the slit, and its rigidity must suffice for rotating the screw against the resistance of the material into which it penetrates. The blade need not, however,

[6] For scientific physics they do, but the effects of mutual attraction of mass are not accessible to human perception. There are other deviations of intuitive physics from real physics which would be accessible to naïve observation but nonetheless persist uncorrected in the majority of normal persons (McCloskey, 1983; Zago & Lacquanti, 2005).

necessarily be part of a screwdriver. Any other object providing a blade with the same properties can replace it. One can screw with a coin or a knife.

Mechanical problem solving and categorical apprehension

The segmentation of tools and objects into functionally significant parts resembles the segmentation of the human body into body parts which we discussed in Chapter 7 as a crucial component of body part coding and imitation of gestures. In this discussion we emphasized that segmentation is based on categorical apprehension. It concentrates on the presence of defining features and disregards variations of other features as long as the defining conditions are fulfilled. This also applies to mechanical relationships. For example, for inserting a hook into a ring, the ring must be closed and the hook open, and the thickness of the hook must be smaller than the diameter of the ring. As long as these categorical conditions are fulfilled, transfer of motion from the hook to the ring will work regardless of additional variations of their size and shapes. For screwing, the screwdriver's blade must be inside the slit of the screw, and the axis of the screwdriver must be in line with the axis of the screw. Insertion of the blade into the slot and congruence between the axes of screwdriver and screw are a categorical feature of their functional interaction. As long as they are maintained, rotation of the screwdriver can be achieved by a considerable variety of hand shapes and motor actions (see Figure 8.3).

The similarity between body part coding and mechanical problem solving goes even further. Like body part coding, mechanical problem solving constitutes an instance of a generative system. A multitude of mechanical devices can be constructed by combination of a limited number of functional parts and their properties. The combinatorial nature of technical reasoning has been particularly emphasized and elaborated by Osiurak et al. (2009, 2011).

Mechanical problem solving can replace manipulation knowledge

Mechanical problem solving results in the formation of a mechanical chain combining functionally significant parts of objects. This chain bridges the cleavage between the body and external objects. Manual grips and movements are integrated into the mechanical chain leading from the proximal body to the recipients of tool actions. Mechanical problem solving optimizes the transmission of proximal movements to the hand, the application of the hand to the tool, and the action of the tool on its recipient. It takes into account both the biomechanical constraints of the connections between hand and proximal body parts as well as the mechanical constraints determining the transmission of manual movements to the tool and its recipient (Jacobs et al., 2009). There is no need for additional manipulation knowledge specifying the configuration and movement of the hand. Not only can mechanical problem solving replace manipulation knowledge, it is also more efficient and flexible. Because of its combinatorial nature it can cope with constellations which have not yet been experienced and for which no appropriate manual actions have yet been acquired.

Clinical disturbances of the two sources of tool use

We are left with only two major sources of knowledge about tool use: functional knowledge retrieved from semantic memory, and mechanical problem solving. The following sections will discuss their clinical disturbances. This discussion is divided into two parts: First I will review group studies and what they tell us about the laterality of both sources, and then single cases demonstrating the clinical appearance and cerebral substrate of dissociations between them.

Laterality of lesions interfering with functional knowledge and mechanical problem solving

Retrieval of functional knowledge can be probed by asking subjects to match the picture of a tool with the picture of another tool serving the same purpose or with a picture of the typical recipient of its action. For example, if the target tool is a pencil subjects have a choice between notebook, newspaper, file folder, and punch for the recipient of its action, and between pen, adhesive tape, paint-brush, and crochet-hook for an alternative tool serving the same purpose (Hodges et al., 2000; Bozeat et al., 2002; Buxbaum & Saffran, 2002; Spatt et al., 2002; Boronat et al., 2005; Hartmann et al., 2005; Goldenberg & Spatt, 2009). Studies comparing functional knowledge between patients with unilateral left or right brain damage agree that failure occurs only in patients with left brain damage and aphasia (Tranel et al., 2003; Hartmann et al., 2005).

Mechanical problem solving can be probed by confronting patients with novel tools and asking them to find out the way they can be used. For example, in the "Novel Tool Test" (Figure 8.4; Goldenberg & Hagmann, 1998b; Hodges et al., 2000; Spatt et al., 2002; Hartmann et al., 2005; Goldenberg et al., 2007a; Goldenberg & Spatt, 2009) patients were presented with cylinders accompanied by an array of novel tools. Each cylinder had a part to which one of the tools fitted (see Figure 8.5). For example, there was one cylinder with a ring at its top and a tool with a hooked end which could be inserted into the ring, and another cylinder with a perforation and a tool with a straight end which could be inserted into the perforation. Patients were asked to select the suitable tool, to attach it to the cylinder, and to lift the cylinder out of the socket. In a similar approach, Heilman et al. (1997) presented mechanical puzzles to patients which had as their goal the retrieval of a wooden block. Each of the puzzles required a different mechanical action such as pushing, twisting, pounding, and lifting. Rather than ready-made tools, small blocks with bendable wire protruding from both sides were provided and patients were asked to adapt this device for extracting the block.

Another approach consists of presenting objects together with an array of tools but without the tool usually employed and asking patients to choose the tool that would best complete the task (Heilman et al., 1997). For example, when given a partially driven nail but no hammer, a correct selection would be pliers whereas selection of a needle would count as an error. An ingenious variant of this task was introduced by Osiurak et al. (2009). They presented objects paired with tools which usually are not employed for their use, and asked patients to show how the prototypical action associated with the object could nonetheless

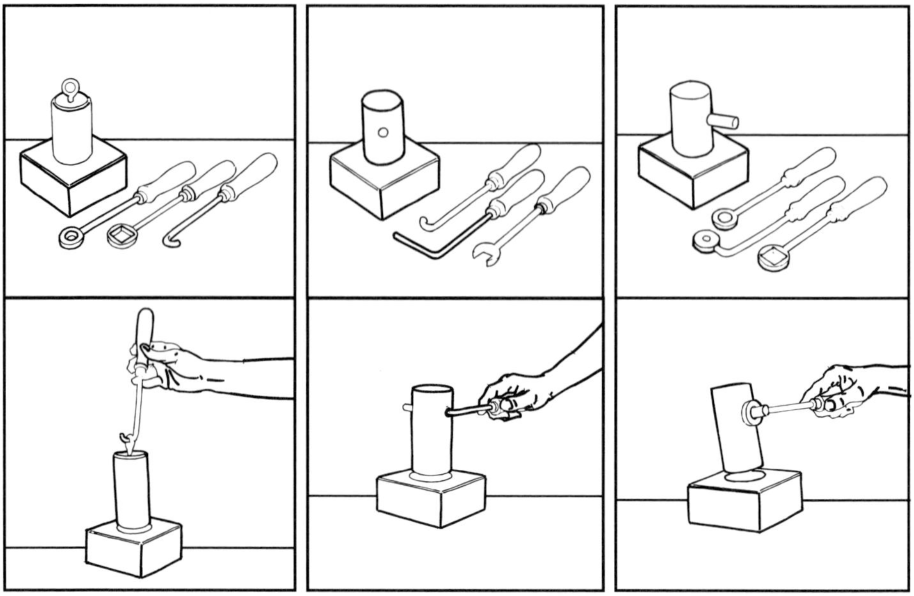

Figure 8.4 Three items of the Novel Tool Test (Goldenberg & Hagmann, 1998b; Goldenberg & Spatt 2009). The test consists of cylinders and tools. Each cylinder has a part to which one of the tools fits. One cylinder at a time is placed in a socket and three tools out laid out beside it. The patients are asked to select the suitable tool and to lift the cylinder out of the socket. Selection of the correct tool and its application to the cylinder are evaluated separately. If the patients fail to select the correct tool it is pointed out to them and they are asked to demonstrate its application. Reprinted from *Neuropsychologia*, *36* (7), Georg Goldenberg and Sonja Hagmann, Tool use and mechanical problem solving in apraxia, pp. 581–9, Copyright (1998), with permission from Elsevier.

be achieved by employing the tool in an unusual way. For example, they presented a pot of yogurt with a fork. Eating of the yogurt could be achieved by turning the fork around and using the handle as a provisional spoon.

Performance of all of these tests was impaired in patients with left brain damage and normal in those with right brain damage.

The conclusion from this short review is quite straightforward: only left brain lesions interfere with both components of tool use. This corresponds to the clinical observation that in patients with unilateral brain damage misuse of single tools and objects is bound to left-sided lesions and usually accompanied by aphasia while raising the question of whether there are clinical dissociations between mechanical problem solving and retrieval of functional knowledge that are both based on left-hemisphere integrity.

Loss of functional knowledge but preserved mechanical problem solving

Some 20 years ago, Angela Sirigu et al. (1991a) published a seminal case report of a young man who had suffered bilateral damage of the temporal lobes from herpes simplex

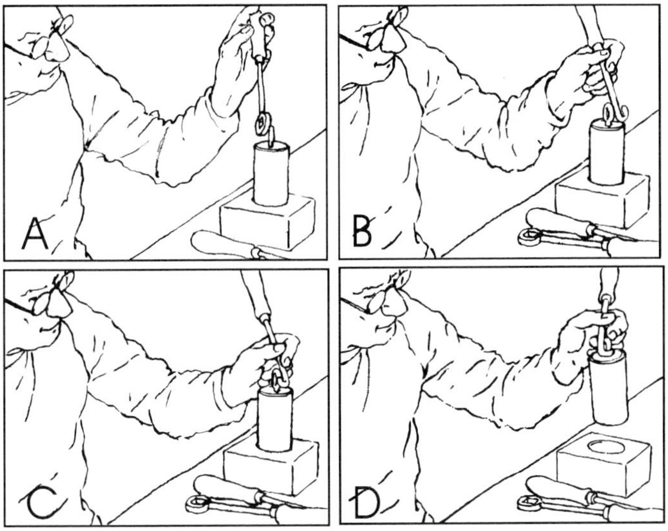

Figure 8.5 Attempts of a patient with left brain damage and severe aphasia to solve the Novel Tool problem that is shown as the leftmost of Figure 8.4. A: He takes a tool with a ring rather than the one with a hook and approaches it to the ring of the cylinder. B: The examiner indicated the correct tool. The patient approaches the hook to the ring. C: He aligns the hook with the ring rather than inserting it. D: With his fingers he presses the hook against the ring and lifts them together.

encephalitis. This had left him with a severe memory problem not only for the acquisition of new information but also for recall of old memories and semantic knowledge. Not only was he unable to name many common objects he also:

> behaved inappropriately with objects, mistaking shaving cream for toothpaste or vice versa, failing to find objects that he was asked to bring from the kitchen, or wearing clothes that were at odds with conventions or seasonal temperature. He was very confused with foods and was found eating a raw potato and frozen fish. (Sirigu et al., 1991a, p. 2557)

His apparently complete loss of knowledge about the things of everyday life contrasted with an astonishingly good ability to deduce their functional properties and facultative uses. For example, when shown a safety pin he commented: "You open on one side, stick something on it, close it, and it stays in. I can tell you how it works, but I don't see its exact use. I don't think I have seen one like this before, it is not a very common object" (Sirigu et al., 1991a, p. 2555), and when shown pliers: "It is used manually; when you pull apart here [points to handle] it opens up at the other end. Perhaps to hold several pieces of paper together" (p. 2566).

Sirigu et al. attributed the patient's "precise analysis of mechanical properties" to preserved somato-sensory representations of their manipulation. It seems to me that preservation of mechanical problem solving would be sufficient, and that there is no compelling necessity for employment of modality-specific motor memories.

The observations of the patient's difficulties in daily living demonstrate the limits of mechanical problem solving. In a way they are the reverse side of its strength. The liberty to detect unusual and novel modes of object use makes it difficult to decide which of these possibilities is appropriate with respect to social conventions and other non-mechanical constraints. A toothbrush can be used for cleaning shoes, and putting on winter clothes is not more difficult in summer than in winter.

Following Sirigu et al.'s seminal paper, relative preservation of tool use contrasting with severe loss of semantic knowledge has become a regular observation in patients with semantic dementia. (Buxbaum et al., 1997; Lauro-Grotto et al., 1997; Hodges et al., 2000; Negri et al., 2007a; Silveri & Ciccarelli, 2009). Semantic dementia is a degenerative disease which, similar to herpes simplex encephalitis, predominantly affects the anterior temporal lobes. The conclusion that temporal lobe damage impairs retrieval of functional knowledge from semantic memory but spares mechanical problem solving is endorsed by the finding of completely normal performance on the Novel Tool Test contrasting with severe impairment on a test of functional associations in a group of patients with semantic dementia (Hodges et al., 1999; 2000).[7]

Dramatic manifestations of loss of functional knowledge occur also in patients with unilaterally left sided vascular lesions (see Figure 8.1) but their contrast to preserved mechanical problem solving is rarely as striking as after bilateral temporal lobe damage from encephalitis or semantic dementia. However, a group study of lesion locations confirmed that lesions causing loss of functional knowledge show maximal overlap in the anterior temporal lobes (Tranel et al., 2003). We (Goldenberg & Spatt, 2009) found that out of 38 patients with left sided lesions and aphasia 5 scored below the group median on a test of functional associations but above the median on Novel Tools. All of them had lesions overlapping in the middle temporal gyrus (see Figure 8.6).

Loss of mechanical problem solving but preserved functional knowledge

In 1995, another seminal single case report was published by Angela Sirigu and her coworkers (Sirigu et al., 1995). They reported a woman who had bilateral posterior parietal dysfunction following an episode of cerebral anoxia. She could reach for objects accurately and take and transport them but complained of difficulties doing such things as cutting her nails, brushing her teeth, locking a door, cutting meat with a fork and a knife, etc. Examination of these and other skills revealed that her difficulties concerned

[7] As we have just discussed with respect to Sirigu et al.'s patient, complete loss of functional knowledge would impair coping with activities of daily living also in cases of complete preservation of mechanical problem solving. If patients with semantic dementia are indeed capable of leading independent lives they must have some additional resource from which they can retrieve basic knowledge about the goals to be achieved by tool use. However, discussion of the specific constellation of symptoms in semantic dementia is beyond the scope of this book.

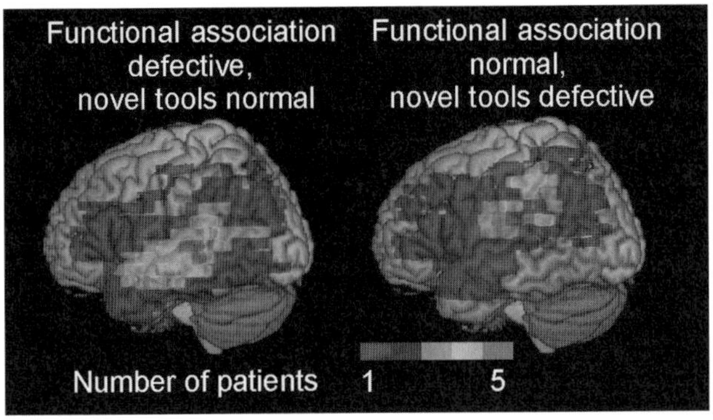

Figure 8.6 Left: Lesion overlap of five patients with intact mechanical problem solving but defective retrieval of functional knowledge. Right: Lesion overlap of five patients with the reverse dissociation. Adapted from Goldenberg, G. and Spatt, J. The neural basis of tool use. *Brain, 132*, p. 1650, by permission of Oxford University Press. (See Plate 8.)

exclusively the adaptation of the hand to the functional requirements of the tool. For example, rather than holding the spoon between the thumb, the index and the middle fingers, with the palm of the hand turned slightly upwards to secure maintenance of its horizontal orientation, she would take the spoon with the whole hand and leave the determination of its orientation to chance. In contrast to this apparent loss of any notion of the appropriate function of the instruments, however, she transported them to the correct place of their application. She moved the spoon back and forth between table and mouth and moved the nail clipper toward the other hand, albeit with a grip which made cutting impossible. When the examiner correctly positioned her fingers on the object before she started moving, subsequent transport and use became completely normal.

Sirigu et al. interpreted the pattern of preserved and defective performance as indicating "damage to or loss of specialized representations of manual postures," that is, manipulation knowledge. It seems to me that the pattern of preserved and defective aspects of tool use would be equally compatible with a severe disturbance of mechanical problem solving in combination with preserved functional knowledge. According to this account, functional knowledge suffices for selecting the recipient of tool action, like the mouth for eating or the hand for nail cutting, but not for analysis of the mechanical relationships between the hand and instrument.

The crucial role of parietal lesions for disturbance of mechanical problem solving has been confirmed by analysis of lesions underlying defective performance on the Novel Tool Test (Goldenberg, 2009). Five patients, who scored below the median on Novel Tools but above the median on functional associations, had overlapping lesions in the inferior parietal lobe. Across the whole group of 38 patients, lesions that were significantly associated with lower scores on Novel Tools extended from the supramarginal gyrus through the inferior to the superior parietal lobe (see Figures 8.6 and 8.7).

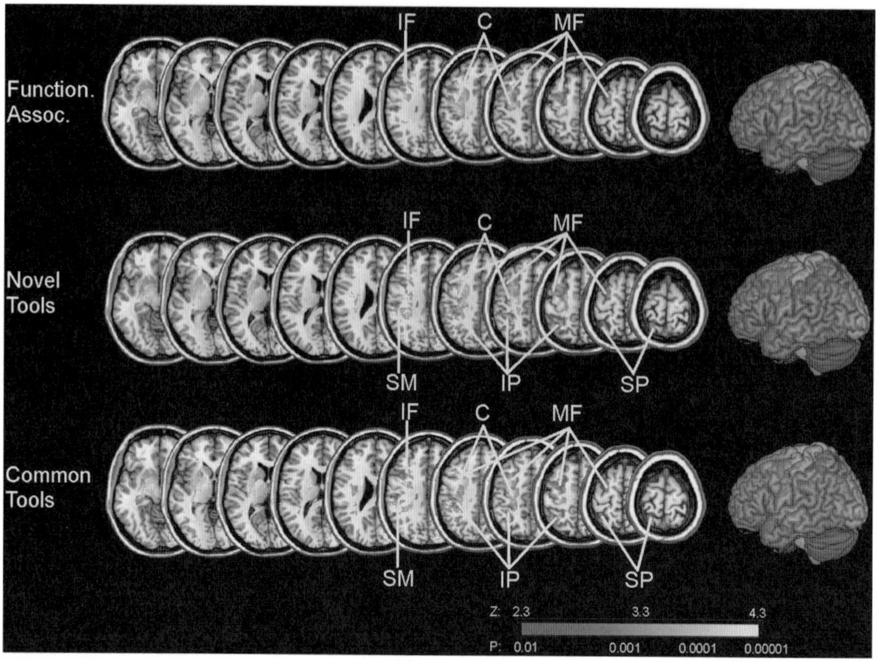

Figure 8.7 Micro study of lesions responsible for defective retrieval of functional knowledge ("functional associations"), defective mechanical problem solving ("novel tools"), and defective use of common tools ("common tools"). IF: inferior frontal; MF: middle frontal; C: central; SM: supramarginal; IP: inferior parietal; SP: superior parietal. The color scale indicates the strength of the influence of lesions in the colored region on test results. Note that parietal lesions disturb mechanical problem and use of common tools but not retrieval of functional knowledge. Adapted from Goldenberg, G. and Spatt, J. The neural basis of tool use. *Brain, 132*, p. 1649, by permission of Oxford University Press. (See Plate 9.)

Putting sources together again

We studied the components of defective tool use in patients with left brain lesions and aphasia (Goldenberg & Hagmann, 1998b; Goldenberg & Spatt, 2009) and found that only patients who failed both, tests of functional knowledge and tests of mechanical problem solving, had significant problems with the use of single conventional tools. We concluded that for mechanically transparent and familiar tools like scissors, hammer, and screwdriver, preservation of either functional knowledge or mechanical problem solving can compensate for the loss of the other component of tool use (Goldenberg & Hagmann, 1998b).[8] Across the whole group, however, defective use of common tools was associated with parietal lesions that overlapped largely with the lesions responsible for Novel Tools,

[8] The restriction of deficits of common tool use to patients who have lost both components of single tool use stands in apparent contrast to Sirigu's patients and to patients with semantic dementia (Hodges et al., 2000) or corticobasal degeneration (Spatt et al., 2002) in whom difficulties in common tool use

whereas there was no noticeable influence of temporal lesions (see Figure 8.7). We concluded that a weakness of functional knowledge is a prerequisite for defective use of common tools, but that deficits of mechanical problem solving are more influential.

The cognitive side of tool use

In the context of single tool use the opposition between high and low level of control is most conspicuous in the discussion of whether manual actions of tool use are determined mainly by manipulation knowledge or by mechanical problem solving. Manipulation knowledge consists of modality-specific motor programs, and it is confined to familiar actions. By contrast, mechanical problem solving is supramodal in that it applies equally to movements and configurations of external objects and the own body, converting both of them into elements of one mechanical chain leading from the proximal body to the recipients of tool actions. Mechanical problem solving enables the construction and use of novel tools as well as unusual ways of using familiar tools rather than being confined to routine actions. Supramodal functioning and the capacity to cope with novelty characterize mechanical problem solving as a cognitive component of tool use and oppose it to the motor representations of manipulation knowledge.

were caused by selective deficits of only one of the two components. A possible source of the apparent discrepancy could be that lesions in our patients were caused by strictly unilateral circumscribed infarctions, whereas patients in the other studies had bilateral lesions from general anoxia or degenerative disease. The finding that in patients with unilateral brain damage deficits of functional knowledge and mechanical problem solving are bound to left brain damage does not exclude the possibility that integrity of the right hemisphere provides some alleviation of their symptoms. Aggravations of hemisphere-specific deficits by additional lesions of the apparently uninvolved other hemisphere are quite common in clinical neuropsychology (Lambon Ralph et al., 2010).

Chapter 9

Naturalistic action

Steinthal's and Pick's seminal descriptions of apraxia for tool and object use were based on observations of everyday behavior. By contrast, most of the evidence considered in the Chapter 8 was derived from experimentally controlled examinations. Typically, patients were handed a tool and asked to demonstrate its use with a fittingly prepared recipient. For example, a hammer was presented together with a block containing a half-way inserted nail (Heilman et al., 1997). Even if the range of possible errors has been augmented by presenting several tools or several recipients for selection, the experimental arrangement remained a highly restrained and artificial excerpt from the manifold of factors determining tool and object use in daily living.

In everyday life, tool use is usually part of multistep actions involving several tools and objects. Their disturbance formed the core of Pick's concept of "ideational" apraxia, but modern research preferred Morlaas' classification, and identified "ideational" apraxia with misuse of single tools and objects. Difficulties with everyday life, multistep actions were re-baptized "action disorganization syndrome" (Humphreys & Forde, 1998; Forde et al., 2004) and "naturalistic action impairment" (Schwartz & Buxbaum, 1997).

Coordination of multiple actions

In experimental testing of single tool use the goal of the action is the demonstration of the prototypical use of the tool. By contrast, in naturalistic multistep actions, there is a superordinate goal transgressing the individual goals associated with each of the tools. The superordinate goal determines the selection of tools and the nature and timing of their contributions to the action chain. An action which is entirely correct when considered in isolation may become detrimental when inserted at the wrong position of the action chain.

Whereas demonstration of the use of single familiar tools and objects by healthy people is virtually errorless, slips of action are a common experience even in routine multistep tasks like dressing, grooming, or preparing food and beverages. It will be difficult to find people who have never switched on the kettle before filling it with water, never brushed their teeth after returning to the bathroom to get their watch, and never driven to their work place when intending to go to the movies.

Errors of brain damaged patients sometimes resemble the slips of actions of healthy persons, but exceed them both by quantity and by severity. Consider, for example, the following protocol of using an electric drip coffee maker by a patient with an extensive left hemisphere lesion and severe aphasia:

> The coffee machine and the necessary ingredients and utensils were placed on the table before the patient. Beside the machine there were three electric sockets. The machine happened to be oriented so that its cable with the plug was situated behind the machine and hence hidden from direct view by the patient. The patient arranged the sockets and looked for the plug but did not find it. He pressed the switch of the coffee machine and looked whether the control light lighted up. As this was not the case he continued looking around for a plug and finally detected an electric kettle equipped with a cable and a plug standing on a shelf. He rolled there with his wheelchair, took the kettle, carried it back to the working place, put it down and inserted the plug into the socket. He switched on the coffee machine again and looked for the control light. It did not light up. He inspected the switch and in the course of this inspection his gaze happened to fall upon the cable and the plug of the coffee maker. He exclaimed a swearword (actually the only word he could say), inserted the plug into one of the sockets and verified that switching on the machine now activated the control light.
>
> In another trial of making coffee he correctly filled water into the machine and inserted the paper cone in the filter, but poured the coffee grounds into the carafe rather than into the filter. He switched on the machine and hot water began to drip through the empty filter cone into the carafe where it mixed with the coffee grounds. The therapist pointed out to him that this procedure will not result in drinkable coffee. The patient recognized the error. He took the filter out of the machine and placed it on the table. Then he took the carafe and poured the mixture of water and coffee grounds into the filter. It ran through the filter on the table. He took up the filter again, placed it upon the carafe and inserted both of them into the machine which could now function regularly. The manoeuvre had left a puddle of water and coffee grounds on the table. The patient took a cloth and wiped the puddle up. Then he lifted the cloth and squeezed it without removing it from its place so that the puddle was reconstituted. (Goldenberg, 2007, p. 163)

A striking feature of these observations is the intimate tangle of correct and wrong features of actions. There is virtually no single action completely wrong or aberrant. For example, the nonsensical action of squeezing the wet cloth upon the table differs from correct repair of a previous error only by the place of execution which should be the sink rather than the work table. Other errors differ from correct action only by their temporal position in the action sequence. Switching on the boiling of water is a regular part of coffee making but produces a mess when done before coffee is in place in the filter. Finally, errors may arise from interaction between intended actions and unrelated objects in the environment. The use of the electric kettle as provider of a plug was contingent upon the detection of this device in the close proximity of the working place.

Other than errors of single tool use those occurring in naturalistic multistep actions cannot be understood in isolation. Their analysis must take into account their position in the temporal and spatial ordering of the action sequence and their effect on the achievement of the global goal. Integration of these interacting factors into a coherent theory of normal and faulty naturalistic actions poses a challenge that mirrors the challenge posed by their swift and errorless performance.

Error classification

An obvious first step for ordering the complexity of disturbed naturalistic action is the reduction of the various kinds of errors to a limited number of basic error categories. Indeed, error classification has become the backbone of most attempts to understand faulty performance of multistep actions (Buxbaum et al., 1998; Schwartz et al., 1998; Feyereisen et al., 1999; Schwartz et al., 1999; Cooper & Shallice, 2000; Goldenberg et al., 2001a; Rumiati et al., 2001; Cooper et al., 2005; Sunderland et al., 2006; Sunderland, 2007).

Table 9.1 gives an overview of systems of error classifications. Error types proposed by different groups have been arranged so that each row of the table enumerates similar error descriptions. The number of proposed error types ranged from four (Sunderland et al., 2006) to 16 (Feyereisen et al., 1999), but the two studies with the extreme values are not included because both of them were narrowly tuned to the analysis of dressing and listed errors that are idiosyncratic for this task.

On first sight, Table 9.1 looks promising. The correspondence between error classifications along the rows of the table suggests agreement on a small number of error types. Differences between authors seem to be confined to the verbal designations of errors and to the granularity of their subdivisions. However, the application of the classifications to the analysis of naturalistic actions turned out to be less unequivocal than expected. Only two studies (Schwartz et al., 1998; Goldenberg et al., 2001a) assessed the inter-rater reliability of error classification. Schwartz et al. commented that "adhering to the coding conventions placed a heavy burden on scorers" (p. 16) and obtained an acceptable inter-rater agreement of 76% only with the help of detailed scoring sheets that enumerated for

Table 9.1 Error classifications

De Renzi & Lucchelli (1988)	Rumiati et al. (2001)	Schwartz et al. (1998)	Humphreys & Forde (1998)	Goldenberg et al. (2001a)
Perplexity				Perplexity Toying
Omission	Step omission	Omission	Step omission	Omission of action Omission of movement
Sequence errors	Action addition Action anticipation Perseveration	Sequence error	Sequence error Action addition Perseveration	
Clumsiness		Spatial misorientation of grasp		Misplacing or misorienting of own body
Mislocation	Mislocation[a]	Spatial misorientation of object	Spatial error	Misplacing or misorienting of objects
Misuse	Misuse[a]	Object substitution Action addition	Wrong object	Wrong object
	Tool omission	Tool omission	Tool omission	
	Pantomiming			

[a] There are 2 variants for each of these error types.

each of the tested multistep action exhaustive descriptions and classifications of possible errors. In this way, agreement between scorers was probed for the recognition of predefined errors rather than for the unconstrained assignment of categories to observations of errors.

In our study (Goldenberg et al., 2001a) classification was based on general descriptions of the error types which had been discussed extensively before. Inter-rater agreement was good for the number of errors (81%) but dropped to disappointingly low values between 47% and 57% for their classification.

To clarify the reasons for this disappointing performance we looked for errors which had received diverging categorizations by two judges. We found that for a substantial portion of them both classifications were defensible. For example, picking up and then putting down again an object not needed at the current stage of the activity could be considered as use of a wrong object (assuming that a useful other object should have been taken), or as an expression of perplexity. To depress a serrated knife into a loaf of bread without slicing could be considered as omission of the sagittal movement of the knife, or as spatial misorientation of the knife with respect to the loaf. To put a filter basket on the carafe without controlling for its alignment with the indentations of the carafe, could be considered as misplacing of the filter or as omission of the additional action of controlling and correcting its exact position.

The ambiguity of error classification does not invalidate any detailed analyses of video-recorded multistep actions. The inter-rater reliability for the number of achieved subgoals was close to 100%, and all studies using error classification agreed that the most frequent type of errors were omissions of action steps. These two results have in common that they quantify the capability of patients to perform the multistep actions but give no further hints as to the particular difficulties causing failure.

Error classification and the cognitive opacity of naturalistic action

The ambiguity of error classification can be interpreted as a further instance of the opposition between high- and low-level approaches to understanding apraxia. The goal of error classification is a reduction of the manifold of possible errors to a limited number of defined error types that can then be combined for a systematic description of the difficulties that patients encounter with naturalistic multistep actions. If successful, this would result in a combinatorial system comparable to that of body parts for imitation or of mechanical properties for use of single conventional tools. This system should not only be useful for spotting well-known and frequent errors. It should be capable of accommodating the whole diversity of possible aberrations from the straight path to the goal of action by combination of the limited set of well-defined error categories. This endeavor failed at the first step of unequivocal assignment of error categories.

Combination of a limited set of elements to a wide diversity of familiar or novel entities is an essential characteristic of high-level, cognitive processing. The failure of its application to the analysis of naturalistic action demonstrates its limits. Error classification does not appear to be a powerful instrument for penetrating the cognitive opacity of naturalistic action.[1]

The cerebral substrate of multistep actions

Pick's descriptions of defective multistep actions in everyday life were derived from observation of demented patients (Pick, 1905a). He did not provide information on the extent and location of their brain damage, but presumably it was diffuse and bilateral in the majority of them. Likewise, some modern case studies describing dramatic impairments of naturalistic action are based on patients with bilateral extensive brain damage (Humphreys et al., 1998; Forde et al., 2004). On the other hand we have discussed in Chapter 8 that errors in use of single familiar tools and objects are exclusively bound to left brain damage. It seems highly unlikely that such errors and hence the presence of left brain damage should not contribute to failure in naturalistic multistep actions. Indeed, studies comparing the number of errors in single tool use and multistep actions of patients with left brain damage documented tight correlations between them (De Renzi & Lucchelli, 1988; Goldenberg & Hagmann, 1998a). Finally, in the historical part (Chapter 4) we mentioned dressing apraxia as a manifestation of right brain damage (Brain, 1941; Hécaen & De Ajuriaguerra, 1945), and contemporary studies confirm that unilateral right brain damage can interfere with dressing (Sunderland et al., 2006). Dressing is a daily living multistep action involving multiple objects. Its impairment in patients with unilateral right brain damage is evidence that right brain damage is sufficient for impairment of naturalistic multistep actions.

There are thus reasons for expecting naturalistic action impairment after bilateral, left-sided and right-sided brain damage. Systematic group studies confirm the low hemisphere specificity. Myrna Schwartz and her coworkers in Philadelphia explored naturalistic actions of patients with circumscribed left (Buxbaum et al., 1998) or right (Schwartz et al., 1999) brain damage as well as with predominantly frontal and bilateral lesions caused by head trauma (Schwartz et al., 1998) and with diffuse damage in dementia of various causes (Giovannetti et al., 2002) by means of a "Multi Level Action Test." Three primary tasks—making a slice of toast with butter and jam, wrapping a present, and packing a lunchbox—were administered under different conditions. Variations between conditions concerned whether patients were given the material for only one task or for two, whether they were presented only the necessary material or also functionally related distracters, and whether all materials were openly presented on the table or some had to be retrieved from a closed drawer.

[1] To be clear I should emphasize that this conclusion refers to the method of analyzing naturalistic actions. It is not meant to suggest that the actions themselves are motor routine that run independently of cognitive supervision and intervention. As I have outlined in Chapter 5, I am looking for the high- versus low-level dichotomy not only in the empirical results but also in the methods used for acquiring them.

The results of the different patient groups were remarkably uniform. All groups committed more errors and completed fewer action steps than controls. Moreover, the variations of conditions had the same effects on all groups. There were more errors when two tasks were combined, when distracters where present, and when parts of the material had to be retrieved from the drawer. The strength of these effects did not differ between groups. Moreover, in all groups omissions were by far the most frequent type of errors, and indeed the only error type more frequent in patients than in healthy controls.[2]

The equal sensitivity of naturalistic action to left and right brain damage was confirmed in a study by our group examining the preparation of coffee with an electric drip coffee maker and the fixing and starting of a tape recorder (Hartmann et al., 2005). In this study, all left brain damaged patients were aphasic and a substantial portion of them also committed errors in examinations of the use of single familiar objects. Their success on the multistep actions was somewhat below that of patients with right brain damage but the difference did not reach statistical significance although right brain damaged patients used single tools and objects flawlessly.

Resource limitations

The uniformity of impairment in different groups of patients and the equal susceptibility to experimental variations led the Philadelphia group to dismiss any "deficit-based" explanation, that is, any explanation postulating selective damage to one specific aptitude necessary for tool and object use. Instead, they proposed that the cause of errors was resource limitation:

> Resource, in this context, refers to a limited-capacity commodity that enables processing to go forward. Related constructs include effort, attention, and cerebral activation. (Schwartz et al., 1998, p. 25)
>
> The dependence on limited-capacity resources has a homogenising effect that obscures any manifestations of underlying neuropsychological deficit, and results in a pattern of naturalistic action performance much like the one seen across patient groups. (Buxbaum et al., 1998, p. 640)

The predominance of omission errors was accommodated with the assumption that carrying out an action presupposes selection of this action among possible alternative actions

> A severe resource limitation may translate into poverty of effort or, more mechanistically, failure to resolve the competition for schema selection such that none of the candidate action schemas reaches threshold. (Schwartz et al., 1998, p. 26)

Finally, since resources are limited also in healthy people, the theory can explain why healthy people whose resources are occupied by other mental activities or external distracters are susceptible to slips of action resembling the errors of patients.

---

[2] The strength of this uniformity is mitigated by the poor reliability of error classification discussed in Chapter 8. Moreover, the absence of more specific errors may also be due to a selection artifact: only two out of 16 patients were aphasic and hence likely to also suffer from apraxia for use of single familiar tools and objects. It would seem likely that the dramatic errors which these patients commit when tested with single tools (see Chapter 8) distinguish aphasic and apraxic patients from other patient groups also in multistep actions. Occupational therapists believe that this is the case but controlled empirical proof is lacking.

Arguably, "resource limitation" and its related constructs "effort, attention, and cerebral activation" are not far away from "clarity of consciousness or, more precisely, attention and its distribution" which Arnold Pick (1905a, see Chapter 2) had suspected as underlying ideational apraxia some 90 years earlier.

Coping with technical devices

In the historical part of this book I have tried to convince you that fundamental questions and ideas have been constant since the beginning of research on apraxia more than 100 years ago. This constancy does not apply to the materials used for examining apraxia of tool and object use. A look in the early literature reminds of objects which were in common use then, but which have vanished from everyday life today, like mechanical coffee mills, door-knockers, washboards, or pen holders. We are presently witnessing the disappearance of technical equipment which had been novel in the last century, such as, for example, telephones dials, gramophones, type writers, or slide projectors, and are forced to cope with the technical affordances of push button phones,[3] MP3 players, computer printers, and scanners. There are even devices which had come into use only in the second half of the twentieth century and which are already vanishing again, like CD players or cassette tape decks. By contrast, simple mechanical tools like hammers, screwdrivers, or door keys have remained largely constant during our lifetimes.[4]

Rapid evolution is one of several properties distinguishing technical equipment from conventional mechanical tools. Another one is their complexity.

Conventional mechanical tools typically consist of a handle and a functional part. To use them the handle is grasped and manipulated in a way that causes interaction of the functional part with the recipient of tool action. By contrast, technical devices typically have a multitude of functional and of manipulable parts, and their functional parts interact not only with external recipients but also among themselves. For example, among the functional parts of a drip coffee maker are a switch, a water container, a filter, and a carafe. Successful use depends on correct placing of the filter on the carafe and on pouring ground coffee into the filter before switching on the water heater. Placing the filter on the carafe is a spatial, and the sequence of pouring in coffee and switching on heating a temporal, interaction between parts of the device. Indeed, the inclusion of technical devices in the discussion of multistep actions with multiple tools and objects is justified by the mere observation that most technical devices are themselves a combination of multiple objects.

---

[3] Since the first draft of this chapter was written, push button phones have begun to give way to smart phones handled by touch screens rather than buttons, and speech control of phones or other devices is already on the way to becoming widespread. Possibly push buttons will be as rare as dials when the book is finally published.

[4] Of course, simple mechanical tools have their history too (Vingerhoets et al., 2011) but their lifecycle is generally much slower than that of technical devices.

A further important difference between conventional mechanical tools and technical devices concerns the transparency of functional relationships. For conventional tools, mechanical interactions between manipulation of the handle and action of the functional part as well as between the action of the functional part and its recipient are observable and provide a basis of mechanical problem solving. By contrast, for technical devices, the interactions of functional parts with external recipients, as well as the interactions between the functional parts themselves, are frequently hidden from view. Thus, the user of a coffee maker sees heated water pouring from the container into the filter, but not the heating coil within the container. Besides, visual observation of the heating coil would not help to understand its function which is electric rather than mechanic.

In Chapter 8 we identified two sources of knowledge about the use of conventional tools: functional knowledge and mechanical problem solving. Both of them change their character when applied to technical devices.

Functional knowledge, instructions for use, and schemas

In Chapter 8 we defined functional knowledge about the prototypical use of familiar tools as consisting of associations between types of tools, their purpose, their recipient, and the action of their use. These associations do not suffice for understanding and handling the spatial and sequential interactions between the multiple parts of technical devices. Semantic knowledge specifying the functions of individual parts of the device and the sequential constraints on their use is rather like the "instructions for use" which usually accompany the purchase of new devices. Frequently, the instructions have been acquired by consultation of such printed instructions.

The transmission by explicit verbal or pictorial presentations makes it possible to acquire knowledge about the use of novel devices without observations of their actual use. Indeed coping with novel devices is presumably the most common cause for consulting instructions for use. It is, however, rarely the case that a device is completely novel to a user. Rather, they will have experience with alternative versions or predecessors of the newly acquired device. This previous experience may have resulted in the storage of a "script" or "schema" in semantic memory (Schank & Abelson, 1977; Shallice, 1988; Cooper & Shallice, 2000; Cooper, 2007).[5] Schemas are abstract descriptions of action sequences. They represent what is shared by different instances of a multistep action but leave open "slots" for filling in specifications of objects or actions that are specific to individual applications of that schema. For example, the schema of making coffee includes that hot water must be brought into temporary contact with ground coffee but leaves open whether this is achieved by letting hot water drip through a coffee-filled filter, as in a drip coffee maker, or by pressing steam through the coffee, as in an Italian espresso maker. Both methods

[5] The difference between the concepts of "script" and "schema" are not relevant for this topic. I follow Tim Shallice's proposal to use "schema" for action sequences concerned with tool and object use (Shallice, 1988; Cooper et al., 2000).

require hot water, but the slot for heating is filled by pushing the on–off switch for the drip coffee maker, and by turning on the stove and putting the coffee maker on the hot plate for the Italian espresso machine.

The sequencing of actions in schemas resembles the sequencing of words in syntactical structures. Rick Cooper, who constructed a computer simulation of schema-based naturalistic action, emphasized the parallel to sentence construction:

> Schemas have "argument slots" that must be filled or bound for any instance of the schema. This situation parallels that of linguistic phrase structure, but where the slots in that structure are filled in with specific words in order convey specific meanings. (Cooper, 2007, p. 323)

The role of schemas is not confined to the mastering of technical devices. There are schemas for multistep actions that employ only conventional tools such as, for example, laying a table or assembling an IKEA book case. I included the discussion of schemas in the section on technical devices because in this context the ability of schemas to assimilate novel devices into the action sequence comes to the fore most conspicuously.

Trial and error

Inference from structure to function which we have identified as the core mechanism for mechanical problem solving is of limited value for finding out how to use unfamiliar technical devices. Mechanical parts and the links between them are frequently hidden from view or replaced by electrical and electronic functions (Norman, 1989, 1993; Goldenberg & Iriki, 2007). The opacity of structure–function relationships forces recourse to trial and error for finding out how the different parts of the device must be manipulated.

Although trial and error is a widespread strategy used not only by mundane humans but also by such an illustrious agent as Darwinian evolution, it is not highly estimated by contemporary psychology and has been neglected by neuropsychology (Robertson, 2001). I was unable to retrieve a single paper treating the cerebral substrate of trial and error problem solving.[6] I will not try to fill this void but emphasize two observations which I consider relevant for understanding the influence of brain damage on the application of trial and error strategies.

A crucial difference between trial and error on the one hand, and insight and planning ahead on the other, concerns the mental representation of the problem. Insight and planning ahead are based on a complete mental representation of the problem that allows examination of possible solutions independently from material interaction with the objects involved. Trial and error alleviates the need to construct a complete and independent mental representation of the problem. The real objects whose arrangement constitutes the problem serve themselves as representations and possible

[6] There is literature on the use of trial and error by patients with brain damage, but it is concerned exclusively with the superiority of errorless learning, and trial and error serve only as the control condition against which the superiority of errorless learning is tested (Wilson et al., 1994; Donaghey et al., 2010).

solutions are based upon them rather than on their mental representation (Zhang, 1997; Rowlands, 2003).

Although it eliminates the necessity of keeping a complete representation of the problem in mind, successful application of trial and error makes substantial demands on supervisory attention and memory. A trial should neither be abandoned before success or failure has been registered, nor continued when the failure is already evident. In order to avoid repetition of unsuccessful trials the actor should keep track of already performed trials and their outcome. The memory load of this registration can be reduced by using systematic strategies for the selection of trials, but it remains significant particularly when there are several potential targets for action and when success depends on the sequence of their manipulations.

Towers and treasure boxes

We explored the difference between planning ahead and trial and error by administration of two multistep problem solving tasks to normal controls and to patients with brain damage. For technical problem solving with a dominant strategy of trial and error we constructed "treasure boxes" (Hartmann et al., 2005), and for multistep problem solving with a dominant strategy of planning ahead we used the "Tower of London" (Shallice, 1982).

Figure 9.1 shows one of the three treasure boxes. They have lids that can be opened after manipulation of several locks consisting of bolts, pins, and rotator disks. Premature opening of one lock can block the opening of another lock, and in one of the boxes a bolt has to be moved temporarily from a non-blocking position into one where it blocks opening in order to get access to another closing device. While some of these constraints are quite obvious from inspection of the device, others are hardly detectable without trying to move the blocking parts leading to a strategy of trial and error.

Figure 9.2 shows a selection of problems from the "Tower of London." Subjects are presented with a device of three sticks with three beads on it. On a second, identical, device the beads are presented in a different configuration and subjects are asked to replicate this configuration on their device. There are two restrictions for legal moves: only one bead must be moved at a time and only one bead must be placed on the smallest, and only two on the middle stick. Like the treasure box the Tower of London presents multistep problems but the conditions and constraints are determined by explicitly given instructions which are supported by obvious features of the structure of the device. The resulting transparency of conditions and constraints enables the construction of a complete mental representation of the problems and their possible solutions and hence planning ahead without recourse to trial and error.

We administered both tests to patients with left and right brain damage and to healthy controls. Before turning to the effects of brain damage it is worthwhile considering an aspect of the normal controls' performance that is relevant to our expectations regarding the importance of trial and error and planning ahead for both tests.

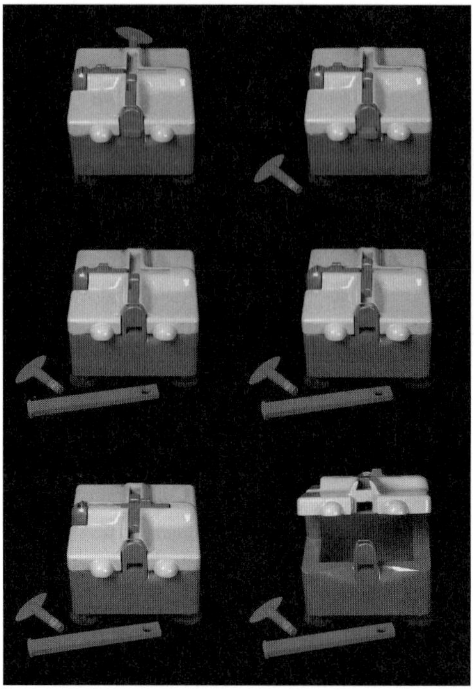

Figure 9.1 A treasure box problem: the pin at the back of the box retains the bolt, the tip of which appears on the front. This relationship is difficult to recognize from inspection. If, however, one manually explores the pin and tries pulling or turning it, it is easy to find out that it can be removed. If one then moves the freed back end of the bolt it becomes evident that the bolt goes through the box and can be drawn out. The two bolts on the top of the box are inserted in hooks and hold back the lid. They can both be removed from their hooks only by first positioning the one aligned sagittally into a middle position so that its central indentation gives way to the other one, aligned in a frontal plane. This sequential constraint can be deduced from inspection of the bolts, but it can also be found out by trial and error. Reprinted from *Neuropsychologia*, *43* (4), Karoline Hartmann, Georg Goldenberg, Maike Daumüller, and Joachim Hermsdörfer, It takes the whole brain to make a cup of coffee: the neuropsychology of naturalistic actions involving technical devices, pp. 625–37, Copyright (2005), with permission from Elsevier.

The minimum number of moves necessary for opening was five for each of the three treasure boxes and ranged from two to seven for the Tower of London problems. We reasoned that solutions with the minimum number of moves can result from trial and error only in the unlikely event that the initial trials happen to consist exclusively of correct moves. By contrast, it should be the regular outcome of correct pre-planning of the whole sequence.

We examined 18 healthy controls. They produced 48 treasure box solutions. Only two of them were achieved with the minimal number of five moves! By contrast, 21 out of 48 five-move, the same number of six-move, and even 14 out of 48 seven-move Tower of London problems were solved with the minimum number of moves. This remarkable difference

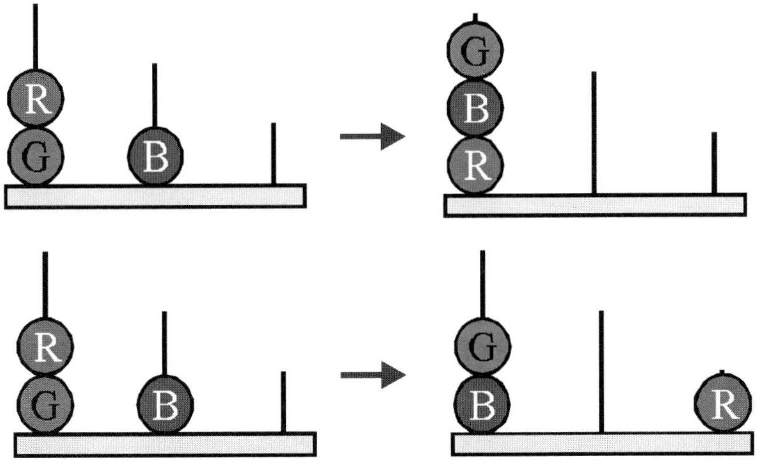

Figure 9.2 Two five-move problems of the Tower of London (data from Shallice, T. (1982). Specific impairments of planning. *Philosophical Transactions of the Royal Society of London, B, 298*, 199–209). The intuitive beginning by moving the red bead to the empty stick leads into the correct sequence for the first example but into a dead end for the second. Avoidance of the trap necessitates planning ahead of the subsequent moves. (See Plate 10.)

between Tower of London and treasure box problems fits well with our assumption that planning ahead was the dominant method for the Tower of London, and trial and error for the treasure box.[7]

The results of the patients were quite straightforward: both left and right brain damaged patients were significantly less successful than healthy controls with both tests, but groups did not differ significantly from each other, and there were not significant differences between their success on the two tests (see Hartmann et al. (2005) for method of scoring and detailed results). In a second study we presented both tests to patients with dysexecutive disturbances from mostly bilateral frontal lobe damage and found essentially the same uniform impairment on both tests as in patients with lateralized brain damage sparing the frontal lobes (Goldenberg et al., 2007a).

Disentangling the uniformity of naturalistic action disturbance

I have already mentioned that neither the Philadelphia group nor our group could find differences between the severities of impairment on naturalistic multistep actions in patients

[7] The opposition of pre-planning and trial-and-error is not as strict as this result suggests. For the Tower of London it has been shown that many normal subjects pre-plan the whole sequence only when explicitly instructed to do so, and that partial planning complemented by on-line updating may be as effective as complete pre-planning (Phillips et al., 1999; Unterrainer et al., 2003). On the other hand, parts of the action sequences for opening the treasure boxes could be planned by consideration of obvious constraints and structure–function relationships (see Figure 9.1). Nonetheless our data supports the assumption that opening of the treasure boxes relied mainly on trial and error, whereas solution of Tower of London problems was more heavily based on mental pre-planning.

with right or left brain damage. This negative finding does not, however, exclude the possibility that the superficially same outcome is caused by different mechanisms Analyses of correlations between success on naturalistic multistep actions, experimental tests of multistep actions, and clinical findings in patients with right and with left brain damage endorse this suspicion.

Right brain damage: Hemineglect and resource limitation

Both the Philadelphia group and our group found significant correlations between the severity of hemineglect and success on naturalistic actions in patients with right brain damage (Schwartz et al., 1999; Hartmann et al., 2005). In our study the influence of neglect extended also to the treasure box and the Tower of London.

The Philadelphia group recorded a preponderance of omissions of action steps for objects placed on the left side of the patient, whereas we did not observe such an asymmetry. However, they admitted that the lateral deviation of attention cannot account for all difficulties, and that a substantial portion of errors is rather due to the non-lateralized reduction of sustained attention that has repeatedly been demonstrated in patients with severe hemineglect (Heilman et al., 1978; Robertson, 1990; Husain & Rorden, 2003; Sunderland et al., 2006). This non-lateralized reduction of attention appears as a convincing instantiation of the "resource limitation" postulated by these authors.

The correlations between severity of hemineglect and non-lateralized errors of naturalistic and experimental multistep actions reminds of defective imitation of meaningless gestures. Remember that in patients with right brain damage there was a negative correlation between severity of hemineglect and imitation of finger configurations that transgressed the lateralized effects of hemineglect and pointed to a non-lateralized narrowing of the focus of attention. A non-lateralized weakness and narrowing of attention seems to be a pervasive source of difficulties for tests of apraxia in patients with right brain damage.

Left brain damage: Schemas and trial and error

Results of patients with left brain damage were more complex and could not easily be subsumed in the effects of general resource depletion. In order to facilitate keeping track of the results let us briefly recapitulate the criteria for patient selection and the study design. All patients with left brain damage had aphasia and were administered the complete Aachen Aphasia Test (Huber et al., 1983, 1984). Naturalistic action was probed for the preparation of coffee with an electric drip coffee maker and for fixing and starting a cassette tape recorder. In addition, all patients tried to solve the treasure boxes and the Tower of London problems. Finally, functional knowledge concerning single tools and objects was assessed by a test of functional associations, and mechanical problem solving by the Novel Tool Test (see Chapter 8).

Analyses of correlations between these tasks suggested fundamental differences between the cognitive processes underlying the two naturalistic multistep tasks. Success of coffee making was significantly correlated with all subtests of the aphasia test as well as with the test of functional association but not all with the treasure boxes, whereas fixing the tape recorder showed the opposite pattern: correlations to aphasia were close to zero and those to functional associations not significant, but there was a significant correlation with the treasure boxes. Tower of London and Novel Tools did not significantly correlate with any of the naturalistic actions.

We interpreted this dissociation as indicating that coffee making depended strongly on semantic knowledge whereas problem solving by trial and error was crucial for fixing the tape recorder. A closer analysis of the task demands of the two naturalistic action sequences is compatible with this interpretation.

Both the coffee maker and the tape recorder put mechanical constraints on their manipulation. For example, in both of them insertion of an implement is possible only after opening of the appropriate compartment (e.g., the battery compartment for the batteries; the filter basket for the filter). The locks of the battery and the tape compartment of the tape recorder were, however, less obvious and more difficult to overcome than the locks of the water tank or the filter compartment of the coffee maker. Presumably, trial and error were the most efficient method for opening the container of the tape recorder. On the other hand, the drip coffee maker is susceptible to sequential errors which lead to dangerous situations or have irrecoverable consequences as, for example, heating the water container without having filled it with water or pouring in coffee without having inserted the filter. By contrast, the sequence of inserting batteries and the tape in the cassette recorder is arbitrary, and premature pushing of the start button is ineffective but has no dangerous or irreparable consequences. Schemas specifying constraints on the sequence of actions are thus more important for the coffee maker than for the tape recorder. As we have discussed before, schemas form part of semantic memory. They may emerge from verbally acquired instructions for use and their structure resembles the syntactical structure of language. The correlations between success of coffee making, tests of functional knowledge, and severity of aphasia reflect these communalities. The absence of correlations with Tower of London and Novel Tools suggests that insight and planning ahead did not make a major contribution to coping with our naturalistic tasks.

Multiple objects, multiple steps, multiple sources of failure

Disturbances of everyday multistep actions have been central to the concept of apraxia since their early description and classification as "ideational apraxia" by Pick and Liepmann, but their theoretical understanding and the exploration of their neural substrate has not made much progress. A main reason for the paucity of unifying theories could be the heterogeneity of possible sources of failure. We have identified three components whose impairment may interfere with naturalistic multistep actions above and beyond the mechanisms already interfering with use of single conventional tools and objects:

Non-specific attentional resources and cognitive effort are necessary for maintaining attention to the multiple steps and the ultimate goal of multistep actions. Weakness of this component seems to be the major reason for difficulties of patients with right brain damage, but may contribute also to errors of patients with other lesions.

Other than mechanical problem solving, technical problem solving cannot rely solely on the inference of function from structure, because in technical devices decisive mechanical structures are frequently hidden from view or absent. Alternatively, functions may rely on electric and electronic relationships which are not transparent for inspection. Trial and error may be the only feasible strategy for solving technical problems. Problem solving by trial and error is about equally impaired in patients with lesions in either hemisphere.

Instructions for use and schemas are particularly important when multistep actions involve technical devices. They may be formulated and acquired verbally or in a language-like abstract format. Their close proximity to linguistic abilities suggests a left hemisphere basis and indeed their influence upon the success of naturalistic actions became evident only in the analysis of patients with left brain damage and aphasia.

Coping with novelty and autonomy of action

The multiplicity of factors that are at stake in naturalistic multistep actions offers multiple points of departure for discussion of their position on the high- versus low-level dimension of action control.

Disturbances of naturalistic multistep actions formed the core of Pick's original descriptions of "ideational apraxia." The term "ideational" implied that the disorder affects the creation of mental images preceding motor execution and hence the high level of action control. In our analysis of modern evidence, the putative mental images could be identified with action schemas. Their suspected loss in patients with left brain damage and aphasia would then count as affecting a high level of action control.

In the holistic tradition, the high level of action control was characterized by autonomous and voluntary action as opposed to conscious planning and creativity as opposed to the automatic execution of routine action. The position of disturbed naturalistic action in this version of the high- versus low-level dichotomy is ambiguous. Hécaen and De Ajuriaguerra noted that "dressing apraxia," which certainly qualifies as disturbance of a naturalistic multistep action, affects a "very automatic action for civilized man" and thus defies "Jackson's doctrine, that the severity of apraxia is inversely correlated to the degree of automatization of the afflicted functions" (Hécaen & De Ajuriaguerra, 1945, p. 132; see Chapter 3). This characterization may still be valid for dressing but in many other domains of everyday life we are confronted with rapidly changing technical devices that demand flexibility and ingenuity for finding out their proper handling. Moreover, even when no novel devices are included, the multiplicity of factors that contribute to swift performance of naturalistic actions raises the probability that their coordination goes astray and that the routine is interrupted by obstacles or action slips. Flexibility and problem solving are thus frequently needed for successful completion of naturalistic multistep actions. Their impairment would qualify as affecting a high level of action control.

However, successful problem solving in naturalistic multistep action does not necessarily lead to the autonomy of mind that the holist considered as a further crucial component of high-order action control. Other than mechanical problem solving for use of single conventional tools, technical problem solving is frequently based on trial and error. It remains dependent on the material interaction with the devices rather than being based on the manipulations of purely mental representations (Rowlands, 2003). In the high- versus low-level dichotomy this dependency relegates trial and error to the lower level.

Chapter 10

Communicative gestures: Pantomime of tool use

The observation that brain damage can interfere with the production of communicative gestures was made by Paul Broca (1861). In his seminal description of patient Tantan who had lost articulated speech after a left frontal lesion, Broca reported that gestures of the patient were frequently incomprehensible, and that "some questions to which a man with normal intelligence would have found a means to respond by gesture remained unanswered" (see Chapter 1). The degradation of gestural communication was also central for Finkelnburg's (1870) suggestion that aphasic patients suffer from a general "asymbolia." Liepmann integrated faulty performance of communicative gestures in his system of apraxias but changed the focus of interest from their communicative value to their motor execution (see Chapter 2). This change went hand in hand with a major modification of the assessment of communicative gestures. Whereas Broca and Finkelnburg had based their conclusions on observation of spontaneous gestures, Liepmann introduced their production on command which has remained the standard procedure for diagnosing apraxia of communicative gestures until today.

The decision to test the correctness of communicative gestures on command rather than in spontaneous conversation has consequences for selection of the type of gestures examined. The examination must be limited to gestures with a fixed meaning that can be unequivocally designated in the command. To enable evaluation of gestures independently from aphasia, their comprehensibility should not depend on accompanying speech. Finally, the spatial structure of the gesture should be complex enough to provide opportunity for conspicuous and unequivocal errors, and conventional enough to decide unequivocally whether individual variations are within the normal range. We will discuss classification of communicative gestures in more detail in Chapter 11 but retain now, that there are two classes of gestures which fulfill these demands and which are traditionally used for probing the integrity of communicative gestures in apraxia: emblems and pantomimes of tool use.

Emblems are gestures with a fixed shape and a conventional meaning like "okay," "be quiet," or "I am alert" (Morris et al., 1979; McNeill, 1992; Kendon, 2004).[1] Liepmann called them "expressive" or "symbolic" movements, while Goodglass and Kaplan (1963) used the

[1] A considerable proportion of these gestures are obscene or aggressive. This corresponds to their role in everyday communication: they permit the signaling of messages which, for fear of consequences, one tries to avoid saying in face-to-face communication.

term "conventional gestures." They have also been named "intransitive" because, in contrast to pantomime of tool use, they make no reference to tools and objects.

In pantomime of tool use the manual actions of using the tool are demonstrated with the empty hand. In neuropsychology, pantomimes of tool use have been classified as "transitive" because they demonstrate an interaction with an imaginary tool or object. However, this can lead to confusion with actual tool use where the hand interacts with a real tool. I will use the terms "emblematic gestures" and "pantomime of tool use".[2]

The examination of communicative gestures

A first prerequisite for assessing the production of gestures on command is comprehension of the instruction specifying the task in general and the gestures to be demonstrated in particular. With few exceptions, apraxia for communicative gestures on command is associated with left-hemisphere lesions and aphasia. The association with aphasia affects the examination of communicative gestures on command more than the imitation of gestures or the use of tools and objects. Whereas instructions for imitation or tool use refer to demonstrated actions and presented objects, instructions for communicative gestures ask the patient to pretend the use of imagined tools or send gestural messages to pretended opponents. There are thus no situational cues to the nature of the required action.

Pantomimes of tool use are frequently preferred over emblematic gestures because for them defective verbal comprehension can be partly compensated. The examiner can illustrate the general instruction by demonstration of pantomimes and the identity of the individual objects by showing the object or a picture of it. By contrast, for emblematic gestures patients must understand both the general instruction and the name of the individual gestures from verbal explanation only. Since the purpose of examination is the assessment of gestures and not of verbal abilities, pantomimes are preferable. This chapter shares the general preference and will concentrate mainly on pantomimes. In the course of their discussion I will propose further arguments as to why pantomimes of tool use are of particular interest for understanding apraxia of communicative gestures.

Circumvention of defective verbal comprehension is not necessarily sufficient for securing adherence to the instruction. Behind the verbal comprehension deficit lurks a conflict between the situational context of testing and the nature of the required actions. This conflict had already been addressed by the holists, notably Kurt Goldstein (1928) and Derek Denny-Brown (1958; see Chapter 3). According to these authors, patients with brain damage and particularly those with aphasia are "directly anchored in reality." They are unable "to imagine fictional events nor can they fake actions" (Goldstein, 1928, p. 238). Denny-Brown's assertion that "the more hypothetic the nature of the request, the more imaginary the circumstances,

---

2 In the UK, the word pantomime primarily refers to a theatrical entertainment performed around Christmas. The use of "pantomime" for the miming of tool use goes back to the seminal study by Goodglass and Kaplan (1963; see Chapter 4) and is now predominant in the neuropsychological as well as in functional imaging literature.

and the more the requested movement is a mimesis of the real thing, the more vulnerable it is to such disease" (Denny-Brown, 1958, p. 10) fits perfectly with the request to demonstrate the use of a tool without taking that tool in the hand, or to make an expressive gesture whose meaning has no relationship to the current social and communicative situation.

Aphasic patients who are unable to pretend the use of presented objects may try to name or describe them rather than pantomiming their use. The tendency for naming may be enhanced by habit. Patients who are in regular therapy for aphasia are certainly more used to naming pictures than to demonstrating their use. Goodglass and Kaplan (1963) termed this behavior "verbal overflow." Verbal overflow can occur in aphasic patients with severely reduced or incomprehensible verbal output and may be accompanied by spontaneous gestures which, however, accentuate parts of their speech rather than simulating the use of the tool.

Analysis of errors in pantomime of tool use

Figure 10.1 shows examples of faulty pantomimes of tool use made by aphasic patients. Remarkably, none of them is completely wrong. They correctly display some features of the tools and their use but omit or distort others. For example, all patients displayed in Figure 10.1 led their hand to the mouth for the pantomime of tooth brushing, and made movements near or upon the table for the pantomime of ironing. Some wrong gestures would be quite efficient for identifying tool and action, but constitute errors because they violate the instruction which emphasizes that the patient should imagine holding the tool in the hand and using it. Consequently only hand shapes and movements that also occur during actual tool use are accepted. This excludes the strategy of drawing the outlines of the tool in the air, although drawing in the air can constitute a valuable and efficient strategy for conveying the identity of an object whose use is demonstrated. Another quite efficient strategy that infringes the restriction of permitted hand shapes is the demonstration of the "body part as object" (BPO; Goodglass & Kaplan, 1963). Rather than demonstrating the grip of the pretended tool, the hand is configured and moved as if it were the tool itself. A very common example of this strategy is the demonstration of cutting with scissors by opening and closing the angle between index and middle finger. The two moving fingers depict the blades of the scissors. Normal subjects use such strategies too. They sometimes even prefer them over correct demonstration of the grip when pantomime is used for communicating their needs to someone whose language they do not speak rather than for satisfying the demands of an examination.[3]

[3] There are arguments against the radical conclusion that denying scores to BPO pantomimes is an arbitrary exclusion of an efficient strategy in favor of a more difficult but less efficient one. The first is developmental: pre-school children produce nearly exclusively BPO. A preference for showing the hand shape associated with holding the imaginary tool develops only between six and nine years (O'Reilly, 1995; Njiokiktjien et al., 2000; Takashi, 2003). The second argument is the clinical observation that healthy subjects who spontaneously produce BPO pantomimes can switch to demonstrating the grip of the imaginary tool when explicitly asked to do so whereas patients with apraxia fail (Duffy & Duffy, 1989; Heilman & Rothi, 1993). This argument is weaker than the developmental one, because the failure to adapt the grip according to a verbal reminder could have its source in deficient verbal comprehension.

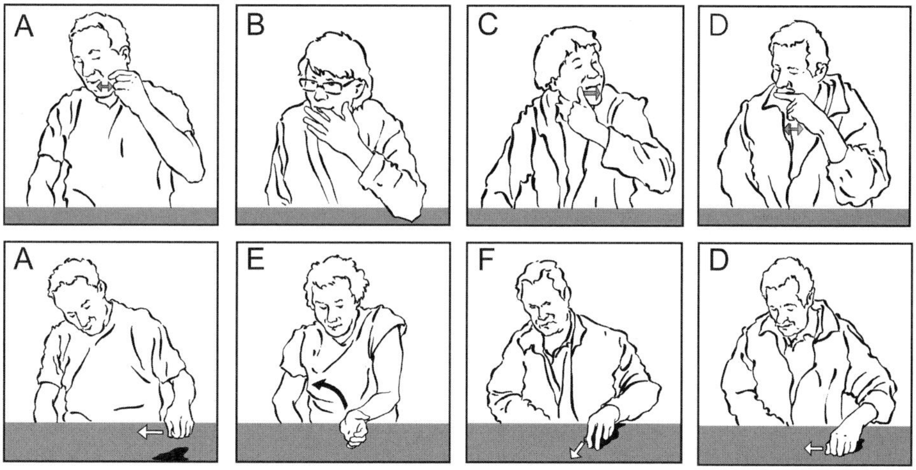

Figure 10.1 Pantomimes of tool use made by patients with left brain damage and aphasia. Top row: Brushing teeth. A makes a correct pantomime: the hand is formed to a precision grip, the distance between the hand and the mound corresponds to the approximate length of a toothbrush, and the hand is moved parallel to the mouth. B only points to the mouth. C moves the hand parallel to the mouth but neither the shape of the hand nor its distance to the mouth consider the imaginary tooth brush. D shows "body part as object" and moves the index as if it were the tooth brush. Bottom row: Ironing. Again, A shows a correct pantomime. The hand is shaped as if it would rest on the handle of the flat-iron, the distance to the table corresponds to the height of the iron, and it is moved in parallel to the table. E demonstrates the approximate shape of the flat-iron rather than pantomiming its use. F slides the hand across the table as if it were the flat iron. D shows the correct grip and the correct movement but disregards the distance between the hand and the table. Reproduced from Goldenberg, G. *Neuropsychologie—Grundlagen, Klinik, Rehabilitation. 4. Auflage*, p. 160, by permission of Elsevier.

The diversity of possible strategies for creating a comprehensible gestural representation of the tool and its use and the insecurity of the border between strategic variants and pathological deficits raise doubts on the existence of a finite "action output lexicon" that lists the correct forms of pantomimes (Rothi et al., 1991). They would be more compatible with the assumption that the shapes of pantomimes are created only when they are needed (Osiurak et al., 2011).

The double nature of pantomime

Creation of pantomimes requires transformation of knowledge about the tool and its manipulation into empty-handed gestures that communicate the identity of the tool and the manner of its manipulation to other persons. The manual movements of the pantomime refer to the manual movements of actual use. Arguably, the great interest of pantomimes for both clinical examination and theoretical understanding of apraxia is due to this double nature. Pantomime of tool use is a communicative manual action that refers to an instrumental one. It thus bridges the cleft between instrumental and communicative functions of the hands. In the next two sections I will discuss both sides of pantomime. First I will analyze the relationship between pantomime and real tool use, and then between pantomime and other modes of communication.

Pantomime and real tool use

As an introduction to discussing differences between motor programs for real use and for pantomime I propose a little experiment: Imagine a glass standing on the table some 30 centimeters in front of you and pantomime the act of taking that glass and leading it to mouth for drinking. You may also put a real glass on the table and pantomime the grasp beside it. Watch carefully the configuration of your hand when it approaches and takes up the imaginary glass. Now, repeat that act but this time actually grasping and lifting the glass and observe again the configuration of the hand. Did you note the difference? For the pantomime you opened the hand approximately to the width of the glass and then moved to the imaginary glass without further changing the aperture of the grip. At the target location the hand stopped and then moved upward to the mouth, still preserving constant aperture. By contrast, for actually grasping the glass your hand initially opened wider than the diameter of the glass and closed again when approaching it (Goodale et al., 1994; Laimgruber et al., 2005). The sequence of opening and closing was finely tuned to the transport of the hand so that the combined movements of whole hand and fingers coincided in a smooth grip of the glass (Jeannerod, 1986). If a pantomime is considered correct only when it faithfully replicates the motor action of actual use you must consider yourself apraxic, because you omitted a central feature of the act of grasping. Of course you are not apraxic. You replaced the complicated but highly automatized movements of real grasping by a simpler non-routine movement sequence that sufficed for indicating drinking from a glass. The constant aperture of the hand indicated the width of the glass, the stop of the transport its location and the subsequent change of its direction toward the mouth the purpose of drinking. Your pantomime conveyed the meaning of the action rather than replicating its exact motor features.

We examined kinematic features of real and pretended drinking from a glass in patients with left or right brain damage and healthy controls (Laimgruber et al., 2005). Patients used the hand ipsilateral to their lesions. Right-handed performance of patients with right brain damage was somewhat slower than that of controls but otherwise undisturbed. Real grasping of patients with left brain damage did not differ from that of controls acting with the left hand but during pantomime the aperture of their grip was significantly smaller (see Figure 10.2). Some of these patients did not open the hand at all and moved to the location of the imaginary glass and further to the mouth with a closed fist. Given that the same left hand mastered the adaptation of grip aperture to the grasping of the real glass the failure to open the hand for pantomime cannot plausibly be referred to lack of deftness or to a general inaccuracy of scaling grip width. It seems rather that the patients omitted from their pantomime the demonstration of the width of the glass by the width of their grip. The pantomime thus lacked a feature which is central for communicating its meaning.

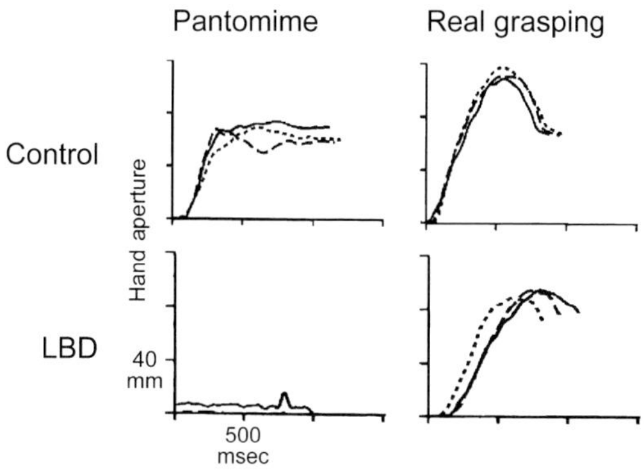

Figure 10.2 Kinematic recording of the hand aperture during pantomiming or real execution of grasping a glass by a normal person and a patient with left brain damage and apraxia: both use their left hands. Real grasping does not significantly differ. Both open their grip wider than the diameter of the glass and close the grip around the glass when they have reached it. Pantomime differs from real grasping in both subjects, but in different ways. The normal person opens their hand to the width of the imagined glass at the beginning of its transport and omits demonstration of closing the grip when their hand has reached the location of the pretended glass. Halting of the hand at this location is sufficient to indicate that the glass has been grasped. The patient with left brain damage transports the hand to the pretended location of the glass without opening it at all. The pantomime still indicates the target location of the transport moment but gives no clue as to the object that is being grasped there. Reprinted from *Neuropsychologia*, *43* (5), Kerstin Laimgruber, Georg Goldenberg, and Joachim Hermsdörfer, Manual and hemispheric asymmetries in the execution of actual and pantomimed prehension, p. 687 Copyright (2005), with permission from Elsevier.

The conclusion that insufficient selection of significant features is a core deficit of apraxia for communicative gestures was endorsed by a significant correlation between grip aperture during pantomime and the score of an independent examination of other pantomimes of tool use. Decreasing quality of pantomime of tool use was associated with decreasing aperture of the grip for pantomiming taking the glass. The specificity of this association was confirmed by the absence of significant correlations between grip aperture and the error rate of imitating meaningless gestures.

What is the crucial difference between pantomime and real tool use?

Defective pantomime of tool use is a frequent symptom of left hemisphere damage. Depending on the refinement of testing it is diagnosed in about one-half to two-thirds of aphasic patients. However, about one-half of afflicted patients can demonstrate tool use normally when they hold the real tool and apply it to its recipient (De Renzi et al., 1982; Goldenberg & Hagmann, 1998b). This raises the question as to which properties of pantomime and real use are decisive for their differential sensitivity to brain damage.

A conspicuous difference between pantomime and actual use is the provision of tactile feedback about the shape, weight, and other properties of the tool in real use and its absence in pantomime. Another potentially important difference concerns the relation of the tool action to its recipient. Whereas in real use the tool interacts with an actually present recipient, pantomime relates to an imaginary target.

In a seminal study De Renzi et al. (1982) systematically varied the modality of feedback for demonstrations of the motor act of tool use. They compared three conditions: pantomime on mere verbal instruction, pantomime with the tool in sight, and blindfolded demonstration of use with the tool in hand. There was no difference between the exactitudes of pantomimes made to purely verbal command and to the sight of object, but tactile presentation without sight led to a marked improvement. A superior role of tactile feedback for eliciting correct tool actions was supported by single case and small group studies showing dramatic improvement of pantomimes even when subjects performed the pantomime holding an object with no structural relationship to the pantomimed tool such as, for example, a stick (Graham et al., 1999; Wada et al., 2000).

In order to analyze the specific influence of tactile feedback on pantomime we (Goldenberg et al., 2004) compared three conditions of pantomime of tool use. In the first condition patients saw a picture of the tool but performed the pantomime empty-handed. In the second condition the picture was also visible, but in addition patients held a piece of wood whose shape and thickness resembled the handle of the tool. For example, a hemi-sphere of eight centimeters in diameter was used to demonstrate eating an apple, squeezing a lemon, and screwing in an electric bulb. This modification had no consistent effect on the exactitude of pantomimes whereas all patients improved markedly when they demonstrated use with the real tool and its recipient. We concluded that tactile feedback per se is not sufficient to evoke motor programs of correct tool use, but that the combined presentation of the real tool and its recipient is necessary for calling into play the mechanisms underlying the use of single familiar tools (see Chapter 8). This conclusion is endorsed by single case studies of patients with left temporal lesions who failed pantomime as well as demonstration of use with the tool in hand but improved to normal skill when the recipient of the action was presented in addition to the tool (Dumont et al., 1999; Hayakawa et al., 2000; Osiurak et al., 2008b). Further support comes from a group study examining the pantomime of scooping soup from one bowl to another by patients with left brain damage and aphasia (Randerath et al., 2011). In this study, the most frequent error of pantomime was omission of the rotation of the hand at the end points of transport that indicates the tilting of the ladle for taking up and pouring out the soup. Performance of the pantomime with a ladle in hand induced only moderate and inconsistent improvement, but when the filled and the empty bowl were actually present, no patient failed to tilt the ladle for taking up and pouring out soup.

These observations qualify the facilitation of pantomime by tactual feedback. The crucial factor seems to be the provision of additional information on structural and functional features of real tool use rather than the tactual or visual presentation of this information. Presumably the presence of recipients enables the employment of mechanical problem solving for determining the correct movements of the manipulated tool and hence the correct movements of the hand[4] (see Chapter 8). By contrast, the absence of recipients changes the task from an instrumental interaction with external objects into the communicative task of transmitting information about the nature and the use of tools.

Subtle differences with important implications

The emphasis on apparently minor variations of experimental conditions for assessing pantomime may appear over-subtle but relates to profound theoretical controversies. The postulate that tactile sensations elicit stored motor program of tool use is easily recognizable as a descendent of the associationist tradition (see Chapter 1). A "short circuit" from local sensation to motor commands had already been proposed by Liepmann as an explanation for correct performance of a limited repertoire of highly practiced actions by the imperial counselor (see Chapter 2). In a similar vein, De Renzi et al. (1982) followed Geschwind's emphasis on disconnections between modality-specific areas as a major source of errors. Considering the dissociation between actions elicited by tactile or visual stimuli they concluded:

> The intermodal dissociation cannot be accounted for except by assuming that apraxia can be modality specific, namely, contingent upon the selective severing of the pathways linking one sensory association area with the centre where the movement is programmed (p. 310).

The alternative position that pantomime differs from real use because it is based on communicative rather than instrumental skills looks for the decisive differences between visual and tactile input not in their sensory modalities but in the information they convey. If this information is sufficient for appreciating structural and functional relationships between hand, tools and recipients it enables the derivation of manual actions from requirements of real use. If such information is absent, subjects must create communicative gestures that are sufficient for indicating the nature of the tool and its action without recourse to elements of real tool use. The adverse effect of this deprivation reminds of Denny Brown's statement about production of communicative gestures in apraxia: "The more hypothetic the nature of the request, the more imaginary the circumstances, and the more the requested movement is a mimesis of the real thing, the more vulnerable it is to such disease". (Denny-Brown, 1958, p. 10).

Are there double dissociations between pantomime and real tool use?

Until now, we have concentrated exclusively on the dissociation between preserved real tool use and disturbed pantomime, but both of the alternative accounts of such dissociations predict the existence of the inverse dissociation between preserved pantomime and defective use of real tools. From the associationist standpoint such dissociation would be expected as the result of lesions severing the pathways from tactile sensation but sparing the pathways from visual areas to motor programs. The position emphasizing the communicative nature of pantomime would expect such dissociation to result from disturbed

4 Mechanical problem solving was probed in one of the reported cases where the success of pantomime depended on the presence of the recipient (Osiurak et al., 2008b) and was found intact.

communicative but preserved instrumental functions. Clinical evidence for the reality of the expected dissociation is rather scanty, but exists. There are two single case reports of patients with biparietal lesions who had severe problems and committed errors when trying to use everyday tools and objects but could pantomime their use much better (Fukutate, 2008) or even perfectly (Motomura & Yamadori, 1994). One of them commented that "he could understand neither the relation of the objects and their spatial elements (direction, position, etc.) nor the timing of the actions" (Fukutate, 2008, p. 49).

While better performance of pantomime than of real use seems to be exceptional as a symptom of brain damage, it is a common experience in normal life. For example, most persons are able to pantomime playing a violin or a trumpet but only a small minority of them can actually play the instruments. It is even possible to pantomime actions which are out of the range of human motor competence. For example, rhythmical up and down beat of both arms beside the body will be recognized as a pantomime of flying but attempts to translate this pantomime into a real action may have dangerous outcomes. The existence of actions which normal subjects can pantomime in spite of being unable to perform them in reality constitutes a strong argument in favor of the independence of communicative motor actions from the instrumental actions to which they refer.

Pantomime, aphasia, and asymbolia

The hypothesis that pantomime is a communicative gesture and the observation that defective pantomime is regularly associated with aphasia lead back to Finkelnburg's (1870) postulate of general asymbolia (see Chapter 1). The asymbolia hypothesis claims that the adverse effect of linguistic impairment on pantomime is not confined to insufficient comprehension of the instructions for pantomime but reflects the common influence of asymbolia on both verbal and non-verbal communicative abilities.

Is association of defective pantomime with aphasia obligatory?

An obvious statistical approach for assessing the strength of the postulated association between defective pantomime and aphasia is the calculation of correlations between scores on tests of pantomime and of language in aphasic patients. A number of studies have looked at this (Picket, 1974; Duffy & Duffy, 1981; Wang & Goodglass, 1992; Duffy et al., 1994; Roy et al., 1998; Goldenberg et al., 2003; Goldenberg et al., 2007b).[5] Two studies found correlation coefficients between 0.8 and 0.9 between scores on pantomime and the Porch Index of Communicative Abilities (Picket, 1974; Duffy & Duffy, 1981), but the tightness of this correlation may be due to the inclusion of tests of pantomime in the Index of Communicative Abilities. In all other studies the correlation coefficients ranged between 0.5 and 0.7 which is statistically significant but certainly not sufficient to support the conclusion that one and the same basic disturbance, asymbolia, completely accounts for both deficiencies of language and of pantomime.

[5] The results from Goldenberg et al. (2007b) were not included in the original publication.

In order to pin down the specificity of the relationship between disturbed pantomime and aphasia, Duffy and Duffy (1981), Wang and Goodglass (1992), and Goldenberg et al. (2003, 2007b) also investigated correlations between pantomime on command and the imitation of gestures. They reasoned that apraxia for imitation depends on left-hemisphere lesions too, but should not be victim to asymbolia, particularly when examined for meaningless gestures. Nonetheless correlations between pantomime and imitation of meaningless gestures were in the same range as those between pantomime and aphasia. More sophisticated multivariate statistical procedures confirmed that aphasia and imitation disturbance are independent predictors of the severity of pantomime impairment. The presence of a second predictor is difficult to reconcile with the assumption that defective pantomime is exclusively due to a general asymbolia shared with aphasia.

Analyses based on dichotomous distinction between normal and defective pantomime or, respectively, the presence and absence of aphasia, yield stronger arguments in favor of a common basic disturbance underlying aphasia and disturbed pantomime. In two studies we looked for the proportion of aphasic patients with preserved pantomime of tool use (Goldenberg et al., 2003, 2007b). There were three out of 40 in the first study and 15 out of 44 in the second. The apparent increase was presumably due to a revision and new standardization of the pantomime test. Although these results concur that only a minority of aphasic patients perform pantomimes of tool use normally, they are not sufficient for claiming a mandatory decline of pantomime in aphasia. However, the relationship becomes closer when only patients with global aphasia are considered. Global aphasia is the most severe form of aphasia. It is characterized by massive reduction of verbal output and deficits in all modalities of language. In the first study none of 13 patients with global aphasia, and in the second study only two out of 19 such patients scored in the normal range on the pantomime test. Since we examined only aphasic patients our results cannot show whether the apparently obligatory presence of pantomime disturbance in severe aphasia also works the other way round, that is, whether all patients with disturbed pantomime are also aphasic. I could not find any study investigating this question.[6] We will come back to this in the discussion of apraxia and handedness (Chapter 12), but I may already relate that in left-handed patients dissociations between defective pantomime and normal linguistic abilities do occur.

The creation of pantomimes

I have argued that pantomiming the use of a tool cannot be reduced to activation of motor programs of real use, and that defective pantomime in patients with aphasia cannot be reduced to being a consequence of aphasia or general asymbolia. Pantomimes are

6 Kertesz et al. (1984) found no single case of apraxia for communicative gestures without aphasia in 17 patients with left brain damage, but the interpretation of this observation is ambiguous, because the authors gave full credit to gestures that were failed on command but correct on imitation. It is thus possible (though unlikely) that non-aphasic patients whose gestures were counted as normal had, in fact, defective pantomime on command but their deficit was masked by the successful imitation (see Chapter 6).

autonomous gestures that communicate the identity of the tool and the way it is used so that they can be comprehended by other subjects. This leads to the question as to how such demonstrations are constructed and which particular difficulties they pose.

I propose that creation of pantomime is based on a combination of selected features of tool use. Only features related to shape, position, and movement of the hand are eligible for combination to pantomimes. Features of the tool must be expressed by corresponding features of the holding hand.

Figure 10.3 exemplifies this idea for the combinations of rotational movement of the hand with different directions of the axes of rotation and different hand shapes. Combinations of three different types of grip and of three different axes of rotation yield nine possible gestures, six of which correspond to pantomimes of common tools.

We may speculate that creation of a pantomime starts with the retrieval of a mental image depicting the object together with the hand acting on it. As we have elaborated with the example of pantomiming to play a violin or to fly like a bird,[7] the mental image need not be based on motor experience with the real execution of the action. It only requires some knowledge about the action or, respectively, some memory of having witnessed this action before. Conversion of that knowledge into pantomimes requires segmentation of the compound image of hand, tool, and action into distinct features and the selection of only those features that can be demonstrated by the configuration, the movement, and the position of the hand. These restrictions may lead to the selection of features that in real tool use are hardly attended to because they are automatically determined by mechanical interactions. For example, in real ironing the distance of the hand from the ironing board

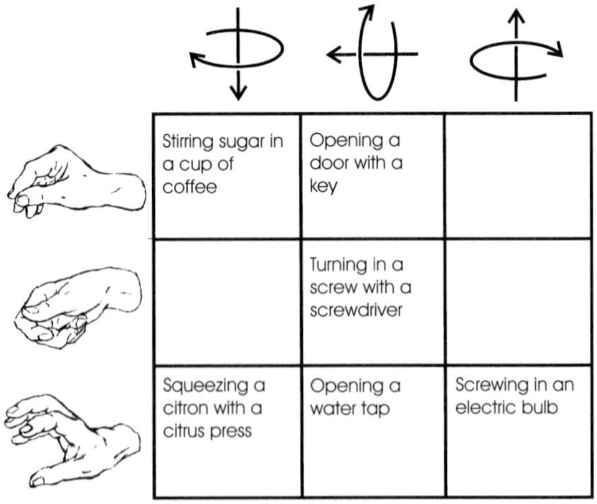
Stirring sugar in a cup of coffee
Opening a door with a key
Turning in a screw with a screwdriver
Squeezing a citron with a citrus press
Opening a water tap
Screwing in an electric bulb

Figure 10.3 Combination of three types of grip with three orientations of rotational movement yields nine gestures, six of which correspond to correct pantomimes of tool use.

7 For the pantomime of flying, the object is the air. It is indicated by the shape and posture of the hand. The hands are held horizontally with the flat palms facing downward. The flatness and extension of the hand are intended to indicate maximal exploitation of the resistance of air and hence refer to a property of the object air.

is determined by the height of the iron, but in pantomiming it must be selected as an attribute of hand position in order to distinguish ironing from wiping the table.

Selected features must then be combined to a continuous movement sequence of the hand. This movement sequence constitutes the pantomime. It resembles the manual motor sequence of real tool use, but the mechanism of its creation is fundamentally different from the generation of motor actions for real tool use. Whereas the motor actions of real tool use result from the incorporation of manual configurations and movements into a mechanical chain that leads to the tool and its recipient, the generation of pantomime results from selection and combination of distinctive features extracted from a mental image of tool use. The apparently minor differences between manual actions of real use and of pantomime that we discussed in the preceding sections are visible indications of the fundamental differences between the mechanisms of their generation.

Laterality of lesions causing apraxia for communicative gestures

Liepmann's postulate that defective performance of emblems and pantomimes on command and defective imitation of gestures are both symptoms of "ideo-kinetic" apraxia has led many researchers to combine results from both modes of examination to sum scores, or to test only imitation to circumvent the influence of accompanying aphasia on the comprehension of verbal commands. Fortunately, the few studies that looked specifically for the lesions interfering with communicative gestures on command agree on the main results. Defective production of communicative gestures on command is bound to left brain damage. Patients with right brain damage perform them either like healthy controls (Goodglass & Kaplan, 1963; Duffy & Duffy, 1981; Lehmkuhl et al., 1983; Goldenberg & Hagmann, 1998b; Goldenberg et al., 2003; Hartmann et al., 2005) or have very mild impairment that becomes apparent only with meticulous scoring of the spatial accuracy of pantomimes (Haaland & Flaherty, 1984; Barbieri & De Renzi, 1988; Roy et al., 1998; Hanna-Pladdy et al., 2001a).

Emblems and pantomimes

Generally, emblems are less affected by left-hemisphere lesions than pantomimes of tool use (Goodglass & Kaplan, 1963; Kertesz & Hooper, 1982; Raade et al., 1991; Roy et al., 1991; Heath et al., 2001; Hanna-Pladdy et al., 2001a; Buxbaum et al., 2007; Stamenova et al., 2010). There are reports of patients with apraxia for pantomime of tool use and intact production of emblems but not of the converse dissociations between intact pantomime and defective emblems (Rapcsak et al., 1993; Dumont et al., 1999). Healthy controls also make more errors with pantomimes than with emblems, indicating that the greater error proneness of pantomimes is due to their inherently greater difficulty (Goodglass & Kaplan, 1963; Kertesz & Hooper, 1982; Rapcsak et al., 1989; Mozaz et al., 2002). Whereas comprehension of the command for pantomimes can be facilitated by showing the tool, comprehension of the command for emblems depends fully on verbal designation. The observation that aphasic patients have nonetheless more problems with pantomime provides support for independence of defective pantomime from the effects of accompanying aphasia. At the same time it raises the question as to what factors underlie the relative preservation of emblematic gestures.

A possible answer could be found in the creative demands of pantomimes and emblems. Other than pantomime, emblems need not be composed by extraction and combination of distinct features of tools and actions. They are stored in long-term memory as unitary manual actions. Their relative sparing in patients with left brain damage and aphasia thus indicates that the inability to produce gestures by selection and combination of significant features is more important for the vulnerability to left brain damage than their closeness to language.

This interpretation has, however, been challenged by a recent study of Carmo & Rumiati (2009). They asked healthy subjects to imitate under time pressure pantomimes and emblems. Although the demonstration of gestures for imitation alleviated the demands on creativity, subjects made more errors with pantomimes than with emblems. Moreover, the difference of error rates was replicated when the original gestures were replaced by meaningless variants that modified relations between hand, arm, and trunk, but preserved the structural complexity of the gestures. These results would suggest that the greater difficulty of pantomimes results from their greater spatial complexity. The two interpretations are, however, not necessarily mutually exclusive. The greater spatial complexity of pantomime may derive from the necessity to display the combination of multiple features of the tool, the hand, and their action. By contrast, the emblem has only one pre-defined message. According to this speculation, the structural complexity of the manual actions for emblems and pantomimes corresponds with the complexity of their communicative contents. Pantomimes convey more elements of information and are composed of more spatial elements. Insufficient selection and combination of multiple elements manifests itself in both spatial and communicative aspects of the gesture.

Intra-hemispheric location of lesions disturbing pantomime

We have explored the intra-hemispheric location of lesions causing defective pantomime in four group studies including a total of 151 patients. In three of them lesions were classified according to whether or not they encroached upon the parietal, the temporal, and the frontal lobes (Goldenberg & Hagmann, 1998b; Goldenberg et al., 2003; Hartmann et al., 2005). Comparison between patients with and without parietal lobe affection confirmed selective impairment of imitation of hand postures and of the Novel Tool Test in patients with parietal lesions (Goldenberg & Hagmann, 1998b; Goldenberg et al., 2003) but failed to show significant influences of parietal lesions on pantomime. One of the studies (Goldenberg et al., 2003) revealed better production of pantomimes in patients whose lesions spared the temporal lobes. Encroachment of the lesion upon the frontal lobes had no significant effect on pantomime.

The forth study was the lesion subtraction study that has already been presented in the discussion of imitation of gestures (see Chapter 7). The patients of this study were also tested for pantomime of tool use. The maximum difference of lesion density between patients with disturbed and preserved pantomime was located in the inferior frontal gyrus and adjacent portions of the insula and precentral gyrus, whereas the frequency of parietal lesions did not differ between patients with or without defective pantomime (Figure 10.4; Goldenberg et al., 2007b). Defective pantomime was associated with larger lesions and with greater severity of aphasia, but the results remained essentially the same when these confounding factors were controlled by excluding patients with extreme values from both groups until there were no statistically significant differences of language comprehension or lesion size between patients with normal and defective pantomime. Nonetheless there is reason to doubt a narrow localization of pantomime impairment in the inferior frontal lobes. Inferior frontal lesions are frequently due to occlusions of the stem of the middle cerebral artery and form part of rather large infarctions that also affect subcortical structures. Indeed, the critical lesions in our study extended into white matter underlying inferior frontal and central regions. Possibly this combination or other associated brain damage, for example, in the temporal lobes, is necessary for causing clinically relevant defects of pantomime.

In spite of these limitations the results of the group studies are quite consistent in demonstrating that parietal lesions do not play a central role for disturbances of pantomime of tool use. This conclusion finds support in a recent lesion–symptom mapping study that investigated the location of lesions underlying defective pantomime in a large sample of otherwise quite heterogeneous patients and which found that in patients with vascular lesions critical lesions are located in inferior frontal but not in parietal lobes (Manuel et al., 2012). Finally,

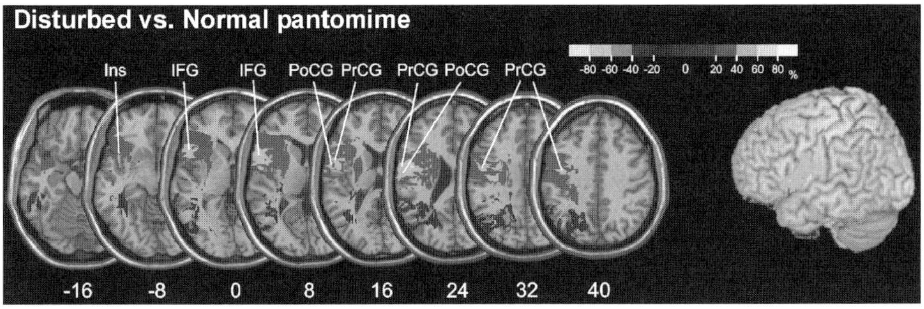

Figure 10.4 Subtraction of lesions of patients with intact pantomime from those of patients with disturbed pantomime: all patients had left brain damage and aphasia. The two groups did not significantly differ with respect to severity of language comprehension deficits or to size of lesion. The colors indicate the difference between the frequencies of lesions in both groups. IFG: inferior frontal gyrus; Ins: insula; PoCG: postcentral gyrus; PrCG: precentral gyrus. Lesions in inferior frontal and central regions are more frequent in patients with disturbed pantomime. By contrast, parietal regions lesions are even slightly more frequent in patients with intact pantomime. Reproduced from Goldenberg, G., Hermsdörfer, J., Glindemann, R., Rorden, C., and Karnath, H. O. Pantomime of tool use depends on integrity of left inferior frontal cortex. *Cerebral Cortex*, *17*, p. 2773, Copyright (2007) by permission of Oxford University Press. (See Plate 11.)

the preservation of pantomime in spite of parietal lesions is demonstrated by cases of "visuo-imitative apraxia" where selective damage to the parietal lobe leads to a dissociation between defective imitation of meaningless gestures and preserved production of communicative gestures on command (Goldenberg & Hagmann, 1997; Peigneux et al., 2000) and by reports of intact pantomime in single case studies of autotopagnosia resulting from extensive parietal lesions (De Renzi & Scotti, 1970; Poncet et al., 1971).

Location of defective pantomime and the posterior to anterior stream of action control

The conclusion that left parietal lesions do not regularly cause apraxia for communicative gestures on command stands in contrast to the predictions derived from all versions of the posterior to anterior stream of action control (Goldenberg, 2009). In Liepmann's original version, parietal lesions should interrupt the fibers leading from the mental image of the intended action constructed in posterior regions to its motor execution directed by motor cortex. In the versions of Kleist, Geschwind, and their modern followers, the parietal lesion should destroy the stored motor engrams of the manual actions of tool use. The conclusion that parietal lesions do not impair pantomimes of tool use is incompatible with the idea that apraxia is caused by interruption of a posterior to anterior stream of action control.

Parietal contributions to apraxia

The minor importance of parietal lesions for demonstration of pantomimes fits well with their central role for imitation and for tool use. I proposed that in imitation and tool use the parietal lobe is necessary for the categorical apprehension of spatial relationships. This implies that the parietal lobes are concerned with the analysis of external stimuli. Inferior parietal function probably extends to the temporary storage of spatial relationships in working memory, but even this transgression from perception to temporary storage applies predominantly to the analysis of perceived external spatial relationships. In imitation the external spatial relationships are between the body parts of the model, and in tool use between the parts of the mechanical chain leading from own body parts via tools to the recipients of tool actions. In pantomime the role of spatial perception of the surrounding is confined to localizing the sector of space where the manual action takes place as, for example, close to the mouth for demonstrating tooth brushing or close to the table for the end point of pretended pounding with a hammer, but it is uninformative about the shape of the gesture. Configuration of the hand and the exact positions, direction, and velocity of its movements are selected with reference to a mental image of the pretended tool and its action rather than being deduced from spatial properties of objects in the actual surrounding.[8]

[8] The importance of analyzing surrounding space may change when functional imaging is used for assessing cerebral activations elicited by pantomime of tool use. For these studies subjects are lying in a scanner. In order to avoid head movements, they are not allowed to move the arm at the shoulder and consequently have to perform all gestures within the space between chest and waist. These restrictions afford a transposition of movement trajectories into a reference frame centered on the supine trunk of

Inferior frontal contribution to pantomime

The location of the left inferior frontal region that our lesion subtraction study identified as crucial for disturbance of pantomime was very similar to the location that was found to be crucial for disturbed imitation of finger configurations in the subtraction study of imitation. By contrast, we found inferior frontal involvement neither for imitation of hand position nor for tool use (Goldenberg & Karnath, 2006; Goldenberg et al., 2007b; Goldenberg & Spatt, 2009).

Liepmann's version of the posterior to anterior stream of action control ended at the motor cortex in the central regions, but Norman Geschwind displaced its anterior pole into the adjacent premotor portion of the left frontal lobe. Geschwind considered the frontal end of the stream as a relay where the motor engrams received from the posterior origin are distributed to the central motor cortices of both hemispheres (see Chapter 4, Figure 4.1). Geschwind reasoned that destruction of this final relay would render both hands apraxic although the left hand is controlled by the undamaged right hemisphere. Apart from the general questionability of a posterior to anterior transport of motor engrams, this theory has no explanation as to why left inferior frontal lesions affect pantomime and imitation of finger configuration but spare tool use and imitation of hand postures.

Left inferior temporal cortex has also been invoked as being a major site of "mirror neurons" providing a direct link from perception to motor execution of actions (see Chapter 6). This led to the expectation that lesions there should impair imitation. Indeed a number of studies based mainly on functional imaging of cerebral activation in healthy subjects suggested enhanced left inferior frontal activity during imitation (Iacoboni et al., 1999; Binkofski et al., 2000; Tanaka & Inui, 2002; Makuuchi, 2005). Notably, all of them probed imitation of single finger movements. Their results thus mirror our finding of defective imitation of finger postures following left inferior frontal brain damage, but they provide no explanation for the affection of pantomime, nor can they explain the sparing of imitation of hand postures.

The paucity of studies exploring the role of inferior frontal lesions in apraxia stands in contrast to the wealth of studies concerned with other possible functions of this multifaceted region. The belief in its outstanding importance started with Broca's contention that the severe reduction of speech in his patient "Tantan" was due to the externally visible inferior frontal lesion rather than to its subcortical extension into basal ganglia and temporal lobe (Marie, 1906a; Broca, 2006; Dronkers et al., 2007). Since then the emphasis of linguistic investigations has shifted from the articulation of words to syntactical competency (Friedmann, 2006). It has been complemented by descriptions of a wide array of non-linguistic

the own body, whereas in clinical testing actions are directed toward other body parts—for example the mouth and face in tooth-brushing or drinking—or are constructed with reference to the basic coordinates of external space which are indicated by horizontal and vertical surfaces of surrounding objects. The transformations from the spatial frame of the upright person and its natural surroundings to that of a person with restricted motility lying in a scanner is likely to depend on parietal lobe function (Alivisatos & Petrides, 1997; Binkofski et al., 1999), and indeed parietal activation is a consistent finding in functional imaging studies of pantomime (Moll et al., 2000; Rumiati et al., 2004; Johnson-Frey et al., 2005; e.g., Hermsdörfer et al., 2007; Vingerhoets et al., 2012).

disturbances. They include, for example, the understanding and planning of motor sequences (Dabis et al., 2008; Fazio et al., 2009), working memory (Baldo & Dronkers, 2006), retrieval from semantic memory (Cabeza & Nyberg, 2000), selection between competing responses (Thompson-Schill et al., 1998; Gold & Buckner, 2002; Zhang et al., 2004), and the visual recognition of embedded figures (Fink et al., 2006). There is thus ample material for forging an account of the pattern of apraxic impairment following its lesions.[9]

Our version of such an account (Goldenberg et al., 2007b) is based on the assumption that inferior frontal lesions interfere with the ability to make choices between closely related alternatives. We reasoned that such choices are particularly relevant for imitation of finger postures and for pantomime. For finger postures selection is made difficult by the close conceptual and perceptual similarity between the fingers (see Chapter 7), and for pantomime by the restriction to choose only features of tool use that can be demonstrated by continuous movements of the empty hand. By contrast, the body parts involved in hand postures are perceptually and conceptually clearly distinct and for real tool use the instruction poses no restriction on the manual actions that are included in the mechanical chain leading from proximal body to the distal action of the tool.

Pantomime and the levels of motor control

The controversy over whether pantomime of tool use is the empty handed execution of the motor program of actual use or an autonomous gesture that demonstrates the tool and its use has relevance for the debate about the level of motor control afflicted by apraxia. The assumption that defective pantomime results from loss or inaccessibility of motor engrams of tool use is recognizable as a descendant of Kleist's and Geschwind's assumption that voluntary movements are controlled by motor-specific engrams storing kinetic features of learned movements. Its limitation to the replay of formerly established modality-specific representations qualifies it as a low-level account. By contrast, the alternative concept of pantomime as a communicative gesture emphasizes the creative nature of pantomimes. The creation of pantomime by selection and combination of characteristic features need not faithfully replicate previously acquired motor routines. The observation that one can pantomime actions which have been seen but never practiced, like playing the violin, underlines the independence of pantomime from stored motor representations and demonstrates versatile transfer of mental images from one modality to another. Creativity and versatility are properties which identify pantomime as an instance of high-level motor control or, put another way, as a cognitive rather than purely motor entity.

---

9 The abundance of suggestions concerning the role of Broca's area corresponds with the abundance of publications. In PubMed the keywordS "Broca's area" yields 15,184 articles published from 2006 to 2011. By contrast, "inferior parietal lobe" gives only 850 entries during the same time, and apraxia 711, which reduces to 230 when "apraxia of speech" is excluded. Arguably, the interest in Broca's area has to do with its anatomical location on the border between the prefrontal cortex that is traditionally acknowledged as housing the highest achievements of human mind and premotor cortex responsible for motor coordination. The same desire to bridge the cleavage between high-level psychic function and motor control that motivated Liepmann's writings on apraxia may underlie the enduring interest in Broca's area.

Chapter 11

Communicating with gestures

The examination of communicative gestures on command produces a discrepancy between the genuine meaning of the gesture and its communicative function. The examiner instructs the patients which gestures they should demonstrate and records their correctness but does not react to their genuine meaning. The pantomime of drinking from a glass does not incite the examiner to provide water, nor will the examiner come around the table and sit next to the patient when they demonstrate beckoning. The patients do not produce the gestures for expressing their wishes or opinions, but to comply with the examiner's instructions. If there is any message conveyed by the gesture it is something like: "I am ready to comply with the instruction and to produce the gesture you named although it has nothing to do with my current desires or opinions."

Whereas the ecological importance of the production of communicative gestures on command is questionable, use of gestures for communication can be very important for the patient's everyday life. We noted in the last chapter that defective production of gestures on command is a symptom of left brain damage and is regularly accompanied by aphasia. For patients with severe aphasia production and comprehension of gestures might offer a communicative channel that partly compensates the insufficiency of verbal communication. For these patients at least, the question of whether deficient production of gestures on command is regularly associated with deficient production of gestures in natural communication is ecologically relevant. In this chapter we will look at the spontaneous use of gestures for communication in patients with aphasia. Since communication includes both expression and comprehension of messages the chapter will also deal with defective recognition of communicative gestures.

The spectrum of communicative gestures

For diagnosing apraxia, examination of gestures on command is usually restricted to pantomimes of tool use and emblematic gestures. These two classes of gestures do not exhaust the spectrum of communicative gestures produced in everyday communication. There have been several proposals for classifications of communicative gestures. Although they mostly agree on basic principles of organization, they use different terminologies and differ in the fineness of distinction between different types of gestures as well as in the width of the range of gestures included (Ekman & Friesen, 1969; McNeill, 1992; Kendon, 2004). Table 11.1 presents a compilation that is organized along two dimensions that may be of

Table 11.1 Classification of gestures

	Refer to verbally transmitted information	**Transmit information on their own**
Idiosyncratic/creative	Regulators	Pictographs
	Ideographs	Pantomimes
Conventional	Emblems—"Italian" gestures	Emblems
		Deictics (Sign language)

particular importance for the gestures' sensitivity to brain damage: their relationship to verbal communication, and the conventionality of their shapes.

Not included in the table are *adaptors* like scratching or touching oneself during conversation. These gestures may reveal psychic tension or discomfort of the speaker but they are not produced with the intention to transmit messages (Buck & VanLear, 2002). For the same reason I excluded *beats* (McNeill, 1992), that is, rhythmical movements of the hands in synchrony with the prosodic rhythm of accompanying speech. At the other extreme of meaningfulness of gestures, the inclusion of *sign language* into their classification is questionable. In any case, the question whether or not these gestures can deploy their meaning without accompanying speech makes little sense because the gestures are themselves parts of a language (Bellugi et al., 1989; Goldin-Meadow, 2005).

Regulators are gestures that regulate the turn taking during conversation, like raising a hand to demand attention or pointing to the partner to ask them to respond to what the speaker said. *Ideographic* gestures have also been named "metaphorical." They illustrate, underline, or comment on the ideas and opinions that are brought forward by speech. For example, a rapid horizontal movement of the extended hand with the palm facing downward may emphasize the rejection of an idea and the end of its further discussion. Alternating pronation and supination of the hand accompanying a verbal utterance can signify that the speaker considers the utterance as expressing their ideas only approximately and with reservation. There is large variability between individual speakers concerning the frequency and the shapes of these gestures. Therefore they are classified as idiosyncratic, but in the further discussion we will see that they can also consist of conventional emblems.

Pictographs and *pantomimes* have been subsumed under the common denomination *physiographs* because both make reference to external objects. For pictographs the outlines of objects are drawn in the air, and for pantomime their use is demonstrated with empty hands. The shapes of these gestures are derived from the shapes of the real objects and from the motor features of their real use. We discussed in the previous chapter that pantomimes are unlikely to be stored as ready-made engrams or motor routines. They are instead constructed when they are needed by selection and combination of distinctive features of objects and their use. This applies also to pictographs, because drawing in the air results in a recognizable image only when the trace of the moving finger emphasizes features of the objects that distinguish it from competing objects and that can be unambiguously demonstrated by the moving finger. Because there can be individual differences between how subjects cope with these task demands the gestures deserve the classification of being idiosyncratic. It is noteworthy that their idiosyncrasy derives from their creative nature.

Emblems have been discussed in the previous chapter. They have a conventional shape associated with a conventional meaning. The conventionality of their message is borne out by the possibility that the same emblematic gestures have very different meanings in different geographical regions (Morris et al., 1979; Kendon, 1981). The kinds of emblems examined for the diagnosis of apraxia carry messages that are comprehensible without accompanying speech. They include gestures with very simple and often needed messages like the shoulder shrug for "I don't know" and nodding or shaking the head for "yes" and "no." Likewise, *deictics*, that is, pointing gestures, are efficient means for indicating objects of interest without a need for accompanying speech.

Although of rather limited relevance for understanding the function of gestures in aphasia, it may be worth mentioning that there is a subset of emblematic gestures that illustrate and complement verbal expression. Because their use is particularly prominent in Italy they have been referred to as *Italian* gestures (Munari, 2005). They are emblems in that they have a conventional shape and a conventional meaning but their meaning refers to simultaneous verbal conversation. For example, bringing all five fingers together in a point facing upward constitutes the "purse" which signals "precise emphasis" and is used to express a request for more precise explanation or justification of a verbal utterance (Morris et al., 1979; Kendon, 2004).

The classification of gestures according to their relationship to accompanying speech and to their conventionality allows a putative preview of the difficulties encountered by aphasic patients when they want to use gestures for compensating the shortcoming of verbal expressions. I discuss them for both dimensions in turn.

Reference to accompanying speech

In persons with normal linguistic competence the use of gestures replacing speech is restricted to a very limited range of situations. They can be useful for communication in very noisy surroundings or in other conditions that hinder acoustic transmission of speech while allowing visual signaling. Certain emblems are used for sending obscene or aggressive messages from a safe distance, preventing the addressee from physical reaction to the insult. In contrast to the rareness of using gestures for replacing speech, production of gestures accompanying speech is ubiquitous. There is large individual variability of the amount and vividness of gesturing during speech, but there is little doubt that normal speakers produce gestures accompanying speech much more frequently than gestures replacing speech.

Aphasic patients have been normal speakers for many years until brain damage abolished or greatly reduced their possibilities of verbal expression. This loss deprives gestures that normally accompany speech of their function. Some of them may still be useful, as, for example, the alternating pro- and supination for indicating the inaccuracy of a concurrent attempt to formulate a verbal expression, but their abundant production confuses the communication partner rather than illuminating the intended messages. In order to accomplish efficient gestural expression patients must overcome the lifelong habit of producing gestures that accompany and illustrate speech. Persistence of gestures that normally accompany speech can lead to a combination of high frequency with low communicative value of the patients' gestures.

Conventionality of gestures

Idiosyncratic gestures differ from conventional gestures not only by their greater individual variability but also by their greater demands on creativity. These demands are particularly high for idiosyncratic gestures replacing speech, that is, pantomimes and ideographs. Not only must they carry information that is normally provided by speech, they must do this in a way that is unambiguously comprehensible for the communication partner. Since they cannot rely on the familiar shapes and meanings of conventional gestures, pantomimes and pictographs must achieve comprehensibility by a creative act of selection and combination of significant features of the objects, events, and desires that are being addressed. Probably these task demands make production and comprehension of pantomimes and ideographs more error prone and more vulnerable to brain damage than the execution of emblems or of idiosyncratic gestures accompanying speech.

Bearing these general reflections in mind we will now review studies exploring the influence of aphasia and apraxia on spontaneous communicative gestures.

Communicative gestures and aphasia

More than a hundred years after Finkelnburg's descriptions of aphasic patients' inability to compensate their loss of spoken expression by gestures, the conclusion that they suffered from a general disorder of communication affecting both speech and gesturing was revived and elaborated. An influential theory of gesture and speech postulated that "gestures and speech are parts of the same psychological structure" (McNeill, 1985, p. 350) because both derive from "inner speech" which is identical to "thinking" and precedes the overt production of speech and gesture. Gestures are therefore "the overt products of the same internal processes that produce the other overt product, speech" (p. 350).

The hypothesis of a common stage of covert thinking that manifests itself in both speech and gesture leads to the expectation that impairment of this stage will become equally manifest in speech and gestures (Cicone et al., 1979; McNeill, 1985; McNeill, 1992). It thus revives Finkelnburg's contention that in aphasia:

> the deficiency of word production represents only an aliquot part of the total disturbance which extends more or less to all brain processes mediating the manifestation of conceptual ideas by learned sensory signs of any kind. (Finkelnburg, 1870, p. 461; see Chapter 1)

Modern versions of parallel breakdown of language and gesture went beyond Finkelnburg's rather vague postulate of a general deficiency of symbolic thought and made testable predictions concerning the similarities between language and gesture of aphasic patients. Patients with anterior lesions and non-fluent language production should produce few and simple gestures which are unequivocally interpretable, whereas patients with posterior lesions whose language production is fluent but distorted should produce many complex but incomprehensible gestures (Cicone et al., 1979; Behrmann & Penn, 1984; McNeill, 1992). The simplicity of these predictions was seductive but did not withstand scrutiny. On the contrary, Le May et al. (1988) registered a higher frequency of spontaneous gestures in patients with non-fluent than with fluent aphasia and Glosser et al. (1986) reported a significant negative correlation between length of verbal phrases and the number of gestures per words. Since higher fluency of speech is associated with longer phrases, the negative correlation indicates that patients with fluent speech produce fewer gestures than those with non-fluent speech. This is the opposite of the prediction derived from a parallel breakdown of language and gesture. It rather seems that the frequency of gestures depends on the severity of the expressive deficit: the less the patients can express verbally, the more they need gestures. Longer phrases transmit more verbal information and thus alleviate the need for compensatory gestures.

Likewise, the observation that gestures of non-fluent aphasics are less ambiguous than those of fluent speakers can be explained by reference to other linguistic parameters of these patients' speech. The severe reduction of verbal output forces them to have recourse to gestures for replacing speech. Among these gestures they prefer conventional gestures, that is, deictics (Fex & Mansson, 1998) and emblems (Cicone et al., 1979; Herrmann et al., 1988; Goodwin, 2000), because they pose less demands on creativity than pictographs or pantomimes. Herrmann et al. described conversations between such patients and their partners:

> The aphasic patients used significantly more often codified gestures as a mean of communication. This, however, in most instances was restricted to head nodding and shaking as signs of approval and disagreement and to shrugging of the shoulders to demonstrate incapacity of understanding or communicating. (Herrmann et al., 1988, p. 51)

Basic emblems have clearly defined shapes that carry little risk of being misunderstood. Their use secures the clarity and unambiguity of the aphasic patients' expression, but the clarity is paid for by a rigorous restriction of the contents that they can express. Rather than manifesting the preservation of gestural competency, their unambiguous comprehensibility results from the extreme reduction of the gestural repertoire.

In conclusion, similarities and discrepancies between defective language and defective gesturing in aphasia can better be explained by the interaction between their communicative roles than by their common origin. They do not confirm to the hypothesis that disturbances of communicative gestures and of speech are expressions of one and the same internal process.

Communicative gestures and apraxia

Remember that the diagnosis of apraxia for communicative gestures is based on their production on command. In the late 1980s, two studies explored whether this artificial test can predict the spontaneous use of gestures for compensating defective verbal output of patients with apraxia. On first sight their results seemed to be irreconcilable. Borod et al. (1989) found that success in production of gestures on command predicted higher values on a "non-vocal communication score" rated by nurses and therapists. By contrast, Feyereisen et al. (1988) found a negative correlation between the severity of apraxia and the amount of gestures use for transmission of messages in a "PACE" setting.[1] On reflection, however, the apparent discrepancy resolves into an interaction between the severity of aphasia and the amount and comprehensibility of spontaneous gestures. On Borod et al.'s non-vocal communication scale the nurses and therapists rated the frequency of gestures that successfully fulfilled predefined communicative functions as, for example, "uses gestures to greet or to summon attention" or "uses pantomime or drawings to show single things or actions." Classification of gestures along this scale obviously requires recognition of their communicative intent and thus implies rating not only of their frequency but also of their comprehensibility. Feyereisen et al. (1988) rated frequency and comprehensibility of gestures separately and found that the negative correlation between success on apraxia testing and use of gestures in the PACE setting was restricted to their frequency: patients with severe apraxia used more gestures than those with only mild or no apraxia. The obvious explanation of this seemingly paradoxal result was the covariance of the degree of apraxia with that of aphasia. The severely apraxic patients also had severe aphasia which limited their possibilities of verbal expression and forced them to compensate by gesturing. Indeed, the correlation reversed when the score on apraxia testing was compared to the proportion of gestural messages that were immediately understood by the communication partner. This proportion decreased with increasing severity of apraxia indicating that spontaneous gestures of patients with severe apraxia were more abundant but less comprehensible than those with only mild or no apraxia.

The correlation between testing communicative gestures on command and the communicative clarity of spontaneous gestures was corroborated in patients with dementia from Alzheimer's disease (Glosser et al., 1998). Spontaneous gestures were recorded during an interview and in a separate examination production of pantomimes on command was probed. Failure on the test of pantomimes was associated with higher proportions of "referentially unclear and non-specific" gestures.

Pantomime, semantics, and communicative gestures

We (Hogrefe et al., 2012) studied the predictive validity of pantomime of tool use for the communicative efficiency of spontaneous gestures in aphasic patients with very reduced verbal expression. For elicitation of gestures, patients were shown short video-clips of "Mr Bean" and "Tweety and Sylvester." Immediately after having seen a clip they were asked to

[1] PACE is an acronym for "promoting aphasics communication efficiency" (Davis & Wilcox, 1985). It designates a therapeutic method that concentrates on transmitting messages by any possible mean rather than on the linguistic correctness of verbal utterances. The patient and a partner each have pictures that cannot be seen by the other and try to communicate what is being shown on the picture. They may use any channel of communication.

retell what they had seen. Because of the severe reduction of verbal expression, retelling was equivalent to rendering the contents of the video-clips exclusively by gestures.

We used two approaches for analyzing the communicative efficiency of gestures. The first was a direct evaluation of their comprehensibility. Naïve subjects were familiarized with the model video-clips and were shown mute recordings of the patients' retelling. They were asked to guess, for each narration, which story was being told and to register which details of the stories they had recognized.

A second mode of evaluation was based on the consideration that greater structural diversity of gestures increases their capacity for transmitting information. Consequently, patients who produce structurally diversified gestures are likely to give a more informative account of the video-clips than patients whose gestures are more stereotyped. For the analysis of structural diversity, structural features of the gestures were transcribed into a reduced character set from the Hamburg Notation System for Sign languages (HamNoSys; Prillwitz et al., 1989). The transcription specified six features of the gestures, such as, for example, the finger configuration, the orientation and location of the hand, or the manner and direction of movements. As a measure of structural diversity we determined for each pair of gestures the number of diverging features and then the mean diversity across all pairs of the individual subjects (Jones & Jones, 2000; Hogrefe et al., 2011).

The results of both modes of evaluations confirmed the association between defective pantomime on command and insufficient spontaneous gesturing. The scores on pantomime correlated with the comprehensibility as well as with the structural diversity of the gestures produced for retelling the clips.

We also administered a test of non-verbal semantic classification (Glindemann et al., 2002). The test presents displays of four pictures, one of which differs from the others by a semantic feature, and subjects are asked to indicate the one picture that makes the exception (Figure 11.1). In half of the items the difference concerns a main semantic feature and in the other half a subordinate feature. Results on this test were also significantly correlated with the comprehensibility and structural diversity of spontaneous gestures. For the diversity of gestures the correlation with semantic classification was even somewhat stronger than that with pantomime, while for comprehensibility the correlation with pantomime was somewhat stronger.[2]

Asymbolia revived?

Neither the relationship of pantomime of tool use nor that of semantic classifications with the diversity and comprehensibility of spontaneous gestures are self-evident. If produced at all, pantomimes of tool use constituted only a minor proportion of the gestures used by patients for rendering the content of the video-clips. Generally, success of retelling

[2] Patients were also tested with the Aachener Aphasia Test that assesses different modalities of aphasic impairment (Huber et al., 1983). There were no significant correlations to any aspect of the spontaneous gestures, but this negative result might be due to a floor effect since our inclusion criterion of severely reduced verbal expression resulted in selection of only patients with severe aphasia.

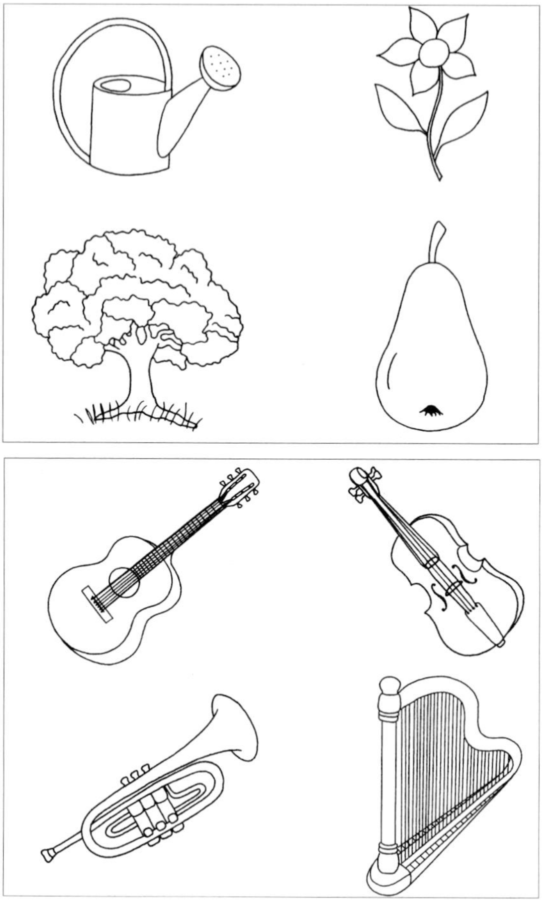

Figure 11.1 Two examples of the test of non-verbal semantic classification (Glindemann et al., 2002). Patients were asked to select the one picture that differs from the remaining three. In the upper example the difference concerns a main semantic feature (natural versus man-made) and in the lower example a subordinate feature (wind versus string instruments). Reproduced from Glindemann, R., Klintwort, D., Ziegler, W., and Goldenberg, G. *Bogenhausener Semantik-Untersuchung BOSU*, Copyright (2002) with permission of Elsevier.

depended not on a single type of gesture, but on the flexible combination of different kinds of "physiographs" in combination with a clever selection of features of the actors and their actions for gestural demonstration. Likewise, the predictive power of semantic classification links two very different motor actions: the production of expressive gestures and the selection of one picture out of an array of four. There is thus little superficial similarity between the predictors of efficient gestural communication and the execution of the communicative gestures. Their connection must be searched at a deeper level than the similarity of motor actions. Arguably it concerns the selection of significant features out of the multitude of properties associated with the objects of gestural demonstration or of semantic classification. In the case of gesturing, there is the additional difficulty of combining such features to a comprehensible demonstration. This particular difficulty is absent in semantic classification, but the necessity to ignore intuitively dominant features in favor of the particular feature that deviates in one out of four otherwise similar exemplars may be sufficiently challenging for invalidating this alleviation of the task.

Selection of significant features is a more mundane and restricted concept than Finkelnburg's "symbolic cognition" or McNeill's "inner speech" but it is recognizable as deriving from the same tradition of theorizing that had given rise to the concept of "asymbolia." We may conclude that the analysis of spontaneous gestures leads to a partial resurrection of the ostracized concept of asymbolia.

Language, gesture, and the left hemisphere

We started this chapter with a critical evaluation of Finkelnburg's claim that disturbances of speech and gesture in aphasia are expressions of one and the same basic deficiency of using symbols. The results were ambiguous. On the one hand we found that the relation between properties of aphasic speech and gesturing are determined by their mutual contributions to communication rather than by their parallel breakdown. On the other hand we found strong correlations of the comprehensibility and diversity of gestures to pantomimes of tool use and semantic classification. In Chapter 10 we concluded that pantomime depends on integrity of the left hemisphere. A substantial number of studies, dating mostly from the last third of the twentieth century, demonstrated exclusive left-hemisphere dependency also for semantic classification (De Renzi et al., 1969; Vignolo, 1990). It thus seems that communicative gestures share with language the vulnerability to left brain damage, but that their impairments are nonetheless distinct and partly independent.

In the following sections we will ask whether the experimental paradigms for assessment of communicative gestures are sufficient to cover the whole range of gestural communication and then discuss possible effects of right brain damage on communicative gestures.

Sharing the load of communication

Using gestures for retelling stories is more similar to everyday communication than producing gestures on command but remains a rather exceptional activity, particularly for patients with severe aphasia. A main difference between retelling and conversation in everyday life concerns the behavior of the communication partner. In the examination of retelling the examiner provides encouraging interjections and occasionally simple, open-ended questions for inciting the patient's production of speech and gestures, but she avoids making expressive gestures herself and does not offer suggestions for better formulations of unclear verbal or gestural expressions. This is different from communication with family or other partners who are willing to support the patient's communicative efficiency. In such settings conversation becomes a joint activity (Goodwin, 2000; Klippi, 2003; Garrod & Pickering, 2004). The conversational partners cooperate to ensure accord concerning the topic that is being negotiated, and they can succeed in structuring the conversation so that the aphasic participant needs only a very few, mostly emblematic, gestures supported by a rudimentary vocabulary of spoken words to convey their opinions and desires.

Division of the communicative load between aphasics and healthy speakers is not the only difference between formal examination of gestural expression and the use of gestures in conversation. Another difference concerns the importance of mimic expressions and whole body attitudes that express emotional responses and disambiguate approval or rejection of suggestions (Duffy & Buck, 1979; Buck & Duffy, 1980). They may support the comprehension of speech and gestures in conversation but are usually not considered for the formal analysis of gestural expressions.

Figure 11.2 presents anecdotic evidence that the correlation with pantomime of tool use that we found for gestural retelling of stories does not necessarily apply to the spontaneous production and comprehension of gestures in conversation. The diagrams are drawn from a video documenting the examination of pantomimes on command. The patient was severely apraxic and failed the pantomime of drinking water from a glass nearly completely. At the same time, however, she and the examiner entertained a quite refined gestural dialogue. Whereas the examination of pantomime had been directed by the examiner's instruction, the gestural dialogue commenting on that task was initiated and directed by the patient who used regulators (holding the hand to the mouth as an invitation to the examiner to explain what he was actually aiming at), ideographs (opening the hand for symbolizing the opening of the stage for the examiner's performance), and emblems (throwing

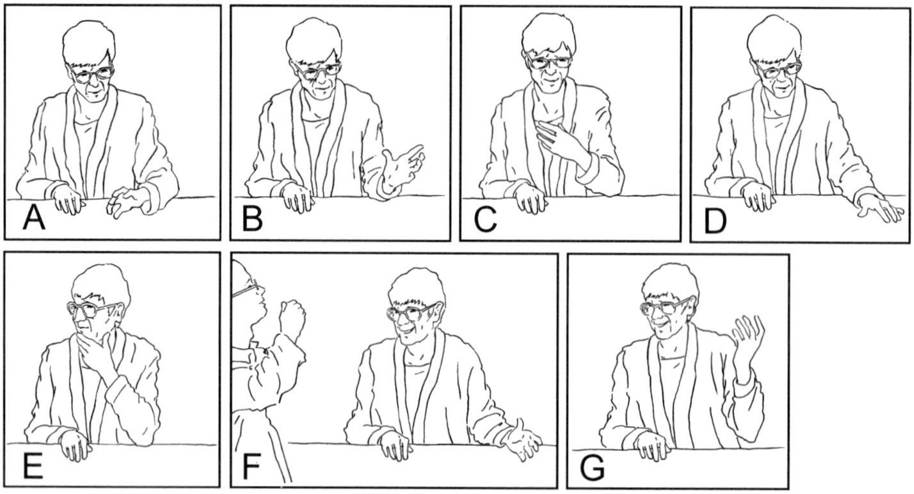

Figure 11.2 Dissociation between pantomime and gestural communication during the examination of pantomime of tool use: The patient had right-sided hemiparesis, global aphasia, and apraxia. She was asked to pantomime drink from a glass. A: The left hand outlines the approximate shape of the imaginary glass. B, C: The hand moves before the chest indicating but not specifying movement of the glass. D: She puts the hand on the table and moves the fingers as if she would bury the imaginary glass in the table. E: She raises the hand to the chin producing a gesture that seems to express a question or a demand for further explanation. F: The examiner reacts to the gestural quest and demonstrates the pantomime. The patient opens her left hand as if opening the space for the examiner's demonstration. G: She raises the hand and makes a movement as if she would throw away the gesture the execution of which is beyond her capacities. The gestural dialogue was detected only when the video was examined afterward. During the examination the examiner was not aware that he participated in a gestural dialogue. Reproduced from Goldenberg, G. *Neuropsychologie—Grundlagen, Klinik, Rehabilitation. 4. Auflage*, p. 161, Copyright (2007) with permission of Elsevier.

something behind her over the shoulder because it is of no use for her) to initiate and comment on a demonstration of the correct pantomime by the examiner.

The gestural dialogue was detected only when the video was inspected after the examination. During the gestural exchange the examiner did not note that in parallel to fulfilling the examination protocol he entertained a gestural communication with the patient. It was as if the examiner and the patient had split their control of gesturing in two independent streams, one following the instructions for pantomime of tool use and the other one engaged in interpersonal communication.

Right hemisphere gestures?

There was a time not long ago when an apparent division between two simultaneous streams of mental processing would have been greeted as a further example of the divide between the left and the right hemisphere (Sperry, 1961; Edwards, 1979; Gazzaniga, 2000; see Chapter 14). Longer ago, this divide was central to Jackson's influential distinction between voluntary and automatic processing that ascribed voluntary action to the left, and automatic processing to the right hemisphere (Jackson, 1932a; see Chapter 3). With this background it would be credible to ascribe the gestural dialogue shown in Figure 11.2 to right hemisphere activity independent from the left hemisphere's engagement in pantomime of tool use. Indeed, a recent study in patients with complete section of the corpus callosum (see Chapter 14) observed that these patients performed shoulder shrugs predominantly with the left side and pantomimes with the right hand (Lausberg et al., 2007). Since after section of the corpus callosum each hand is controlled exclusively by its opposite hemisphere this asymmetry would indicate that the shoulder shrugs were produced by the right hemisphere and the pantomime by the left. Shoulder shrugs refer directly to a question posed by the partner whereas pantomime describes absent objects and events. One might take this difference as the starting point for elaboration of a variant of Jackson's voluntary versus automatic distinction postulating that the right hemisphere directs gestures that relate to the immediate social interaction while the left hemisphere is responsible for referring to physically absent objects and events.

If the right hemisphere made different contributions to gesturing than the right, right brain damage should lead to clinical symptoms reflecting the loss of this contribution. Studies of gesturing in right brain damage are rare. They consistently report a reduction in the rate of gestures accompanying speech (Hadar et al., 1998; Cocks et al., 2007) but give no unequivocal evidence for qualitative change or impairment of gestures. It might well be that further studies examining larger groups of right brain damaged patients with more refined qualitative assessment of gestures do reveal significant contributions of the right hemisphere to spontaneous gesturing.

Understanding gestures

Communication requires not only production but also comprehension of signs. In aphasia the deficiency of verbal expression is frequently more impressive than that of understanding, but reduced comprehension of speech does constitute an additional obstacle for successful communication. It thus seems a legitimate question whether aphasic patients understand gestures better than language.

During the last 40 years a number of studies have explored the comprehension of gestures by patients with aphasia. All of them tested pantomime of tool use while only a handful also included emblematic gestures (Gainotti & Lemmo, 1976; Seron et al., 1979; Feyereisen et al., 1981; Ferro et al., 1983). Their main result can be summed up very briefly: patients with aphasia make more errors on tests of gesture comprehension than normal controls or patients with brain damage but without aphasia.

In contrast to the exploration of gesture production none of the studies concerned with comprehension of gestures attempted to approach the testing conditions to natural conversation. Most studies displayed pantomimes of tool use either on a cartoon or on videoclips or made by the examiner and asked patients to select from an array of pictures the object whose use was being demonstrated (Picket, 1974; Duffy et al., 1975; Gainotti & Lemmo, 1976; Varney, 1978; Seron et al., 1979; Ferro et al., 1983; Rothi et al., 1985; Varney & Damasio, 1987; Wang & Goodglass, 1992; Bell, 1994; Saygin et al., 2004). Variants of this basic paradigm included the selection of an image depicting a suitable context for emblematic gestures (Gainotti & Lemmo, 1976; Feyereisen et al., 1981), selection of a videorecorded pantomime corresponding to a verbally designated object (Buxbaum et al., 2005; Kalénine et al., 2010), or the verbal naming of demonstrated pantomimes (Negri et al., 2007b).[3]

Further variations of the test paradigm concern the selection of targets and distracters for the choice of the corresponding objects. While most of the studies include items with a semantic relationship to the target (e.g., for the pantomime of playing the guitar a violin) some of them also offer distracters which require similar motor actions as the target (e.g., for the guitar a rifle) (Wang & Goodglass, 1992; Bell, 1994; Saygin et al., 2004). Likewise, when the test requires selection of the pantomime that matches a given object, distracters may be either pantomimes demonstrating the correct use of another object, or pantomimes demonstrating use of the target object with a wrong hand shape or other deviations from the optimal configuration of the motor act (Heilman et al., 1982; Buxbaum et al., 2005).

Finally, correlations can be computed between success on the experimental tests and indices of the severity of aphasia and of apraxia *sensu stricto* that is, the production of gestures on command or in imitation. Last but not least the location of lesions responsible for deficient understanding of gestures can be evaluated by modern methods of structural imaging.

[3] The basic format of most of these tests is remarkably similar to the test of semantic classification that predicted comprehensibility and structural diversity of spontaneous gestures of aphasic patients. Following the argument brought forward in the discussion of the semantic classification test we may speculate whether the aphasic patients' difficulties with matching of gestures are just one more instance of defective selection of significant features (Vignolo, 1990). According to this account, the crucial factor for failure is the format rather than the content of the test.

The combination of these variations gave rise to a considerable number of studies with partly diverging or even conflicting results. I am not going to discuss them in detail nor try to find out which of the conflicting results are valid and which are not. I find it more interesting to follow the theoretical arguments presented in this line of research as they constitute another turn in the debate between high-level and low-level approaches to the understanding of gestures.

Recognition of pantomime: Asymbolia or motor simulation?

The first studies demonstrating defective understanding of gestures by aphasic patients were carried out in the mid-1970s (Picket, 1974; Duffy et al., 1975).They came about ten years after Goodglass and Kaplan's (1963) seminal paper that had reinstated Liepmann's account of apraxia as a disorder of motor control (see Chapter 4). Faulty recognition of gestures was brought forward as an argument against this revival, and as evidence that the:

> Gestural deficit in aphasic patients may be best explained as part of the total communicative deficit and not as a result of limb apraxia. (Picket, 1974, p. 84)

Support for a common basic deficit underlying all modalities of communication was provided by strong correlations between the failure rate on tests of gesture comprehension and indices of the severity of aphasia. Robert Duffy, a leading proponent of the asymbolia hypothesis, concluded from a study of pantomime recognition in aphasics:

> There is a common symbolic competence underlying gestural and verbal communication. Aphasia is an impairment of this symbolic competence. (Duffy et al., 1975; p. 127)

Further studies narrowed down the correlations of impaired pantomime recognition to severity of aphasia by demonstrating that it concerned predominantly language comprehension (Gainotti & Lemmo, 1976; Varney, 1978; Seron et al., 1979; Wang & Goodglass, 1992). This series of studies did not invoke the capacity for motor execution of the gestures as crucial for their understanding. A study which found that defective comprehension of pantomimes is predominantly caused by posterior temporal and adjacent inferior parietal lesions emphasized that lesions in this location are also associated with defective comprehension of written language but did not even mention the role of parietal lesions for faulty execution of gestures (Varney & Damasio, 1987).

However, the same finding of parietal lobe involvement in defective recognition of gestures was also brought forward in favor of a radically different interpretation of gesture recognition (Heilman et al., 1982; Ferro et al., 1983). It was based on Kleist's and Geschwind's version of the posterior to anterior stream of motor control. It was postulated that the origin of the stream is constituted by left parietal "visuo-kinesthetic engrams" which function as "master control for the kind of representational limb movements impaired in apraxia" (Geschwind & Damasio, 1985, p. 429; see Chapter 4). Destruction of these engrams would impair not only the execution of pantomimes and emblems but also their recognition. Consequently patients with left parietal lesions should commit errors when asked to discriminate correct from incorrect pantomimes of tool use whereas patients with more anterior lesions that interrupt the stream of motor control but do not destroy its origin should be able to recognize whether demonstrated pantomimes are correct or not in spite of being themselves unable to execute them (Heilman et al., 1982; Rothi et al., 1985; Bell, 1994; Buxbaum et al., 2005). We have discussed the evidence for storage of motor engrams in the parietal lobes in Chapter 10 and ended up with severe doubts on its reality. The point I want to make at this place is that the application of the alleged parietal motor engrams to the discrimination and comprehension of gestures assigns a perceptual function to motor representations.

The idea that motor representations support recognition of actions had previously been elaborated as a mechanism of speech perception (Liberman et al., 1967) and gained popularity as an explanation for a wide range of human capacities and behaviors in recent years. The popularity was encouraged by the detection of "mirror neurons" in monkey premotor cortex. They are similarly active when the monkey sees another monkey or human perform an action and when it performs the same action (Di Pellegrino et al., 1992; Rizzolatti & Sinigaglia, 2008). Support for the existence of mirror neurons in human beings was provided by functional imaging and electrophysiological studies showing that mere observation of actions automatically activates motor regions that would be involved in the execution of the same actions (Fadiga et al., 1995; Buccino et al., 2001). We have already discussed the possibility that damage to this "shortcut" from perception to execution of actions underlies defective imitation of gestures in Chapter 6, but found it implausible. This would not, however, necessarily exclude a role for recognition of action. Such a role has been elaborated in the context of a "simulation theory" of action recognition (Rizzolatti & Sinigaglia, 2010). According to this view the observation of other person's actions activates portions of motor cortex that would be appropriate to direct the motor execution of the same actions. Such motor simulation of observed actions should provide insight into the motor goals and intentions of the observed individual. Since motor neurons are located in the anterior part of the brain and since monkey mirror neurons were originally detected in frontal regions, frontal lobe damage would be expected to lead to defective recognition of gestures. Indeed, Giacomo Rizzolatti, the discoverer and leading theoretician of mirror neurons, wrote:

> The same frontal opercular region that appears to contain mirror neurons is also involved in action recognition. It is known that frontal patients with aphasic deficits are frequently impaired in pantomime recognition. (Rizzolatti & Matelli, 2003; p. 154)

As we have already seen, the clinical evidence points to a crucial role of parietal and posterior temporal rather than frontal lesions for defective recognition of gestures (Heilman et al., 1982; Ferro et al., 1983; Varney & Damasio, 1987; Wang & Goodglass, 1992; Kalénine et al., 2010), but there are indications that defective matching of objects to pantomimes could also be caused by inferior frontal region (Ferro et al., 1983; Saygin et al., 2004). Moreover, absence of consistent evidence for defective comprehension of pantomimes following frontal lesions would not necessarily invalidate the mirror neuron account, since mirror neurons have been postulated to also exist in the parietal lobes (Fogassi & Luppino, 2005). A more serious problem is that simulation based on activity of mirror neurons could afford understanding only for actions that are in our motor repertoire, but that the range of actions we can understand is much larger than the range of actions we can execute. A supplementary mechanism would be needed for understanding the multitude of actions that are not in our motor repertoire. Even if theoretically possible, such a duplication of cognitive mechanisms of action understanding would be awkward.

My refusal of a crucial role of mirror neurons for understanding actions goes back to the same basic argument as the refusal of a crucial role of stored motor programs of tool use for pantomime, discussed in Chapter 10. In both instances, the key problem is that the range of actions that we know and understand is much larger than the range of actions our motor system can execute.

Cognitive versus motor mechanisms of action understanding

From a clinical point of view our review of the literature on understanding of gestures was somewhat disappointing. It yielded experimental test results concerned mainly with the matching between gestures and pictures but did not even address the question of whether aphasic patients follow instructions or respond to questions better when they are expressed by gestures than when they are spoken. The doubts on the ecological importance of these results are compensated by their theoretical interest. The controversial accounts of defective understanding of gestures are remarkably clear in their classification of the disturbance as belonging to supramodal high or a motor-specific low level. The most radical variant of high-level accounts is the hypothesis of general asymbolia. The emphasis on the correlation between defective comprehension of gestures and language is a less radical variant that still postulates a supramodal communality between the disturbed functions. By contrast, low-level approaches emphasize the importance of motor representation not only for execution but also for comprehension of gestures. Their most popular version invokes mirror neurons as the neural substrate of a direct link from motor execution to the recognition of action. The classification of mirror neurons as a low level substrate of action recognition is justified by their modality-specific motor character, by their restriction to familiar actions, and by their automatic activation from the mere sight of actions.

Chapter 12

Apraxia in left-handers

Until now our discussion of the hemispheric lateralization of apraxia tacitly assumed that patients are right-handed, and that their left hemisphere is dominant for language as well as for control of the dominant hand. Since apraxia is mainly a symptom of left brain damage its laterality corresponds with both of these functions.

Speculations about a functional communality underlying the common lateralization emphasized either the relationship of apraxia to language or to that of motor control. We have encountered these theories already in the historical part of this book but let me briefly recapitulate them.

Liepmann related the dominance of the left hemisphere for movements made without external support explicitly to right-handedness. He argued that right-handedness implies not only that the right hand is more skillful than the left but also that:

> what the left hand can is to a large part not its (respectively the right hemisphere's) property, but is borrowed from the right hand (respectively, the left hemisphere). (Liepmann, 1908, pp. 34–35)

Liepmann believed that the superior motor competence of the left hemisphere explains why unilateral left-sided lesions cause bilateral apraxia. By contrast he downplayed the significance of the association between apraxia and aphasia. In his seminal group study he detected patients with left brain damage who had apraxia but no aphasia and others who had aphasia but no apraxia. From this double dissociation he concluded that aphasia and apraxia are independent symptoms of left brain damage.

Later, Liepmann tried to reconcile apraxia with aphasia. He advanced a theory of left-hemisphere motor dominance that included language. He speculated that the necessity to make movements without external support which is the core of left-hemisphere motor dominance applies also to articulation of speech and is thus fundamental for the left hemisphere's linguistic dominance too (Liepmann, 1908). He wrote:

> It is only when you withdraw the help from objects and force the patient to make movements wholly from memory that the insufficiency of the right hemisphere comes forward conspicuously. The right hemisphere is inferior to the left for the execution of movements without objects. However, the motor act of speaking is also a movement without objects. During speaking, tongue, mouth, and palate perform only shifts of their spatial relationships, like the hand in expressive movements or in pretending object use. The control that the ear exerts during speaking is not equivalent to the guidance that hand and ear receive from objects: The sound comes too late. The superiority of the left hemisphere for speaking can thus be referred to its general dominance for movements without objects, purely from memory. (Liepmann, 1908, p. 49)

In the modern literature, the Canadian psychologist Doreen Kimura (1982, 1983a) has been the most faithful proponent of Liepmann's ideas on the link between handedness and general motor dominance and also supported his speculations on the origins of language dominance.

The alternative emphasis on the relationship of apraxia with aphasia was implicit in Finkelnburg's concept of asymbolia as a common central disorder underlying defective speech and defective gestural expression. It found an explicit formulation in Steinthal's notion that "apraxia is an obvious amplification of aphasia" (see Chapter 1). Likewise, Goldstein's (1928, p. 238) dictum that aphasic patients' failure on tests of pantomime of tool use is not "a particular symptom of apraxia, but demonstrates a general change of behavior which in apraxia comes to the fore particularly clearly" presupposes aphasia itself as the most prominent manifestation of this change (see Chapter 3).

Emphasis on the correspondence of left lateralization with language or with motor control of the dominant hand can once again be interpreted as opposing a high-level to a low-level account of apraxia. The insistence on aphasia or general asymbolia as permanent companions of apraxia emphasizes the high-level cognitive side and the postulate of a close link to handedness the low-level motor side of apraxia.

Left-handers

Left-handedness is a salient deviation from the typical distribution of bodily asymmetries that has long incited fantasies and prejudices. Since the twentieth century, however, it has engendered a large body of objective scientific research. Paul Broca's (1865) ingenious insight that there is a coupling between right-handedness and the left hemisphere's dominance for speech has remained valid for the majority of right-handed persons, but the logical conclusion that there should be a similarly tight coupling between left-handedness and right-hemisphere dominance for language proved to be wrong. The proportion of right-hemisphere dominance for language is higher in left-handers than in right-handers, but the majority of left-handers have the competency for speech located in the left hemisphere (Hécaen et al., 1981; Kimura, 1983b; Knecht et al., 2000), that is, opposite to the hemisphere directing their dominant hand.

Neither is the brain of left-handers with right-hemisphere speech a mirror, nor is that of left-handers with left-hemisphere speech a faithful replication of the hemisphere asymmetries of functions in the standard right-hander brain. It rather seems as if the absence of right-handedness leads to a reshuffling of asymmetric brain functions resulting in a random distribution of their laterality. It may disrupt the neighborhood of functions that are regularly located in the same hemisphere of the right-hander brain or, conversely, unite in one hemisphere functions that in the right-hander brain are located in opposite hemispheres (Alexander & Annet, 1996; Tzourio-Mazoyer et al., 2004).

Pursuing the metaphor of reshuffling laterality of functions a step further, we note that shuffling cards can tear apart adjoining cards but cannot change the arrangement of different symbols printed upon each of them. We can relate this simple insight to the localization of cognitive functions by identifying the symbols on the cards with components of individual functions. The random distribution of laterality of functions in left-handers can tear apart individual functions but not the unity of their components. It thus becomes a window for looking not only into possible dissociation but also into obligatory associations between apparently independent function. If two of them are in fact subcomponents of one overarching function, they will always be located in the same hemisphere. For the association between aphasia, apraxia, and handedness this means that according to the high-level account apraxia should always be caused by lesions of the same hemisphere as aphasia, whereas on the low-level account apraxia should always be bound to lesions of the hemisphere controlling the dominant hand.

Is lateralization of apraxia weaker in left-handers than in right-handers?

It has been proposed that the left-hander brain differs from the typical right-hander brain not only in the distribution of lateralized functions to the left or right hemisphere, but also in the strength of asymmetry, and that functions that are clearly lateralized in the typical right-hander brain may be distributed across both hemispheres in the left-hander brain. Apraxia has been nominated as a candidate for such bilateral representation (Kimura, 1983b; Hécaen, 1984), but it is difficult to derive predictions of the incidence of apraxia in samples of left- and right-handed patients with unilateral left or right brain damage. On the one hand, the bilaterality of the neural substrate of apraxia in left-handers increases the probability that lesions to either hemisphere have an impact on it and should hence increase the overall incidence of apraxia in left-handers. On the other hand, when the neural basis of apraxia is distributed across both hemispheres lesions to one of them can be compensated by the other, and the clinical manifestations of their destruction will be only temporary or too mild to be detected. According to this reasoning the overall frequency of apraxia should be lower in left-handers than in right-handers. The literature rather favors the second possibility but the empirical support for a lower incidence of apraxia in left-handers is not compelling. For example, Doreen Kimura (1983b) found apraxia for imitation of meaningless gestures in 9% each of left- and right-brain damaged left-handers. This was distinctly lower than a frequency of 30% in right-handers with left brain damage. However, the frequency of apraxia in right-handers with right brain damage was only 3% and hence the mean incidence in right- or left-brain damaged right-handers 16%. Though still higher than the frequency of apraxia in left-handers, the difference has diminished considerably. In a study of our own (Goldenberg, submitted) study we found defective imitation of hand postures in 28% and defective pantomime of tool use in 35% of the left-handed patients. This is clearly below the incidences of 61% for defective imitation of hand postures and 66% for defective pantomime in right-handed patients with left brain damage and aphasia that had previously been examined with the same tests (Goldenberg & Karnath, 2006; Goldenberg et al., 2007b). However, the proportion of right-handed patients with right brain damage who has been classified as apraxic by the same tasks varies around 10% to 15% (Goldenberg, 1996; Goldenberg & Strauss, 2002; Hartmann et al., 2005; Goldenberg et al., 2009). The mean incidence of apraxia in right-handed patients with either left or right brain damage thus comes very close to the 30% observed in left-handers.

For imitation of finger configuration the results were less straightforward. The proportion of left-handed patients classified as apraxic remained some 10% lower than that of right-handed patients even when compared to the mean proportions of right and left brain damaged right-handers. There is, however, considerable variability of the incidence of defective finger imitation across multiple samples of right-handers (Goldenberg, 1996; Goldenberg et al., 2002, 2009), so that the 10% difference does not necessarily exceed the range of chance variation.

Is apraxia in left-handers milder than in right-handers?

A less equivocal consequence of the putative bilateral representation of apraxia in left-handers concerns the severity of apraxia. If the hypothesis of more bilateral organization of the neural substrate of apraxia in the left-hander brain is correct, apraxia should generally be milder in left-handers than in right-handers because in left-handers the undamaged hemisphere also contributes to the neural substrate of apraxia and thus mitigates the consequences of its loss in the damaged hemisphere (Hécaen, 1984).

I probed the validity of this prediction by comparing the mean scores on apraxia testing between left-handed and right-handed patients that had been classified as apraxic because they scored below the cut-off of healthy controls. All right-handers had left-hemisphere lesions whereas laterality of lesions was mixed in the left-handers. The results supported the prediction only partially. For imitation of meaningless hand and finger postures the means of apraxic left- and right-handers were virtually identical, but for pantomime of tool use the impairment of the left-handed patients was significantly less severe than that of the right-handers.

In sum, our results do not allow complete rejection of increased bilaterality but speak against bilaterality as the pervasive and dominant principle of the neural substrate of apraxia in left-handed persons. As in right-handers, apraxia in left-handers is essentially a bilateral disturbance caused by lesions of only one hemisphere.

Dissociations of apraxia from handedness and from aphasia

There is a substantial body of single-case reports of left-handed patients with right-sided lesions who were apraxic but not aphasic[1] (Heilman et al., 1973; Valenstein & Heilman, 1979; Margolin, 1980; Poeck & Lehmkuhl, 1980; Verstichel et al., 1994). By contrast,

[1] There are several case reports of left-handers in whom right brain lesions produced both aphasia and apraxia (Poeck & Kerschensteiner, 1971; Delis et al., 1983; Archibald, 1987; Ochipa et al., 1989) so that the right hemisphere's organization of laterality of functions mirrored that of the regular right-hander. Though valuable for demonstrating the wide range of possible combinations of functions in left-handers, these cases are not relevant for the question of whether apraxia can dissociate from aphasia and from handedness.

dissociation between apraxia and handedness manifested by apraxia from left-hemisphere lesions has not been considered worthwhile for single-case reports. It was, however, reported in systematic group studies (Kimura, 1983b; Hécaen, 1984).

The dissociation between the laterality of apraxia and aphasia has aroused more interest in case reports of right-handed persons who become aphasic after lesions of the right hemisphere. This variant of aphasia has been termed "crossed aphasia." A substantial number of single-case reports documented apraxia accompanying it (Assal et al., 1981; Basso et al., 1985; Rapcsak et al., 1987; Selnes et al., 1991; Raymer et al., 1999; Bartha et al., 2004). In these cases the laterality of apraxia corresponds with that of aphasia but not with control of the dominant hand.

Splitting up the dissociations

The possibility that the closeness of apraxia to aphasia or handedness differs between different manifestations of apraxias has not been considered by any of the studies discussed so far. Most of them used a combination of performance of communicative gestures on command and in imitation to assess apraxia, while a small minority probed imitation of meaningless gestures (Kimura, 1983b; Archibald, 1987), but none compared both kinds of gestures.

We made this important distinction and examined separately imitation of meaningless hand and finger postures and pantomime of tool use (Goldenberg, submitted) in 50 consecutive left-handed patients who had been admitted to our department for rehabilitation after stroke in either the left or the right hemisphere. Twenty-three out of 28 patients with left brain damage but only six out of 22 with right brain damage were aphasic. The preponderance of left-hemisphere dominance for language also in left-handers contradicts the idea that their brain is a mirror of the right-handers brain but accords well with previous systematic studies (Hécaen et al., 1981; Kimura, 1983b; Knecht et al., 2000).

When looking for dissociations between apraxia on the one hand, and aphasia or handedness on the other, we must bear in mind that in spite of its dependence on left-hemisphere integrity, apraxia is not an obligatory consequence of left brain damage even in right-handers. Lesions may affect the responsible hemisphere but miss the critical regions within the hemisphere. Consequently, the absence of apraxia does not constitute a strong argument against its localization in the affected hemisphere. Stronger evidence for dissociations between the laterality of apraxia and that of aphasia or of dominant motor control is provided by patients who have apraxia but either no aphasia or no damage to the hemisphere directing the dominant hand.[2]

[2] For the dissociation between aphasia and apraxia even apraxia without aphasia does not mandatorily imply different laterality of their substrates. There are cases of apraxia without aphasia following lesions to the left hemisphere of right-handed persons. However, these cases are rather rare and typically confined to visuo-imitative apraxia (see Chapter 6), whereas we have not yet found evidence for pantomime disturbance without aphasia in right-handers (see Chapter 10).

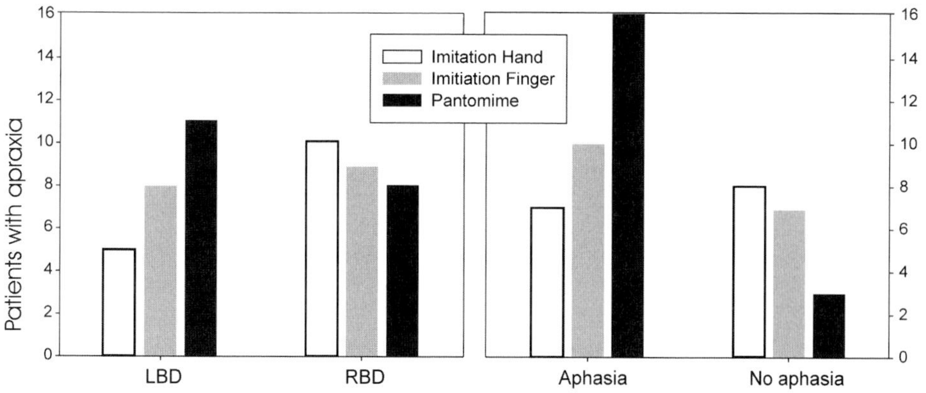

Figure 12.1 Frequencies of apraxia for imitation of hand and finger posture and for pantomime in 50 left-handed patients: the results of apraxia testing are presented in relation to the laterality of lesions in the left graph, and in relation to the presence or absence of aphasia in the right one. Apraxia resulting from left brain damage indicates dissociation from handedness, whereas apraxia in patients without aphasia indicates dissociation from language. Both kinds of dissociations occur for each of the three variants of apraxia, but the dissociation between defective pantomime and preservation of language is rare. The three patients showing this dissociation had right brain damage.

Figure 12.1 demonstrates that both types of dissociations occurred with considerable frequency. There was no unequivocal instance of dissociation from both aphasia and handedness as would be constituted by apraxia without aphasia from a left-sided lesion. The equivocal exceptions were two patients with a left-sided lesion but no aphasia, one of which scored slightly below the normal range only on imitation of finger postures and the other on imitation of hand postures.

Closer inspection of Figure 12.1 reveals interactions between the frequency of dissociations and the type of gestures. The most striking deviation from a random distribution is the rareness of dissociations between aphasia and pantomime. Only three out of 19 patients with impaired pantomime had no aphasia. The strong tendency for co-occurrence of defective pantomime and aphasia fits well with previous studies showing significant correlations between pantomime of tool use, subtests of the Aachen Aphasia Test, and tests of functional association (Goldenberg, 2003b; Goldenberg et al., 2003; Hartmann et al., 2005). We may speculate that the communality that favors neighborhood of localization is the importance of easy access to semantic memory. At the same time, however, the three left-handed patients whose impairment of pantomime was not accompanied by aphasia (see Figure 12.1) provide the missing piece of evidence for the independence of pantomime from language that we could not unequivocally derive from the analysis of defective pantomime in right-handed patients (see Chapter 10).

A less conspicuous but statistically significant asymmetry concerns imitation of hand postures. Its impairment is more frequent after lesions of the right than after lesion of the left hemisphere. Again, however, the association is not mandatory. There were five patients with defective imitation of hand postures caused by left-hemisphere lesions. Moreover, a detailed analysis showed that defective imitation by right brain damaged patients was associated with the presence of hemineglect. Remember that we found an influence of hemineglect on imitation also in right-handed patients with a right-sided lesion, although for them it was largely confined to imitation of finger rather than hand postures. The correlation with hemineglect points nevertheless to the possibility that the association between right hemisphere lesions and apraxia for imitation in left-handed patients is mediated by spatial and attentional functions of the right hemisphere rather than by its control of the dominant hand.

Coming back to the metaphor of shuffling cards, the observation of the differential relationships of imitation of hand postures and of pantomime of tool use suggest that they are not figures on the same card. Traditionally both of them have been subsumed under the heading of "ideo-motor apraxia." Their differential tendencies for co-localization with aphasia or handedness in the brains of left-handed people are a further argument against the validity of the putative entity "ideo-motor apraxia."

The independence of apraxia

In the introduction to this chapter I argued that obligatory association of apraxia with aphasia emphasizes the high-level cognitive, and a close link to handedness the low-level motor side of apraxia. The empirical results revealed that neither of these associations is obligatory. It seems that the attempt to distinguish the cognitive from the motor side of apraxia by analysis of its co-occurrence with aphasia or motor control of the dominant hand has failed. However, the observation that the laterality of apraxia can vary independently from aphasia or handedness does not alter the basic fact that its cerebral substrate is lateralized at all. Although the evidence is not sufficient for a complete rejection of increased bilaterality of the cerebral substrate of apraxia in left-handers, the main principle is, as in right-handers, that unilateral lesions cause bilateral disturbances of manual actions. In Chapter 15 I will argue that this lateralization is a key to understanding the interplay of high- and low-level mechanism of action control. Before doing so, however, I will try to disentangle apraxia from other instances of bilateral motor disturbances caused by unilateral brain damage. This will be the topic of Chapter 13.

Chapter 13

Approaching apraxia from the motor side

If we had to make an interim assessment of the balance of evidence supporting "high-level" cognitive or "low-level" motor explanations of apraxia it would be in favor of the cognitive side. Regardless of whether we considered imitation, production of communicative gestures, or tool and object use, none of the observations purported to demonstrate faulty motor execution of correctly conceived gestures and actions as being at the core of apraxic errors, withstood critical discussion. Before closing the issue and declaring victory for "high-level" accounts we should consider the possibility that the bias in their favor was due to limits of observation. Most of the evidence was derived from clinical examination: the examiner advised the patients what to do and rated the quality of the gestures or actions produced in response. Quite frequently the reliability of rating was enhanced by video recording enabling later careful analysis by several judges or by preparation of defined criteria for rating, but in all instances the substrate of assessment was the visible movement of the patient's limbs. Limb movements are produced by coordinated movements of multiple muscles and joints, but the smoothness and efficiency of their coordination is not necessarily transparent to observation of the resulting limb action. As a further restriction, the temporal resolution and the attentional capacity of human vision are limited. It might be the case that visual observation misses significant features of motor actions because the actions are too fast or happen outside of the focus of attention.

In a way, the visible movements during production of gestures and actions form a macro level that hides a micro level of motor action. It might be conceivable that direct investigations of the micro level bring forward defects of motor coordination that influence or even cause errors at the macro level. Basically, two approaches have been tried for documenting and analyzing motor mechanisms at the micro level that possibly underlie the visible errors justifying a diagnosis of apraxia: kinematic measurement of the gestures and actions produced in the examination of apraxia, and experimental investigation of more simple and "elemental" motor actions such as pointing and grasping by patients with brain damage and apraxia. We will discuss them in turn.

Kinematic analysis of apraxic motor actions

Kinematic analysis of movements is based on high-resolution recording of the temporal and spatial trajectory of limbs or their parts in three-dimensional space. Typically, markers are fixed on selected points at arms or hands. Coordinates of their position are transmitted to a central recording device where they are sampled for reconstruction of their spatial and temporal trajectory. Depending on the technical properties of the device, spatial accuracy of the recording is in the range of less than a millimeter and temporal accuracy may be below ten milliseconds (100 Hz), both surpassing by far the capacity of the naked eye.

In a seminal series of studies, Howard Poizner and colleagues (Poizner et al., 1990; Clark et al., 1994; Poizner et al., 1995, 1998) applied kinematic recording to pantomime of tool use and to real tool use by a few patients with apraxia and compared them to healthy controls. The patients produced obvious apraxic errors during the kinematic recording. For example, they made a chopping rather than a slicing motion when pantomiming the cutting of bread. Kinematic analyses revealed abnormalities beyond the obvious aberration of the location and direction of the moving hand. In particular, the coordination between shoulder, elbow, and wrist movements was not well synchronized, resulting in irregular rather than fluid movement of the hand. It also appeared that patients immobilized their elbow and wrist and performed movements that normally result from synergy of shoulder, elbow, and wrist movements from only the shoulder.

The authors interpreted their results in the tradition of Kleist, Geschwind, and Heilman (who was member of the group) as indicating a loss of "visuo-kinesthetic motor representation of learned movements." Since these engrams are believed to specify both the spatial course of gestures and the coordination of joint actions producing them, their breakdown should affect both aspects of the gesture equally. Consequently the authors did not consider the possibility of dissociations between defective joint coordination and defective spatial course of actions.

Is the association of kinematic abnormalities with apraxic errors mandatory?

The mandatory association of kinematic abnormalities with apraxic errors was called into doubts in a study by our group, led by Joachim Hermsdörfer (Hermsdörfer et al., 1996). We examined the velocity profiles of movements of the hands ipsilateral to the lesioned hemisphere in patients with right or left brain damage during imitation of meaningless hand postures like those discussed in Chapter 7. The analysis was based on the widely recognized distinction between a transport phase and an adjustment phase of goal-directed limb movement (Woodworth, 1899; Meyer et al., 1990). The transport phase brings the hand in close proximity to the target. It consists of an initial acceleration that leads to a single peak of maximum velocity followed by deceleration. The subsequent adjustment phase is slower and has no distinct velocity peak. Its length varies depending on the accuracy of the transport phase and the resulting need for further adaptation of the hand location. Though not uncontroversial, there is a widespread agreement that transport relies more on ballistic open-loop and adjustment on feedback-dependent closed-loop motor control (Brooks, 1986; Jeannerod, 1988).

In addition to the kinematic measurement we recorded whether or not the path of the imitating hand ended at the correct posture, that is, whether imitation was correct or apraxic.

On first sight the results were quite clear-cut: only patients with left brain damage showed kinematic abnormalities consisting of reduced maximal velocity, additional velocity peaks during the transport phase, and prolongation of the adjustment phase. The rating of the spatial accuracy of the final position of the hand confirmed our previous finding (see Chapter 7) that difficulties with imitation of these meaningless hand postures are also restricted to patients with left brain damage. Thus, patients with left brain damage displayed both kinematic abnormalities and apraxic errors of imitation. There was, however, no correlation at all between the severities of both deficits. There were left brain damaged patients in whom both measurements yielded pathological results, but there were also patients who produced kinematically aberrant movements ending in correct final positions and others who made kinematically flawless movements to wrong positions. A recent study confirmed the dissociation between kinematic abnormalities and apraxic errors for pantomime of tool use (Hermsdörfer et al., 2012).

There are two possible explanations for the common occurrence of apraxic errors and kinematic abnormalities in patients with left brain damage. The first one would be that the kinematic abnormalities were indirect consequences of apraxic errors. Patients may have realized their difficulties in translating the decisive features of the demonstrated gesture to their own body and reacted to their insecurity and helplessness by hesitating and searching movements. Such a reactive change of movement style could also explain some of the abnormalities found in the kinematics of pantomime by Poizner et al. An alternative explanation would be that apraxic errors and kinematic abnormalities are independent sequels of left brain damage. Indeed, some support for the existence of two parallel but independent impairments was provided by a later study that used the same paradigm for assessment of imitation, but combined it with kinematic analysis of precise pointing to a labile target. There was again no correlation between kinematic abnormalities and spatial accuracy of imitation, but a significant correlation between the velocity profiles of imitation and of pointing (Hermsdörfer et al., 2003).

Experimental investigations of pointing, reaching, and grasping

This approach aims to get closer to the micro level of motor control by reducing the complexity of the tasks that are investigated. In the majority of studies they are variants of pointing, reaching, and grasping, that is, the most elemental goal-directed motor acts. This reduction of complexity enables tight control of task performance and exact measurement of movement parameters. It is, however, paid for by substantial differences between experimental conditions and the clinical diagnosis of apraxia (for critical discussion see Iestwaart et al., 2006).

In the typical clinical examination of apraxia the patient faces the examiner who either verbally or by demonstration or by provision of tools and objects invites the patient to perform a defined gesture or action. If the patient fails there may be a second trial, and eventually even a third, but never more. Then another gesture or action is probed. The diagnosis thus essentially rests on examination of multiple different gestures or actions, each of which is probed once or twice. Repetitive performance of one gesture or action is not a regular component of apraxia testing. As already discussed at the beginning of this chapter, the evaluation of apraxic errors is made by observation with the naked eye and is thus limited by the temporal resolution and the attentional capacity of human vision.

By contrast, in the typical setting of experimental investigations of pointing, reaching, and grasping, the patient is confronted with a more or less abstract target (e.g., a light diode, a cylinder, etc.) and has to perform one type of action upon this target repeatedly. There may be changes of single parameters of the action, such as, for example, the angle of reaching to a target, between repetitions but each setting of the parameters is itself repeated multiple times. Most importantly, the patient's motor actions remain the same and practice trials guarantee that they are performed correctly. For example, when the motor act is pointing with a stylus to targets of different width (Haaland et al., 1987; Winstein & Pohl, 1995; Haaland et al., 1999) there is no question of apraxia manifesting itself by "grasping the pen upside down" (Steinthal, 1871; see Chapter 1).

Evaluation of performance is based on exact measurement and statistical sampling of multiple trials rather than on direct observation of single trials. The multiplicity of trials can make even very small differences statistically significant. Experiments frequently include more than hundred trials and significant differences between groups or between conditions rarely surpass one second for temporal, and one centimeter for spatial parameters (Winstein & Pohl, 1995; Hermsdörfer et al., 2003; Haaland et al., 2004; Schaefer et al., 2007; Mutha et al., 2011). The generalization from these statistical group differences to clinical manifestations of apraxia in individual patients is not necessarily obvious.

With a single exception (Mutha et al., 2011), all experimental studies examined motor actions of the hand ipsilateral to the brain lesion. Most of them compared left brain damaged patients with right brain damaged patients or healthy controls using the left limb, and only some of them also compared left brain damaged patients with and without a clinical diagnosis of apraxia or looked for a correlation between experimental findings and severity of apraxia.

Repetitive pointing and tapping

In 1975, Heilman and collaborators reported that repetitive tapping on a single lever was slower in patients with aphasia and apraxia in comparison to patients with aphasia but without apraxia, and that the degree of slowing correlated with the severity of apraxia (Heilman, 1975). A number of subsequent studies by other groups failed to replicate this finding (Kimura, 1977; Haaland et al., 1980; Haaland, 1984; Hanna-Pladdy et al., 2002), but two more recent studies replicated the correlation between velocity of finger tapping and severity of apraxia as assessed by imitation of meaningless hand postures in patients with left brain damage (Hermsdörfer & Goldenberg, 2002; Iestwaart et al., 2006). In both of these studies the correlations were mainly due to the extreme results of few (two out of seven in Iestwaart et al., and four out of 39 in Hermsdörfer et al.) patients with very severe apraxia. Possibly, reduced velocity of finger tapping was a sign of general slowing related to the global size and severity of brain damage which, in turn, are correlated with the severity of apraxia. However, in view of the many differences between simple finger tapping and imitation of complex gestures the correlation awaits further replications before being accepted as reliable.

More consistent abnormalities were found in studies exploring alternating tapping on two spatially distant targets. The average movement time from one target to the other depends on the proportion between their distance and their width. It increases with increasing distance and with decreasing width (Fitts, 1954). It is a generally accepted presumption that motor control for tapping relatively wide targets at small distances relies mainly on open-loop ballistic movements whereas tapping narrow targets at larger distances depends more on feedback controlled adjustments at the end of the movement path. Several studies documented that patients with left brain damage gained less speed with increasing target width than right brain damaged patients or controls (Haaland et al., 1987; Haaland & Harrington, 1994; Winstein & Pohl, 1995). This led to the hypothesis that left brain damage interferes specifically with open-loop ballistic motor control (Winstein & Pohl, 1995).

The relevance of this hypothesis for the clinical manifestations of apraxia is not obvious. Our finding that increased reliance on feedback-controlled slow movements for imitation of hand positions did not at all correlate with the error rate indicates again a decisive role of the mode of motor control for apraxic errors. Moreover, during clinical examination for apraxia a majority of motor actions including, for example, the pantomime or tool use, actual tool use, and imitation of finger configuration, enable visual control by the patients, and examiners do not usually exert pressure on speed that could motivate the patients to prefer fast ballistic over slow feedback-controlled movements. Their errors arise in spite of the possibility to compensate for an isolated degradation of ballistic movements by feedback control. Finally, the demonstration that patients who make errors on imitation of hand postures are also impaired when asked to replicate them on a manikin (see Chapter 6) is hardly compatible with a selective disturbance of open-loop ballistic movements, because manipulation of the manikin is performed mainly under visual and tactile feedback and hence should not be severely affected by degradation of open-loop ballistic movements.

Simple grasping

The clinical impression that grasping objects with the left hand is preserved in patients with left brain damage is confirmed by the few experimental studies devoted to this ecologically important aspect of motor control (Hermsdörfer et al., 1999b; Iestwaart et al., 2001, 2006). It may be mildly slowed down in relation to normal controls but is not slower than grasping by patients with right brain damage. Like normal controls, the patients scale grip width to the size of the objects and adapt grip strength to its weight when lifting them (Iestwaart et al., 2006; Dawson et al., 2010; Li et al., 2011).

Accuracy of reaching and scaling of grip width to location and size of objects remain perfect when their sight is withdrawn and patients are allowed to start their action only five seconds later based on their memory of the preceding presentation (Iestwaart et al., 2001). All subjects of this experiment had severe apraxia for imitation of hand postures.

Their preserved reaching and grasping from memory contradict Liepmann's statement that apraxic errors come to the fore most conspicuously when movements are to be performed "purely from memory" (see Chapter 2).

Overhand versus underhand grip

The definition of apraxia as a disorder of higher levels of motor control invites looking for variants of grasping where the choice of the grip is not exhausted by adaptation of the grip to the presented object but also demands planning ahead of the actions to be performed with the grasped object. A paradigm that demands planning ahead of future actions for the selection of hand movements was introduced by Rosenbaum et al. (1990). It is illustrated in Figure 13.1. Subjects have to grasp a horizontal bar and place it perpendicularly into a hole. In the control condition they are free to choose which end of the bar they put into the hole, while in the experimental condition one end of the bar is marked, and subjects have to put this end into the hole. The starting position of the hand is always palm down. Subjects are free to choose whether they prefer to grasp the bar with an underhand or an overhand grip but must not change the grip between grasping and inserting the bar. In the crucial condition the mark of the bar points medially from the acting hand, that is, to the right when subjects use the left hand and vice versa. In this arrangement the overhand grip is more comfortable because it does not require rotation of the hand, but this initial comfort is paid for by a biomechanically strained final rotation of the hand for inserting the marked end (see Figure 13.1). In this conflict normal subjects opt for the final comfort. They grasp the bar with the less comfortable underhand grip in order to maximize the final comfort. Since this choice demands planning ahead, it can be conceived as constituting an instance of "higher-level" action control.

We used this paradigm for exploring the planning ahead of movements in patients with left or right brain damage and healthy controls (Hermsdörfer et al., 1999a). We recorded not only grip choice but also the kinematic parameters of the hand movements. We expected that left brain damaged patients, particularly when apraxic, would fail on the crucial condition where the immediate comfort of grasping the bar in conflict with the final comfort of its insertion, but the actual results were less straightforward. Abnormal performance characterized by disregard of the final comfort and perseveration of overhand grip was seen in patients with right brain damage who were also slower than the other groups.[1] Patients with left brain damage selected the ultimately comfortable grip as reliably as controls. Apparently planning ahead of one movement step for making a dual choice between two possible orientations of the same type of grip was not sufficient for bringing into play left lateralized mechanisms of bilateral action control.

While the selection of the optimal grip was not affected by left brain damage, kinematic recording of movement paths leading to the underhand grip revealed an unexpected

1 Osiurak et al. (2008a) conducted a very similar experiment. They replicated the prevalence of suboptimal grip selection by patients with right brain damage but found some reduction of optimal choices also in patients with left brain damage.

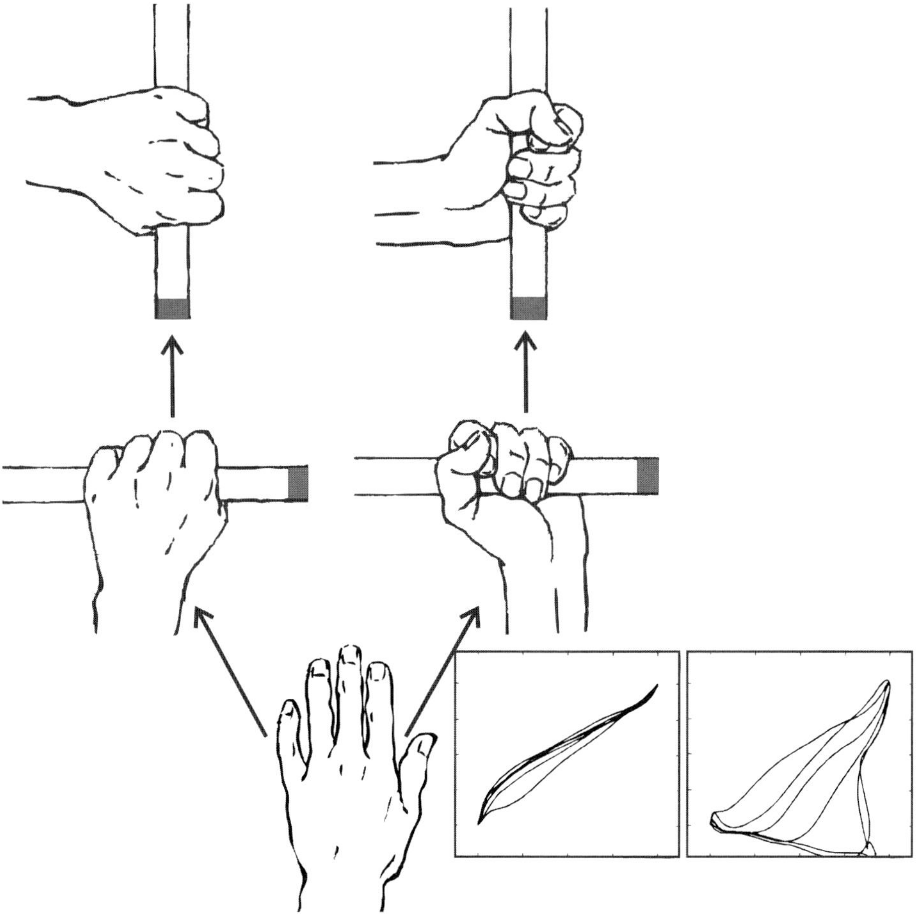

Figure 13.1 The schema illustrates the alternative paths of the hand for overhand or underhand grip in the Rosenbaum paradigm (data from Rosenbaum et al., 1990). Left: The overhand grip is less strained and the path to it is simpler because the starting position and grip are both palm down. However, insertion of the shaded end of the bar into the hole results in an uncomfortably strained final position. Right: The path from the starting position demands not only transport but also a rotation of the hand and the grasping position is strained, but the final position is comfortable. Insert: Both controls and patients with left brain damage prefer the underhand approach, but the movement to the grip differs. Whereas controls combine the transport of the hand from the starting position to the bar and the rotation from the palm down to the palm up position into one smooth movement path, patients with left brain damage tend to split the two components into two consecutive movements. Cartoon based on description of task in Rosenbaum, D. A., Marchak, F., Barnes, H. J., Vaughan, J., Slotta, J. D., & Jorgensen, M. J. Constraints for action selection: Overhand versus underhand grips. In M. Jeannerod (Ed.), *Attention and Performance XIII Motor Representation and Control* (pp. 321–342). Copyright (1990), Lawrence Erlbaum. The inserts are adapted from Hermsdörfer, J., Laimgruber, K., Kerkhoff, G., Mai, N., & Goldenberg, G. (1999). Effects of unilateral brain damage on grip selection, coordination, and kinematics of ipsilesional prehension. *Exp.Brain.Res.* 128:41–51, by permission of Springer.

deviation. The starting position of the hand was with the palm down. For reaching overhand grips the hand had to make both a forward movement and a rotation. Controls and patients with right brain damage combined both elements to one straight smooth movement. By contrast, patients with left brain damage tended to split the trajectory of the hand into two consecutive phases. They first moved the hand close to the bar and only then rotated it to the underhand grip posture (see Figure 13.1).

It seems worthwhile to remain a bit longer on the splitting of directional elements of grasping in left brain damage. The forward movement is mainly driven by anteversion of the upper arm in the shoulder and the adaptation of the hand to the angle of the bar by rotation in the elbow. The splitting of both elements is thus associated with a reduction of the number of simultaneously moved joints. This reminds of the apraxic patients examined by Poizner et al. (1995) who immobilized elbow and wrist and performed movements that normally result from synergy of shoulder, elbow, and wrist only from the shoulder. However, in our study neither the discontinuity of the movement path for grasping nor any other kinematic features of the left brain damaged patients' movements correlated with the severity of apraxia as assessed by imitation of meaningless hand postures.

Experimental variations of pointing

A recent series of studies took up the topic of accurate pointing again, but this time with a technical device that permitted rapid changes of the visually perceived location of targets as well as manipulations or withdrawal of visual feedback from the subject's moving hand, and combined fine-grained measurement of accuracy of movements with kinematic analysis of their velocity profile.

Schaefer et al. (2007) compared rapid pointing to one of two possible targets between patients with left and right brain damage. The sequence of both targets was randomized so that subjects could plan their movement only immediately before the start. As soon as their hand left the home position to reach for the target, visual feedback from the moving hand was withdrawn so that patients could not themselves evaluate the accuracy of their pointing. The left hands of left brain damaged patients nonetheless hit the targets as accurately as the left hands of controls, but the right hand of right brain damaged patients was less accurate than the right hands of controls. In a follow-up experiment (Schaefer et al., 2009) the number of possible targets was augmented to three, and one of them was placed medial to the shoulder putting high demands on multijoint coordination. Again, accuracy of reaching was reduced only in patients with right brain lesions but this time the movement trajectories of the left brain damaged patients displayed conspicuous abnormalities. Particularly for the medial target the trajectories were curved rather than straight. Patients partitioned the medially and anteriorly oriented straight connection from the start to the target position of the hand into two consecutive trajectories, the first leading medially and the second anteriorly. The similarity of this finding to the distortion of reaching for underhand grip and presumably also to the reduction of simultaneous joint actions in the kinematic analysis of the pantomime of slicing bread is remarkable.

Somewhat surprisingly, in both studies the proportion of patients with a clinical diagnosis of apraxia based on imitation was the same in left and right brain damaged patients. There were no significant differences of any parameter between patients classified as apraxic or not. However, a further study using the same apparatus and experimental design for a comparison between apraxic and non-apraxic left brain damaged patients confirmed that the deformation of the path to the medial target was more marked in apraxic patients than in left brain damaged patients without apraxia (Mutha et al., 2010).

A further study from the same group (Mutha et al., 2011) exploited the possibilities of the experimental device for distortion rather than withdrawal of visual feedback. Subjects pointed in a randomized sequence to eight circularly arranged targets. In a first run they received unaltered visual feedback of their moving hand. In a second series of trials feedback deviated 30 degrees from the actual movement direction, while in the final series it was veridical again. The deviation of feedback has the same effect as the well-known paradigm of prism adaptation (Hay et al., 1965; Rossetti et al., 1998). Subjects first miss the target, then add a final correction to their movements and finally adapt the transformation of visual location in motor action so that their movements lead straight to the visible locations of the targets. When vision is normalized again, subjects show an after-effect of adaptation and their pointing deviates to the opposite side of the primary deviation, but after several trials normal visuo-motor coordination is re-established.

Mutha et al. examined adaptation to the shift of visual feedback from the moving hand in patients with left and right parietal brain damage and healthy controls. Differing from the usual practice, however, they examined the hand contralateral to the lesion. When the deviation of feedback from the moving hand was introduced all groups reacted with the addition of final corrective movements. In the further series, however, controls and patients with right parietal lesions integrated the deviation into their motor planning and reached the targets with straight movements without additional corrections. By contrast, the patients with left brain damage remained dependent on final corrections even after more than 200 trials of reaching with feedback distortion. The inflexibility of their visuo-motor coordination paid off when the distortion was removed again. In contrast to the other groups they had no after-effect and pointed straight to the targets without a need for re-adaptation.

Revisiting handedness

Throughout this review I have repeatedly mentioned relationships between experimental abnormalities of motor control and the clinical diagnosis of apraxia but I discussed them in detail only for the dissociation between kinematics and spatial accuracy of imitation. I will now sum up the evidence from the experiments of repetitive pointing, reaching, and grasping.

A majority of these studies compared right and left brain damaged patients. Even when they reported the proportion of patients classified as apraxic, no additional comparisons were carried out between apraxic and non-apraxic left brain damaged patients (Haaland &

Delaney, 1981; Haaland et al., 1987, 2004; Haaland & Harrington, 1994; Winstein & Pohl, 1995; Hanna-Pladdy et al., 2002; Schaefer et al., 2009; Mutha et al., 2011). A handful of studies compared left brain damaged patients with apraxia to those without and found more deficits in the apraxic patients (Harrington & Haaland, 1992; Haaland et al., 1980; 1999; Mutha et al., 2010). In one study (Haaland et al., 1994) the influence of apraxia was completely different from the main effect of lesion laterality. Whereas the main effect of laterality was that repetitive pointing of left brain damaged patients gained less speed with increasing target width than that of right brain damaged patients or controls, apraxic patients differed from other left brain damaged patients by less accurate pointing to the smallest targets.

Finally, there are several studies that calculated correlations between repetitive motor performance and the severity of apraxia. With the sole exception of the controversial correlation between speed of finger tapping and severity of apraxia (Heilman, 1975; Hermsdörfer & Goldenberg, 2002; Iestwaart et al., 2006) they failed to reach statistical significance (Haaland, 1984; Hermsdörfer et al., 1999a; 1999b; 2002; 2003; 2012; Iestwaart et al., 2006; Schaefer et al., 2007).

In sum, statistical support for a tight or even causal relationship between defective motor execution of repetitive movements and apraxia is equivocal. The evidence would be better compatible with damage to two independent mechanisms that are both located in the same hemisphere.

A role for ipsilateral motor control

A possible candidate for a mechanism that could contribute to the influence of left brain on motor control of the ipsilateral hand could be the combination of ipsilateral projections from motor cortex to the limbs with handedness. The existence of ipsilateral motor efferences had already been a central argument for Geschwind's theory of apraxia. However, Geschwind believed that these projections derive from brain regions outside the motor cortex and influence only proximal limb movements (Geschwind, 1975; see Chapter 4). By contrast, modern studies using functional imaging and transcranial magnetic stimulation have provided ample proof for the involvement of primary motor and adjacent premotor cortex in the control of ipsilateral motor actions of the whole limb including the control of individual finger actions (Chen et al., 1997; Verstynen et al., 2004). Activity related to ipsilateral actions is stronger for the subdominant hand, that is, for right handers in the left hemisphere[2] and increases with increasing complexity of the motor action as indicated by the number of different muscular actions involved (Verstynen et al., 2004). Importantly, ipsilateral activity does not wear off when the same movement is executed repeatedly, which suggests that it is necessary for the execution rather than for the planning of movements.

[2] Ipsilateral control could be exerted either by pyramidal or extrapyramidal fiber tracts that descend without crossing to spinal motor neurons or via transcallosal connections to the contralateral motor cortex. This anatomical difference is not important for the present discussion but may be relevant for intermanual conflicts after lesions of the corpus callosum (see chapter 14).

On the basis of these findings it may be speculated that the effects of brain damage on motor skill of the hand ipsilateral to the lesion are at least partly due to encroachment of the lesions on the neural substrates of ipsilateral motor control. The analysis of the conditions and nature of errors presented earlier would fit quite well with this hypothesis. Generally, left-sided lesions impair the combination of multiple muscular actions to achieve integrated swift hand movements whereas right-sided lesions disturb the accuracy of the finally achieved position. This division corresponds well with the division of labor between the dominant right and the subdominant left hand. In bilateral movements such as, for example, threading a needle or carving, the dominant hand takes the fast and active part whereas the subdominant hand secures the accurate positioning of the target (Beaton, 2003). One might speculate that the left motor cortex directs primarily the dynamic action of the dominant right hand but also exerts control of the subdominant left hand when it must make movements of the kind that are usually assigned to the dominant hand. Lesions of left-sided motor cortex would thus impair actions of the left hand that require those aptitudes that are dominantly exerted by the right hand (Tretriluxana et al., 2009). Conversely, right-sided lesions would impair the exactitude of the final positions not only for the left but also for the right hand.

Apraxia and the micro level of motor coordination

We started this chapter with the consideration that analysis of clinically imperceptible features of apraxic actions might reveal that symptoms of apraxia are emergent manifestations of defective micro level motor coordination. Indeed our review demonstrated the existence of clinically imperceptible disturbances of motor coordination that fulfill a crucial criterion for a diagnosis of apraxia in that they affect the limbs ipsilateral to the damaged hemisphere. Like apraxia, they are predominantly caused by left brain damage.

There is no convincing evidence that the clinical symptoms of apraxia derive from these abnormalities at the micro level of motor coordination. It rather seems that they are an additional but in principle independent sequel of left, and for some aspects also right, brain damage. They demonstrate that unilateral brain damage can cause bilateral disturbances of motor coordination, but not that apraxia is one of them. Apraxia retains its place at the cognitive side of motor control.[3]

[3] Apraxia is not a protected trade mark. One might consider the classification of ipsilateral disturbances of motor execution as a further variant of apraxia. A main disadvantage of this inclusion would be that apraxia loses its status as a clinical syndrome that can be diagnosed by the naked eye in a clinical examination, because these abnormalities become evident only by repeated and technically supported measurement. Moreover, the available results are all on the group level and it is doubtful whether they would permit a reliable distinction between normal and abnormal performance in individual patients.

Chapter 14

Callosal apraxia and intermanual conflict

Liepmann and Maas' (1907) short report of unilaterally left-sided apraxia caused by a lesion of the corpus callosum had been followed by a surge of similar reports which, however, ebbed away when the dominance of associationist concepts gave way to holistic doctrines. Geschwind and Kaplan's (1962) publication of a new case of callosal apraxia heralded the beginning of a new era of localizing function (see Chapters 3 and 4). Like Liepmann and Maas' first report this one was followed by reports of similar cases, and this time the causal role of the callosal dissection remained uncontested (Hécaen & Gimeno-Alava, 1960; De Ajuriaguerra & Tissot, 1969). Presumably part of this success was due to the progress of radiology. The increasingly exact delineation of responsible lesions lent no support to speculations that undetected right-hemisphere lesions were the true causes of left-hand clumsiness.

In the course of these reports, callosal apraxia emerged as a clinical syndrome with several consistent features.

The clinical syndrome of callosal apraxia

Lesions causing callosal apraxia must affect the middle-third of the corpus callosum (Kazui et al., 1992; Giroud & Dumas, 1995). They usually encroach upon neighboring frontal cortex. It has been suggested that this extension is necessary for the emergence of callosal apraxia (Goldenberg et al., 1985; Kazui et al., 1992), but there are single reports of patients with left-sided apraxia from callosal lesions with no radiological evidence for encroachment upon adjacent frontal lobe (Graff-Radford et al., 1987; Lausberg et al., 1999).

Callosal apraxia is usually associated with other symptoms betraying the interruption of information flow between the linguistic competence of the left hemisphere and right-hemisphere control of left hand sensory and motor functions. The patient's left hand cannot write (see Figure 14.1). Blindfolded patients cannot name objects held by the left hand nor say which finger of their left hand is touched. Because there is also disconnection between the sensory–motor regions of both hemispheres, patients are unable to replicate with one hand movements or postures passively induced on the other hand. There is, however, at least one report of callosal apraxia without any other symptoms of callosal disconnection (Kazui & Sawada, 1993). In most cases left-hand apraxia affected execution of meaningful gestures on command as well as imitation of gestures. Actual use of objects is generally less affected.

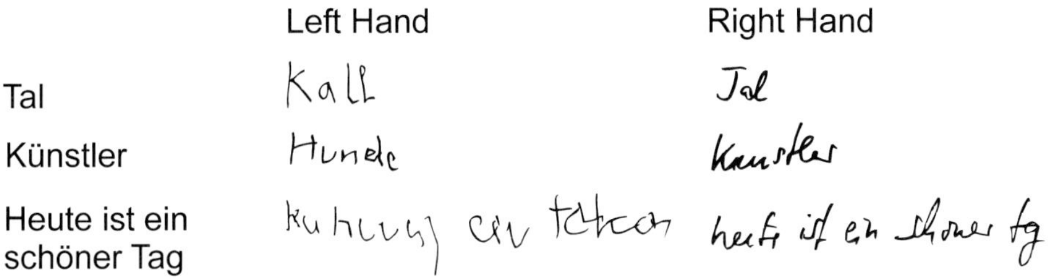

Figure 14.1 Writing to dictation with the left and the right hand by a patient with a lesion destroying the anterior two-thirds of the corpus callosum: Tal: valley; Künstler: artist; Heute ist ein schöner Tag: Today is a beautiful day. Writing by the right hand is faultless except for the omission of dots above the u in "Künstler" and above the o in "schöner." By contrast the left hand produces a meaningless sequence of letters for "Tal" and an aberrant word (Hunde: dogs) for the artist. When trying to write the short sentence the left hand produces a mixture of arbitrary letters and shapes that resemble letters but cannot be identified as regular letters. Reproduced from Goldenberg, G. *Neuropsychologie—Grundlagen, Klinik, Rehabilitation. 4. Auflage*, p. 164, Copyright (2007) with permission of Elsevier.

The revival of callosotomy

Belief in the reality of callosal apraxia was endorsed by a re-evaluation of the consequences of surgical callosotomy. Nearly 20 years after the first surgical sections of the corpus callosum the American neurosurgeon Joseph Bogen revived the technique for relief of pharmacologically uncontrollable epileptic seizures. The operations were successful for reduction or even abolishment of seizures. As in the first series, patients did not display obvious symptoms of callosal disconnection. However, this time Bogen invited an experimental neurobiologist rather than a clinical psychiatrist to investigate possible sequels of the callosal dissection. This neurobiologist was Roger Sperry, who was later to win the Nobel Prize in Physiology or Medicine. Sperry had already performed experiments investigating the effects of corpus callosum section in cat or monkey. He realized that under naturalistic conditions the disconnected hemispheres receive the same environmental input and can cooperate for constructing the response even in the absence of a direct connection via the corpus callosum. Together with his graduate student Michael Gazzaniga he developed experimental methods for restricting visual or tactile input selectively to only one of the disconnected hemispheres (Sperry, 1961; Bogen & Gazzaniga, 1965). This allowed them to assess the capabilities of each hemisphere separately. They found that the left hemisphere is fully competent for language, whereas the right hemisphere's linguistic competence is confined to comprehension of a limited repertoire of high-frequency words. By contrast, the right hemisphere has superior visuo-spatial competency.

These conclusions were not fundamentally novel in comparison with already established clinical knowledge (see Chapter 3). The more exciting aspect of their experiments was the demonstration that the hemispheres could exert their capabilities independently from each other. With appropriate experimental manipulations they could even be induced to produce conflicting responses to the same stimuli. Thus, when the left hand palpated an object out of sight, the tactual information would come to the right hemisphere but could not be forwarded to the left hemisphere because of the absence of callosal connection. The right hemisphere could demonstrate recognition of the palpated object by selecting with the left hand the same object from an array of distracters. When, however, the patient was asked to name the palpated object, only the left hemisphere could formulate a verbal response, and it produced the name of some other, unrelated, object rather than confessing its ignorance. It thus appeared as if the two halves of the cerebrum harbored two independent minds. When their connection was severed each of them continued to construct images of the external world and to make decisions based on them without caring about what was going on in the other half's mind. Seen against this background, Liepmann's contention that one hemisphere's motor output could be cut off from the other hemisphere's knowledge appeared a modest claim.

The experimental investigations of the split-brain patients endorsed the general validity of disconnection as an explanatory principle, but they failed to replicate symptoms of callosal apraxia that had been established by examination of patients with natural lesions of the corpus callosum. Apparently the deficit caused by surgical section was confined to an inability to move the left hand according to verbal instruction. This symptom was not more than a fragment of the whole clinical picture shown by patients with natural lesions of the corpus callosum. Michael Gazzaniga summarized the results of his investigations into apraxia in patients with surgical section of the corpus callosum:

> The overall picture of praxic disturbance in these selected cases was mild and resembled that described by Akelaitis and co-workers in the early 1940's in contrast to the more severe symptoms outlined by Liepmann and others. (Gazzaniga et al., 1967, p. 611)

We will discuss the differences between surgical and natural section of the corpus callosum separately for imitation and for communicative gestures on command.

Imitation

Clinical observations and systematic studies of patients with surgical section of the corpus callosum agreed that the patients were unable to move or configure the left hand according to verbal commands but could readily imitate the same movements or postures (Gazzaniga et al., 1967; Zaidel & Sperry, 1977; Volpe et al., 1982). By contrast, with two notable exceptions (Geschwind & Kaplan, 1962; Goldenberg et al., 2001b), left-handed imitation of gestures was defective in all patients whose apraxia was caused by natural lesions of the corpus callosum (Watson & Heilman, 1983; Goldenberg et al., 1985; Graff-Radford et al., 1987; Tanaka et al., 1990a; Boldrini et al., 1992; Kazui et al., 1992; Kazui & Sawada, 1993; Giroud & Dumas, 1995; Tanaka et al., 1996; Marangolo et al., 1998; Lausberg et al., 1999). Scrutiny of the case reports, however, suggests that the imitation deficit in natural lesions depends on the length of the interval between the onset of callosal disconnection and the examination. The time between the causal accident and the diagnosis of callosal apraxia was six months in one patient (Goldenberg et al., 1985) but less than three months in the other patients with defective imitation. Patients who were tested repeatedly showed marked improvement or even normalization of left-handed imitation (Watson & Heilman, 1983; Goldenberg et al., 1985; Graff-Radford et al., 1987; Tanaka et al., 1990b; Boldrini et al., 1992; Kazui et al., 1992; 1993; Tanaka et al., 1996; Lausberg et al., 1999). Apparently, imitation recovers during the months after callosal damage. The two exceptions could also be due to recovery. Patient P. U. (Goldenberg et al., 2001b), who was of the exceptional cases with preserved imitation, came to our observation only two years after the bleeding that destroyed his corpus callosum. Extrapolation from the time course of recovery in the other patients makes it plausible that two years had been sufficient for complete recovery of imitation. Sparing of imitation in Geschwind and Kaplan's patient is less easily explainable. Since he had a slow-growing tumor, it was hypothesized that gradual destruction of the corpus callosum had allowed for the simultaneous development of compensatory mechanisms (Andersen et al., 1990). However, the destruction of his corpus callosum was supposed to be due to a vascular occlusion during tumor operation, and the examination took place only two months after this acute event (see Chapter 4). Possibly, infiltration by the tumor had altered callosal function and already initiated compensatory mechanisms before the vascular incident.

Recovery would also be a plausible explanation for intact imitation by patients with surgical sections in the chronic stages after surgery, but the strength of this speculation is weakened by Gazzaniga et al.'s (1967) report of preserved imitation contrasting with missing reactions to verbal commands in the first week after operation. However, the movements that Gazzaniga et al. listed as examples of preserved imitation (e.g., raise your arm, make a fist) were definitely less complex than gestures usually applied for the diagnosis of apraxia and would probably also be imitated correctly by patients with unquestionable apraxia from hemisphere lesions.

Imitation by isolated hemispheres

In the clinical examination of imitation both hemispheres can see the model. In this condition successful imitation may be a product of collaboration between the hemispheres via subcortical connections that function despite the absence of callosal connections. To tell apart the capabilities of the isolated left and the right hemispheres the visual input must be presented separately only one of them. Depriving the other hemisphere from the visual input received by the other prevents it from collaborating with the other hemisphere's attempts to imitate. Since the visual cortex of each hemisphere receives input only from the opposite half of both eyes' visual fields, restriction of input to one hemisphere can be achieved by presenting images exclusively to the opposite visual field. The most widely used procedure for this purpose consists of placing subjects before a screen and asking them to fixate a central mark. Visual stimuli are then flashed to either the right or the left visual field for durations that are too short for eye movements to bring the stimulus into the other visual field (see Figure 14.2).

Both visual cortices are connected by the posterior part of the corpus callosum, called the splenium. If the splenium is intact, the visual information received by one hemisphere will immediately be transferred to the visual cortex of the other hemisphere enabling it to

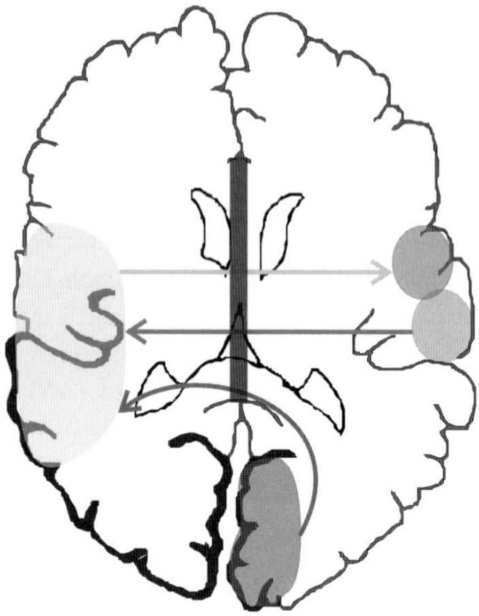

Figure 14.2 Section of the corpus callosum interrupts the link between left hemisphere linguistic competence and right hemisphere functions. Yellow: left-hemisphere language area. Green: verbal motor disconnection disables movements of the left hand to verbal command. Blue: disconnection between right somatosensory cortex and left hemisphere language areas leads to tactile anomia. Patients palpate objects put into the left hand skillfully and may even be able to demonstrate their use but produce aberrant responses when asked to name them. Red: section of the posterior portion of the corpus callosum causes visuo-verbal disconnection. Patients are unable to name objects and to read letters and words in their left visual hemifield. Beyond these clinical manifestations callosal disconnection can be experimentally exploited for examining the capabilities of isolated hemispheres. For this purpose disconnection between left and right visual cortex is particularly important, because it allows restriction not only of tactile but also of visual input to only one hemisphere. (See Plate 12.)

collaborate for the response to the visual stimulus. Restriction of visual input to only one hemisphere necessitates severance of the splenium. This is regularly included in surgical callosotomy but is rare in natural lesions causing callosal apraxia, because the vascular supply of the middle part of the corpus callosum, section of which causes apraxia, is different from that of the splenium. P. U. (Goldenberg et al., 2001b) is one of the rare patients in whom callosal apraxia from a natural lesion was associated with destruction of the splenium. This gave us the opportunity to compare imitation by isolated hemispheres between a patient with a natural lesion and published patients with surgical split brains (Gazzaniga et al., 1967; Zaidel & Sperry, 1977; Volpe et al., 1982; Lausberg & Cruz, 2004).

On clinical examination with unrestricted vision P. U.'s left hand was, like the left hand of surgical patients, apraxic for pantomime to verbal command but not for imitation.

The basic experimental set-up for assessing the capacities of each hemisphere on its own was the same in the surgical split-brain studies and our examination of P. U.: pictures of gestures were flashed to either the left or the right visual field and the patients were asked to imitate them either with the left or with the right hand.

All surgical patients and P. U. were severely handicapped though not completely lost when trying to imitate with the hand opposite to the visual field that received the visual input. In this arrangement the hemisphere that sees the stimulus must direct the hand that is normally under control of the opposite hemisphere. The error rates were higher in the combination of left visual field with right hand than vice versa, suggesting that control of the left hand by the left hemisphere is more efficient than control of the right hand by the right hemisphere. The following results all refer to imitation with the hand on the same side as the visual input. In this constellation the same hemisphere receives the visual information and directs the hand. The performance thus reflects the aptitudes of only one isolated hemisphere.

The accuracy of imitation of finger configuration differed between surgical patients and P. U.: whereas it had been reported to be only mildly impaired or even normal in surgical patients, it was severely defective in P. U. Nevertheless there were no significant differences between the right and the left hemisphere either in P. U. or in the surgical patients.

Thus far it appears that both hemispheres have equal capacities for imitating meaningless gestures. The picture changed, however, when imitation was probed for postures of the hand relative to the head and face (see Figures 7.1 and 14.3). P. U.'s left hemisphere imitated them perfectly whereas his right hemisphere, at best, achieved a coarse approximation of the target gesture (Petreska et al., 2010). The original studies of imitation by surgical split-brain patients had not examined similar hand postures, but some 25 years later Lausberg and Cruz administered our hand postures to three of the original patients and replicated the asymmetry in favor of better imitation by the left hemisphere (Lausberg & Cruz, 2004).

You may remember that in patients with unilateral lesions we replicated the different sensitivity of whole hand postures and finger configuration to left and right brain damage in a perceptual matching test (Goldenberg, 2001; see Chapter 7). We adapted this experiment for separate examination of P. U.'s hemispheres. Drawing of the target gestures were flashed into either the right or the left visual field and P. U. was subsequently asked to select the same gesture among four gestures made by different persons and photographed under different angles of view. This selection was made in free view, but since only one hemisphere had seen the target, the selection revealed the capacities of only this hemisphere. For hand postures presented to the right visual field, the proportion of P. U.'s correct choices was above the mean of controls who had been examined with the same procedure. By contrast, it was far below the control range when the target posture had been flashed to the left visual field and hence the right hemisphere. Matching of finger configurations was mildly reduced in both visual fields.

In sum our experiments and their replication by Lausberg disproved the claim that after section of the corpus callosum both hemispheres are equally capable of imitating visually presented gestures. The apparent support for this claim from previous studies was due to

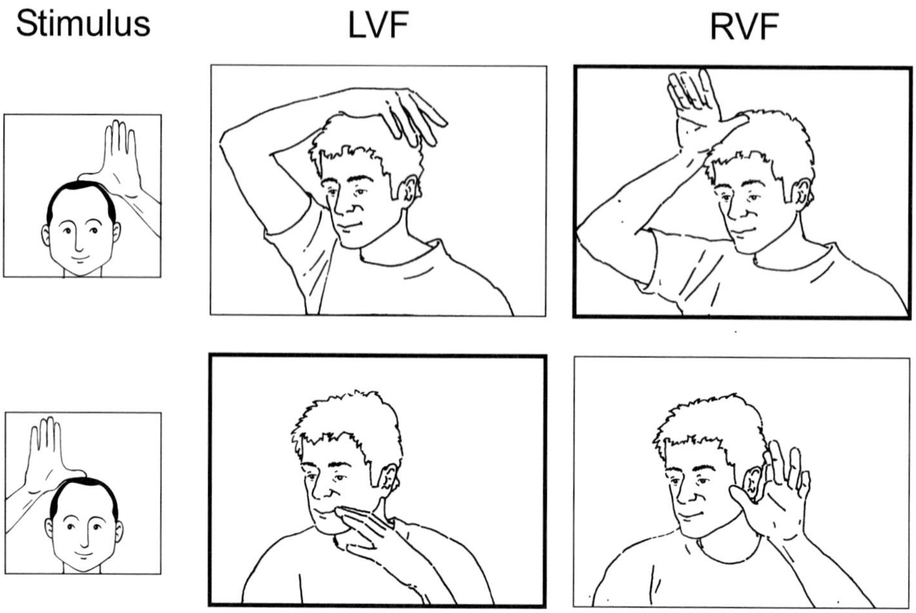

Figure 14.3 Imitation by isolated hemispheres: P. U. (Goldenberg et al., 2001b) was presented with models for imitation tachistoscopically in either the left (LVF) or the right visual hemifield (RVF) and was asked to imitate either with the left or the right hand. The top row shows right-hand and the bottom row left-hand performance. The small icon on the left side shows the picture that is presented as the model for imitation. When the laterality of the visual presentation coincides with the laterality of the imitating hand only one hemisphere is in charge. These conditions are marked by bold frames. In the right-hemifield right-hand combination the left hemisphere copies the hand posture swift and correctly. By contrast, the left-hemifield left-hand combination gives rise to a hesitating and ultimately aberrant movement. The other two conditions demanded ipsilateral motor control that was insufficient for correct imitation by either hemisphere. Adapted from *Neuropsychologia*, *39* (13), Georg Goldenberg, Kerstin Laimgruber, and Joachim Hermsdörfer, Imitation of gestures by disconnected hemispheres, p. 1438, Copyright (2001), with permission from Elsevier.

the exclusive examination of finger configurations which are, however, a special class of gestures, imitation of which does not show the strong dependency on left-hemisphere function that determines success in imitation of whole hand postures.

Communicative gestures on command

There is general agreement that in callosal apraxia left-handed execution of communicative gestures on verbal command is defective. Performance deteriorates further when patients are blindfolded during execution of the gestures. Presumably the blindfold prevents the left hemisphere from observing the apraxic errors of the left hand and sending helpful signals via extracallosal connections to the right hemisphere. Patients whose imitation is less severely impaired than production of communicative gestures on command can circumvent the right hemisphere's incapacity to generate communicative gestures by first performing the gesture with the right hand and then imitating it with the left (see Figure 14.4).

Although the clinical appearance is most likely the same in patients with surgical and natural lesions of the corpus callosum, they have received different interpretations. Whereas most clinicians consider defective production of communicative gestures by the left hand as the core symptom of callosal apraxia, authors working with surgical split-brain patients emphasized the verbal nature of the command and considered errors as a manifestation of verbal–motor disconnection (Gazzaniga et al., 1967; Zaidel & Sperry, 1977). The implication that performance of communicative gesture would become normal if instructions were given non-verbally was put to experimental proof by Hedda Lausberg

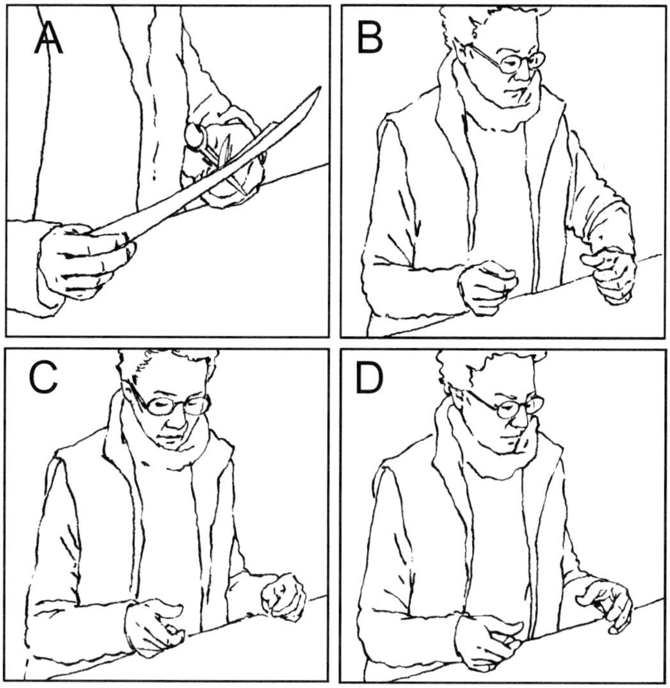

Figure 14.4 A: The same patient as in Figure 14.1 is asked to cut a piece of paper with the left hand. She does so skillfully. B: Immediately afterward she is asked to repeat the movement of the left hand for pantomiming the use of the scissors. She is helpless and searches for correct movements but does not find the correct posture of the fingers. She rotates the hand rather than opening and closing the fingers. C: While the examiner is occupied by preparation of the next test the patient pantomimes cutting with scissors with the right hand and attentively observes that hand's movement. D: The left hand repeats the correct pantomime. Apparently the left hemisphere has demonstrated the correct movement to the right hemisphere which exploited preserved imitation for replicating it.

et al. (2003) with the same patients that had been examined for the imitation of unilaterally presented hand postures. Lausberg and her coworkers elicited pantomimes of tool use by visual presentation of the tools rather than by their verbal designations. Other than in the study of imitation the stimuli were presented in free vision and hence were accessible for both hemispheres. Nonetheless the performances of both hands differed markedly. Right-hand performance did not differ from controls, but left-hand pantomimes were distinctly defective though still recognizable as attempts to demonstrate the use of the object. In sum, the sensitivity of apraxia to the mode of instruction was the same as in patients with left brain damage or with callosal disconnection from natural causes: defective pantomime was not restricted to their execution on verbal command.

A remarkable aspect of Lausberg et al.'s study is the persistence of left-hand apraxia for pantomime. The time elapsed since surgery ranged from ten to 35 years, but the patients still displayed left-hand apraxia for pantomiming the use of objects. Likewise, P. U.'s left hand displayed apraxia for pantomime of tool use two years after severance of the corpus callosum, and in contrast to defective imitation there was no need for lateralized presentation of stimuli to elicit errors of pantomime. Apparently left-hand apraxia for pantomime of tool use is less likely to recover from the effects of callosal disconnection than imitation.

Intermanual conflicts

Thus far we can conclude that dissection of the corpus callosum causes apraxia of the left hand regardless of whether it is due to surgical callosotomy or to natural lesions, and that the symptoms of unilateral callosal apraxia largely replicate those of bilateral apraxia caused by left-sided hemisphere lesions. These results confirm the reality of callosal apraxia and highlight the clinical astuteness of Hugo Liepmann and his contemporaries but they tell us little about apraxia that is not already known from the studies of patients with unilateral hemisphere lesions. The replication is comforting but not exciting.

There is, however, a tradition of more exciting symptoms of callosal disconnection. This tradition started with the disobedient right hand of Liepmann's imperial counselor and was central to Akelaitis' proposal of "diagonistic apraxia." It concerns actions of one hand that are in conflict with the subject's conscious intentions and can lead to struggles between both hands.

The following description of a woman struggling with unwanted actions of her right hand illustrates the weirdness of such intermanual conflict:

> One patient tried to eat a "Wiener Schnitzel" by sitting on her right hand and trying to cut the Schnitzel with the fork she was holding in her left hand. Eventually, the right hand came up and grabbed the knife, but instead of cutting little pieces it shoved away the schnitzel and tried to keep it away from the motor reach of the left hand, which was holding the fork useless above the plate. As in other examples, there is an element that is reminiscent of mischief. (Brainin et al., 2008, p. 251)

The notion of mischief implies a voluntary opposition of the right hand against the actions of the left hand. Since the hands are directed by opposite hemispheres the conflict indicates malevolence between hemispheres.

In the first book summarizing the observations and experiments of the new series of split-brain patients, Michael Gazzaniga related instances of unintended actions explicitly to conflicting character traits and emotional reactions of the hemispheres:

> Case 1 would sometimes find himself pulling his pants down with one hand and pulling them up with the other. Once, he grabbed his wife with his left hand and shook her violently, while with the right trying to come to his wife's aid in bringing the left belligerent hand under control. Once, while I was playing horseshoe with the patient in his backyard, he happened to pick up an axe leaning against the house with his left hand. Because it was entirely likely that the more aggressive right hemisphere might be in control, I discretely left the scene—not wanting to be the victim for the test case of which half-brain does society punish or execute. (Gazzaniga, 1970, p. 107)

In this case aberrant actions were made by the left hand that is under control of the right hemisphere. As in the first example, they were hostile, but in contrast to the first example they were directed against the patient's wife and his examiner rather than interfering directly with activities of his other hand. The conflict between the preferences and goals of the two hemispheres evokes the idea that the two hemispheres house separate minds that can pursue opposite goals. This idea was not new. It had already been elaborated some 100 years earlier under the headings of "dual brain" and "dual mind."

Dual mind and dual brain

The idea that the two hemispheres are the seat of two minds was an influential notion in the nineteenth century and preceded the scientific exploration of functional asymmetries of the hemispheres (Wigan, 1844). The duality of mind was founded upon an opposition between the "light" and the "dark" or, respectively, the "civilized" and the "savage" part of human nature (Harrington, 1987). Robert Louis Stevenson's novel *Strange Case of Dr Jekyll and Mr Hyde* is a fictional version of this conflict between two fundamentally different minds housed in one person (Stiles, 2006). The association of the duality of mind with the duality of the cerebral hemispheres was supported by experiments of "hemihypnosis." The subjects of these experiments were, with very few exceptions, young women. By asymmetric manipulations, like closing one eye during the presentation of hypnotizing stimuli, or whispering commands to one ear during the hypnotized state, or simply rubbing one side of the skull, they were led to assume different postures of the left and the right side of the body (see Figure 14.5) or different mimic expressions on the left and right half of the face. These differences between the right and the left half of the body were believed to express different mental states induced by separate hypnosis of the two minds located in the right and the left half of the brain (Bourneville & Regnarde, 1879; Didi-Huberman, 1982; Harrington, 1987). Although the diverging motor actions of right and left limbs seem not to have included direct fights between them, they can be regarded as early observations of intermanual conflict[1]

[1] To avoid any misunderstanding, let me emphasize that the mechanisms at work in these experiments must have been purely psychic. Probably the women complied with the experimenter and did what he expected. In any case, the procedures used for inducing hemihypnosis have no counterpart in the

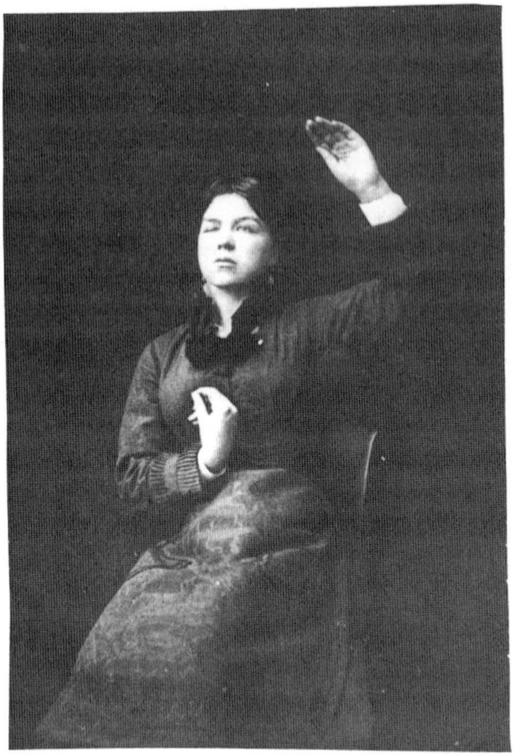

Planche XVI.

HÉMI-LÉTHARGIE ET HÉMI-CATALEPSIE

Figure 14.5 The photograph demonstrates an early experiment that exploited "hemihypnosis" for inducing independent functioning of both hemispheres (Bourneville & Regnarde, 1879). The subject of the experiment was a young in-patient of the Salpétrère Hospital in Paris. The first stage of hypnosis, called catalepsy, was induced by application of a strong sensory stimulus like bright light or loud noise. Then the patient was asked to close only one eye. Closing of the eyes was believed to trigger the second stage of hypnosis, called lethargy. Because the patient closed only one eye, lethargy was supposed to affect only the hemisphere opposite to that eye and manifested itself in motor action of the same side of the body as the closed eye. The other half of the body remained in the cataleptic state (Harrington, 1987). It is noteworthy that in this enactment of an alleged intermanual conflict both hands produce different actions in distant spatial locations. By contrast, intermanual conflicts caused by section of the corpus callosum are mostly caused by similar actions executed by both hands in close vicinity to each other (see Figures 2.2 and 14.6).

anatomy and physiology of the brain. Already the basic anatomical premises are wrong. Both eyes and both ears are connected to both hemispheres, so that confining input to one eye or one ear does not restrict its perception to the opposite hemisphere. The idea that brushing one side of the skull will activate the hemisphere below it neglects the interpolation of the bone skull.

The modern studies demonstrating independent functioning of hemispheres in surgical split-brain patients differed from these nineteenth-century precursors by their solid anchoring in the anatomy of the hemispheres and their connections, but their interpretation reflected the lasting influence of the nineteenth-century ideas on the dual mind in the dual brain. In contrast to the nineteenth century, however, the sympathies of the twentieth-century version were mainly for the dark side of the mind situated in the mute right hemisphere. The right hemisphere was now believed to be the site of creativity and emotion as opposed to the rational and analytical nature of the speaking left hemisphere (Hoppe, 1977; Edwards, 1979).

Dual brain and holism

In the historical part (Chapter 4) we noted that the possibility of independent functioning of isolated hemispheres was a central argument for the resurgence of the localizing approach to mind and brain. Remember, for example, Geschwind and Kaplan's discussion of their case of callosal apraxia:

> It appears to us that the simplest description of this patient's most striking disturbances is that he behaved as if his two cerebral hemispheres were functioning nearly autonomously. (Geschwind et al., 1962, p. 683)

In this reasoning the concept of the dual brain appears as an ally in the effort to overcome holism. On scrutiny, however, the alliance becomes ambiguous. The proponents of the dual brain postulated division of the brain into two independent hemispheres and equipped each of them with a complete mind, but they were not interested in the exploration of anatomical and functional partitions within the hemispheres (Hoppe, 1977). In a way, the dual brain duplicated the unitary structure of brain and mind rather than dissecting them. It replaced one indivisible mind by two but retained their indivisibility. It thus retained a trace of holism.

The attribution of intermanual conflicts to opposite intentions of independent hemispheres has become a minority position in the literature on intermanual conflict. However, we will see later in this chapter that central themes of the holistic stance survive in the heart of newer accounts of intermanual conflict although they are based on fine-grained partition of localized functions within hemispheres rather than on oppositions between whole hemispheres.

Not all anarchists are alien

A regular feature of intermanual conflict is that afflicted patients experience one hand as acting according to their intention and the other as pursuing its own goals that interfere with the patient's intentions. It seems evident that in callosal apraxia it is the apraxic left hand that disobeys and interferes, but clinical observations contradict this expectation and call into doubts the closeness of the link between callosal apraxia and disobedience of one hand. The doubts were initiated by a seminal paper by Goldberg et al. (1981). They reported two right-handed patients with lesions of the left medial frontal cortex who experienced apparently purposeful right-hand actions that did not correspond with conscious volition. Many of these unwanted actions consisted of reaching out and grasping objects, but there were also more complex actions. For example, one patient's right arm came up to keep her glasses on after she had begun to remove them with the left hand. On another occasion the right hand not only picked up a pencil but began scribbling with it.

Although the radiological means of the early eighties did not permit unequivocal exclusion of extension of the lesion into the adjacent corpus callosum, a contribution of callosal apraxia to the unintended actions was unlikely, because the involuntary actions were made by the right hand which is under command of the dominant left hemisphere and should hence be immune against callosal apraxia.

Goldberg identified these involuntary actions of one hand as "alien hand syndrome." This term (French: "main étrangère") had originally been used by two French neurologists (Brion & Jedynak, 1972) for designating the incapacity of patients with parietal lesions to recognize their own hand when it was grasped by the other hand out of sight. By contrast, Goldberg's patients experienced the action of their hand as being out of control but never doubted that the hand performing the actions was their own. To emphasize that the hand is disobedient rather than alien, Sergio Della Sala proposed calling the phenomenon "anarchic hand" (Della Sala et al., 1994; Marchetti & Della Sala, 1998).

Since then, a substantial number of studies confirmed that the anarchic hand can be either the left or the right (McNabb et al., 1988; Della Sala et al., 1991; Lavados et al., 2002; Brainin et al., 2008). Lesions are regularly located in the anterior portion of the interhemispheric fissure where they can encroach either upon the mesial frontal lobe, or the adjacent corpus callosum, or both. In the majority of cases the frontal lobe opposite to the anarchic hand is included in the lesion but there is at least one patient on record who experienced disruptive actions of the left hand that had been rendered apraxic by a purely callosal lesion without any extension into the frontal lobes (Lausberg et al., 1999).

Forced grasping and intermanual conflict

Necessarily, any manual action with an impact on an external object must start by establishing contact between the hand and that object, or, to say it simply, by grasping it. This applies to the involuntary and inappropriate actions of the anarchic hand as well as to any other instrumental manual action. Compulsive grasping of nearby objects may, however, occur as a symptom of frontal lobe damage without being followed by disruptive actions and intermanual conflict. Whereas the anarchic hand is a rare event, forced grasping is a quite common symptom of frontal lesions. We have already encountered it as part of Denny-Brown's "magnetic" apraxia (Adie & Critchley, 1927; Denny-Brown, 1958; De Renzi & Barbieri, 1992).

There is a major difference between grasping by the anarchic hand and the common variant of forced grasping. Whereas the common variant concerns objects in the immediate vicinity of the grasping hand, the anarchic hand preferably grasps for objects that are close to or even held by, the other, obedient, hand. Indeed, this preference is a major source of intermanual conflict. Gazzaniga's example of the patient whose left hand seized an axe that had not been held by the right hand is exceptional. Possibly the axe happened to be near to the patient's apraxic left hand and taking hold of it was due to the common variant of forced grasping but would not have paved the way to more extensive and dangerous actions even if Gazzaniga had stayed by the patient.

Like other patients with frontal lobe damage, patients suffering from an anarchic hand may also display this common variant of forced grasping as an additional symptom of their frontal lobe damage, but intermanual conflict and disruptive actions are regularly initiated by moving the anarchic hand close to the other hand rather than by seizing objects that happen to be in the vicinity of the anarchic hand.

Anarchic hand and the autonomy of action

Based on the prevalence of medial frontal lesions and of forced grasping in patients with an anarchic hand, Goldberg developed a theory that found much approval and readily replaced the reference of intermanual conflict to hemisphere rivalry (Goldberg et al., 1981; Della Sala et al., 1994; Kritikos et al., 2005). He postulated the existence of two distinct systems governing the delivery of motor commands from the primary motor cortex. One is centered on the supplementary motor area at the medial surface of the frontal lobe and the other on premotor cortex at its lateral surface. The medial system is responsible for internally generated intentional movement whereas the lateral system directs motor responses to external stimuli. The anarchic hand is caused by selective damage to the medial system and disturbs the orderly execution of intentional movement. The breakdown of the medial system disinhibits action control by the lateral system. Forced grasping is a manifestation of the subsequently heightened dependency of motor action on external stimuli. Kritikos and colleagues conducted experimental examinations supporting the heightened sensitivity of a patient's anarchic left hand to external distracters and concluded that:

> The essential deficit in patients with anarchic hand syndrome is increased susceptibility to non-relevant cues in the environment and thus impaired selection of appropriate motor programmes. (Kritikos et al., 2005, p. 645)

If you remember Chapter 3, this line of reasoning will sound very familiar to you. It is easily recognizable as a variant of Denny-Brown's "magnetic apraxia" and, more generally, of the distinction between autonomous and externally driven action that was dear to the holists, and that is a particularly straightforward variant of the high- versus low-level dichotomy of motor control.

Mischief or overzealousness?

We have until now discussed two suggestions concerning the mechanisms underlying intermanual conflict and the anarchic hand: one is hemisphere rivalry, and the other one the subjugation of a motor system devoted to intentional actions to an alternative system specialized on reactions to external stimuli. Both suggestions have in common the assumption that the conflict between one hand's actions and the patient's intentions reflects an underlying conflict between two anatomical units pursuing different goals. For the

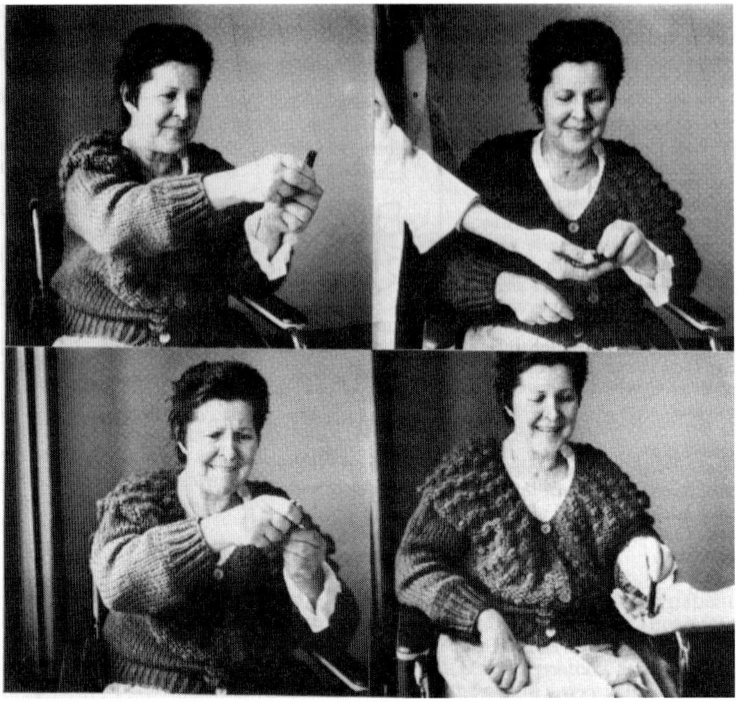

Figure 14.6 Intermanual conflict in a patient with destruction of the anterior two-thirds of the corpus callosum (same patient as in Figure 2.2): the patient tried to take a pen hold by the left hand into the right hand. Left: The left hand withholds the pen. Right: When an examiner approaches her hand the patient's left hand yields the pen readily to the examiner's hand regardless of whether she approaches from the right or from the left side. The patient's mimic expression expresses her discontent with the left hand's stinginess and her relief when the left hand releases the pen. Reproduced from Goldenberg, G, Wimmer, A., Holzner, F., and Wessely, P. Apraxia of the left limbs in a case of callosal disconnection: The contribution of medial frontal lobe damage. *Cortex*, *21*, p. 142, Copyright (1985) with permission of Elsevier.

hemisphere rivalry hypothesis these units are the right and the left hemisphere, and for the anarchic hand hypothesis the medial and the lateral premotor cortex. A closer look at the type of actions committed by the struggling hands casts doubts on the conflict between their goals, because it reveals that the actions of both hands have at least as much in common as they differ.

The tendency of the anarchic hand to grasp objects held by the other hand implies that both hands act at in close vicinity much as they do in coordinated bimanual collaboration. The communality of both hands' actions is not exhausted by their common location. Typically, actions of the disobedient hand are elicited by voluntary actions of the unaffected hand. The disruptive movements may start just before or immediately after the intended movement but always in close temporal coupling with the voluntary initiation of the other hand's action (Tanaka et al., 1996; Lavados et al., 2002). Figure 14.6 shows an example of the dependency of the disruptive actions from the simultaneous voluntary action of the unaffected hand.

Although the actions of both hands are in conflict, they are frequently very similar and differ only in single parameters of the movements, most frequently the direction. Thus a frequent type of disruptive action is grasping an object that the unaffected hand has seized and withdrawing it to the side of the disobedient hand (Goldenberg et al., 1985; Jason & Pajurkova, 1992). The mirrored action may be more complex than merely seizing and pulling. For example, a patient with callosal section of the corpus callosum buttoned up his shirt with right hand but the other hand came along right behind it undoing the buttons (Bogen, 1993). The mirroring of the voluntary action may evoke an impression of mockery as in the following observation of a patient with callosal apraxia following severe head trauma:

> When combing his hair with his right hand, his left hand was noted to grasp a spoon and to simultaneously perform a similar combing gesture over his hair. (Buxbaum et al., 1995, p. 3)

The actions of the disobedient need not necessarily be in conflict with the patient's goals at all. Thus a patient with callosal apraxia attempted to turn on a water tap with this right hand, but his left hand involuntarily came over ahead of the right and turned it on first (Tanaka et al., 1996). I once tried to test imitation of hand postures separately in both hands of a patient with partial callosal disconnection, but in spite of the instruction to use only one hand, both hands tried to execute the demanded action simultaneously, ending up in a mess of correct and incorrect hand postures fighting for a place close to the face. Lavados et al. (2002) made a similar observation and proposed the term "agonistic apraxia" for performance of a command with the hand opposite to the one requested by the examiner.

There are even instances of unintended motor actions of one hand that help the other hand to reach the goal of its intentional activity, such as in the following observation of a patient with callosal apraxia (Goldenberg et al., 1985). A key was given to her left hand and she was asked to open a lock:

> She first held the key without moving it. Then the right hand touched slightly the back of the left hand, and while it rested there the left hand introduced the key and opened the lock. When the right hand was prevented from intervening, the left hand eventually moved the key between the fingers and palpated it but did not bring it to the key hole.[2] (Goldenberg et al., 1985, p. 139)

In sum these observation invite a reinterpretation of obtrusive actions. A majority of them seems to be due to the propensity of the disobedient hand to perform actions that are intended to be performed by the other hand. If we want to ascribe a mental state to the disobedient hand it might be overzealousness rather than mischief.

---

2 Note that in this observation the dominant hand that usually acted in conformity with the patient's intention acted unintentionally and interfered with the intended action of the apraxic hand. The common denominator with usual examples of intermanual conflict is the tendency of both hands to pursue the same goal. This tendency led to conflict in the other observations, but to cooperation in this observation.

Intermanual conflict and ipsilateral motor efferences

At least for patients whose intermanual conflict is due to callosal disconnection, obtrusive actions may have their source in an imbalance between ipsilateral motor control and callosal inhibition. The functions of the corpus callosum are not restricted to the transmission of information from one hemisphere to the other. There are callosal fibers linking corresponding areas of left and right motor cortex that have inhibitory effects. They counteract the effects of direct ipsilateral motor efferences that tend to elicit symmetric movements of the other hand when one hand is intentionally moved (Ziemann et al., 1999). These ipsilateral efferences go predominantly to proximal parts of the extremities directing movements of the whole hand rather than of single fingers (Zaidel & Sperry, 1977). We may speculate that lesions of the corpus callosum and perhaps also of white matter in the adjacent parts of the medial frontal lobe weaken the inhibition of unintended co-movements of the other hand during intentional movements of the dominant hand. Because of the predominantly proximal effects of ipsilateral efferences the distal portion of the co-movements is underspecified. Its features may derive from interactions with external objects at the place of its action among which is the regularly acting dominant hand. These local interactions may happen to result in conflict with the intentionally acting dominant hand and prevent it from carrying out the subject's intentions.

From top to bottom of the mind–body hierarchy

Application of the high- versus low-level or, respectively, mind versus body, dichotomy to theories of intermanual conflicts reveals that they span a wide range from very high to quite low levels of explanations. The "dual mind" modal invokes the top level of the mind–body hierarchy. It posits a conflict between two complete minds that pursue independent goals and may even have independent consciousness. Anatomy plays a role in this theory only as far as the two hemispheres provide separate places for the two minds but it has no further influence on their internal mechanisms, their goals, and their beliefs. Goldberg's proposal of a conflict between two motor systems that occupy different sectors of premotor cortex has an intermediate position. It distinguishes two anatomically defined localized systems of motor control, but the functional properties of these systems reflect the dichotomy between autonomy and external control that was a central issue of the holistic epoch. Finally, the proposal that intermanual conflicts derive from an imbalance between ipsilateral and contralateral motor pathways draws its arguments exclusively from anatomy and physiology and can thus be assigned to the bottom level of the putative hierarchy.

Chapter 15

The cognitive side of motor control

In the preceding chapters I have reviewed 140 years of the history of apraxia and tried to give a fairly complete overview of today's accumulated empirical evidence. During the course of 14 chapters we have encountered many fascinating observations and elegant experiments as well as a wide diversity of ideas and theories purporting to explain them. The aim of the book was, however, more ambitious than a comprehensive overview of apraxia. I wanted to develop and probe the hypothesis that research and theories of apraxia are grounded in a mind versus body dichotomy. This dichotomy was spelled out explicitly by Liepmann and forms the implicit basis for theories that distinguish between higher and lower levels, or between cognitive and motor mechanisms of action control. Different versions of such theories have been introduced and discussed in the preceding chapters. In this chapter I want to propose a new hypothesis addressing the interaction between a high and low level of control in apraxia. Before doing so we should try to define the range of clinical phenomena to which a theory of apraxia should apply.

The core and the limits of apraxia

A popular definition of apraxia characterizes it as a "disorder of skilled movement not caused by weakness, akinesia, deafferentation, abnormal tone or posture, movement disorders (such as tremors or chorea), intellectual deterioration, poor comprehension, or uncooperativeness" (Heilman & Rothi, 1993). A disrespectful paraphrase of this definition would be that apraxia is a name allotted to motor symptoms that cannot be explained by known causes. Reading the definition with a less critical attitude one may note that the exclusion criteria are ordered in two groups, one consisting of motor disorders and the other of cognitive dysfunctions. Apraxia is placed between them. Arguably, this placement constitutes a further example of the intermediate position of apraxia in a mind–body dichotomy.

The absence of an unequivocal definition of apraxia does not exclude the possibility that such a definition exists and waits for adequate formulation, but it may also indicate that apraxia is not a unitary disorder with clearly defined boundaries. The second possibility seems more credible. The insecurity of the borders of apraxia is illustrated by the fate of manifestations that had once been subsumed under its heading but lost this place in its further history, such as, for example, constructional apraxia or dressing apraxia. Nor does general acceptance of the designation "apraxia" guarantee that the designated symptoms are manifestations of one common basic disorder. The heterogeneity of symptoms that are more or less unanimously recognized as apraxia is confirmed by the independence of their occurrence. For example, defective imitation of gestures and production of communicative gestures on command can occur independently from each other, and pantomime of tool use can be impaired although actual tool use is preserved.

You would probably be surprised and somewhat disappointed to learn in the fifteenth chapter of a book on apraxia that the author considers it as an arbitrary collection of unrelated symptoms. Let me reassure you, that this is not my opinion. Indeed, I hope to have achieved a coherent account of most putative manifestations of apraxia by following the central thread of a high- versus low-level dichotomy shining through its symptoms. This could lead to the proposal to make the transparency of an interaction between high and low levels of action control the criterion for recognizing a disturbance of action as apraxia. I am, however, aware that the presence and degree of such transparency may itself be controversial and depend on the theoretical stance of the observer. It is therefore ill suited for defining indisputable limits to the range of symptoms that should be included into the realm of apraxia. I suggest an alternative approach to the definition of apraxia. Rather than looking for the limits of apraxia we may look for its core, that is, for manifestations where cognitive interventions on motor control come to the fore most purely. Identification and interpretation of these core deficits will be more fruitful for understanding the nature of apraxia than the attempt to define its limits by compilation of a list of exclusion criteria.

Unilateral lesions cause bilateral apraxia

My proposal for identifying core manifestations of apraxia starts from two peculiarities of the anatomy of lesions causing apraxia. The first of them is that apraxia manifests itself by bilateral motor symptoms but is caused by unilateral hemisphere lesions. The second peculiarity is that for some manifestations of apraxia causal lesions may be located either in the right or in the left hemisphere, whereas for other manifestations the responsible lesions are strictly lateralized to one hemisphere. In typical right-handed persons this is the left one (see Figure 15.1). For the sake of simplicity, in the rest of this chapter I will neglect the variability of lateralization in left-handers and assume that strict unilaterality of causal lesions is always bound to left-hemisphere lesions. As I have outlined in Chapter 12, the functionally decisive feature is unilaterality and not whether it is to the right or the left side.

Lateralization means that lesions of one hemisphere cause bilateral symptoms whereas lesions of the opposite hemisphere do not cause the same symptoms at all. Arguably, the deviation from the symmetry of the neural substrates of motor control can provide a cue for identifying the manifestations of apraxia where the difference to common mechanisms of motor control comes to the fore most conspicuously and which can hence be considered as core manifestations of apraxia.

I will take this anatomical peculiarity as the starting point for speculating first upon the functional properties that characterize the core manifestations of apraxia, then about the anatomical properties of lateralized function that support them, and finally about the correspondence between anatomy and function.

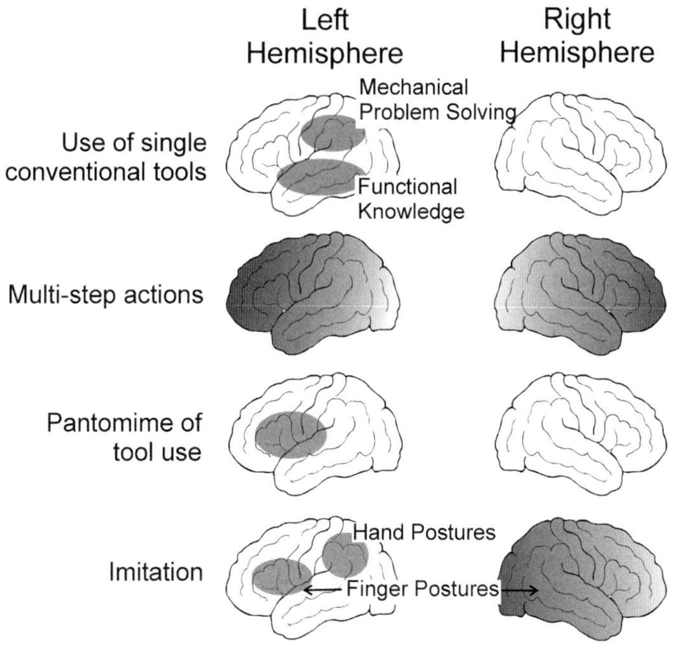

Figure 15.1 A summary of locations of different manifestations of apraxia: shading of the whole hemisphere does not exclude the possibility of more fine-grained localizations within the hemisphere, but indicates that there is no firm empirical data for delimiting the critical areas. Adapted from Goldenberg, G. *Neuropsychologie—Grundlagen, Klinik, Rehabilitation. 4. Auflage*, p. 149, Copyright (2007) with permission of Elsevier.

Segmentation and combination

There are three manifestations of apraxia exclusively bound to left-hemisphere damage: imitation of meaningless hand postures, pantomime of tool use, and use of single mechanical tools. I submit that their functional communality is constituted by a central role of segmentation and combination. I have elaborated these features for each of these manifestations in the respective chapters and will only briefly recapitulate them here. For imitation of hand postures the multiple visual features of the demonstrated gesture are segmented into distinct body parts which are combined for reproducing the hand posture. For use of single mechanical tools the structures of tool and recipient are segmented into functionally significant traits which are combined to form a mechanical chain from the manual action to the ultimate impact on the distal recipient. For pantomime of tool use the compound image of hand, action, and object is segmented into distinctive features of the object and the acting hand which are combined for producing a gesture indicating the pretended object and its use.

The combinatorial nature of the presumed core manifestations can explain the versatility of their application to novel items. Healthy adults can imitate unfamiliar and meaningless hand postures and select and use mechanically transparent novel tools in an errorless way on the first trial (see Chapters 7 and 8). Although pantomime of tool use is somewhat more difficult, healthy subjects usually succeed on the unfamiliar task of producing a comprehensible pantomime of tool use on first trial and without help. The ease of coping with novelty is a hallmark of combinatorial systems. It results from their ability to create a wide diversity of novel entities from a limited repertoire of constant elements.

Segmentation and combination of actions enable subjects to understand and reproduce actions and to create adaptive actions in response to novel demands. I think that this justifies classification of their contribution to action as the cognitive side of motor control.

Other manifestations of apraxia

The proposal that imitation of hand postures, pantomime of tool use, and use of single mechanical tools are the core manifestations of apraxia is based on the assumption that they are particularly pure manifestations of the breakdown of the cognitive side of motor control. It is not intended to suggest that this breakdown does not play a role in other manifestations of apraxia like imitation of finger and foot postures or performance of multistep actions with multiple tools and objects. I rather assume that for these variants of apraxia other factors, like distribution of attention or capacity of working memory, are also important, and that damage to these additional components can cause disturbances even when lesions spare the substrate of the core manifestations.

Apraxia and aphasia

Segmentation and combination are universal mechanisms that confer stability as well as adaptivity to large systems (Abler, 1989). The most highly developed human system of segmentation and combination is language where an infinite number of verbal messages can be created from a limited vocabulary which, in turn, is constituted by combinations of a limited number of phonemes that emerge from segmentation and combination of a limited number of phonetic features (Chomsky, 1957; Jakobson, 1976). The existence of fully developed sign languages demonstrates that an equivalent degree of complexity can be achieved by combinations of manual gestures, but the elements and combinatorial rules of gestures forming sign languages are different from the manual actions affected by apraxia, and cerebral lesions can cause aphasia for sign language independently from apraxia (Marshall et al., 2004). The combinatorial richness of manual actions involved in apraxia is certainly more modest than that of language. The number of possible meaningless gestures, pantomimes, or mechanical relationships is much larger than the number of their constitutive elements but not infinite.

The combinatorial system producing manual actions and gestures thus appears like a slimmed-down version of the system supporting language. Both aphasia and the core manifestations of apraxia are symptoms of left-hemisphere damage. The conclusion that aphasia and apraxia are both results of the breakdown of a common left-hemisphere system for segmentation and combination is, however, refuted by the dissociation of aphasia from apraxia in left-handed patients (see Chapter 12). The essential communality between the neural substrates of aphasia and of the core manifestations of apraxia is not that they are lateralized to the same hemisphere but that they are lateralized at all. Nonetheless the parallel between their neural substrates endorses the essentiality of the link between segmentation and combination on the one side and lateralization of function on the other.

Unilateral control of bilateral motor actions

Unilateral control of bilateral body functions does not alleviate the need for regular crossed control of lateralized body functions by their opposite hemisphere. Lesions of the right motor cortex cause hemiplegia of the left limbs rather than apraxia, but render the left limbs unable to carry out imitation, pantomime, or any other action that could testify its exemption from apraxia. Obviously preservation of lateralized function cannot replace defects of symmetrically organized functions. On the contrary, the deployment of lateralized function presupposes intactness of the symmetrically organized functions for exerting its influence upon them.

The lateralized function guides the regular mechanisms of bilateral control when task demands transgress their competency. Arguably, the interaction between lateralized and bilateral neural substrates can thus be conceptualized as intervention of high-level upon low-level mechanisms of neural control. The severity of the clinical deficit arising from loss of the lateralized function reflects the importance of this intervention or, in other words, the importance of the high-level contribution to action control. It is extremely high for language where unilateral left-sided lesions can lead to pervasive loss of communicative abilities. At the other extreme, it is rather low for the asymmetric control of bimanual coordination between dominant and subdominant hand that we discussed in Chapter 12. Loss of this unilateral contribution to bimanual motor control comes to the fore only in fine-grained measurements of multiple trials of experimental motor tasks. The importance of the unilateral control of bimanual movements at stake in apraxia is not as pervasive as that of language but certainly substantially higher than that of handedness. Manifestations of apraxia are obvious to the naked eye and at least some of them interfere substantially with instrumental activities and communication in daily living.

Diagrams or anatomy?

The conclusion that segmentation and combination depend on the function of left-lateralized cerebral regions says where the neural processes underlying them take place but not how they are accomplished. We discussed the difference between these two aspects of localization of function in their historical context in Chapter 3. We concluded that the contention that analysis of the cerebral substrate of psychological functions can explain their properties is based on a belief of congruence between neural and psychological functions. Thus, for Liepmann, the fiber tracts connecting posterior brain regions with the motor cortex were congruent with the conversion of mental images of intended actions into motor commands. Moreover, his "horizontal schema" (see Chapter 2) depicted a higher number and density of these fibers in the left hemisphere corresponding to the left-hemisphere dominance for this conversion and hence for motor control.

Liepmann did not present any independent evidence for the alleged asymmetry of fiber tracts. The only empirical support for their asymmetry was the very motor dominance that it should explain. In other words, the allegedly anatomical diagram was a functional diagram in anatomical disguise. It would have deserved the contemptuous classification as "diagram making" (see Chapter 3). However, since then anatomical research has collected independent evidence for anatomical differences between the hemispheres that putatively mirror the differences between the functional consequences of left- and right-hemisphere lesions.

Once again, the resuscitation of the associationists' belief of congruence between anatomy and function ideas was initiated by Norman Geschwind. He demonstrated that in the majority of a consecutive sample of post-mortem brains the horizontal surface of the left upper temporal convolution is larger than its right-sided counterpart (Geschwind & Levitsky, 1968). Lesions to this region cause aphasia characterized by fluent but paraphasic and paragrammatic speech, whereas symmetrical lesions on the right side have no influence on linguistic abilities (Wernicke, 1874). The anatomical asymmetry thus seemed to correspond to the lateralization of the neural substrate of linguistic competency. Later studies by other authors demonstrated asymmetry in favor of greater left- than right-sided expansion of corresponding regions not only in the superior temporal lobe but also in frontal and inferior parietal lobes, and converse asymmetry in favor of the right side in posterior parieto-occipital regions (Golestani et al., 2002; Pujol et al., 2002). The parietal and frontal asymmetries are of particular interest for us because it is there that we found the critical locations for the core manifestations of apraxia within the left hemisphere (see Figures 7.2, 8.7, and 10.3). On the other side, lesions to the right posterior parietal regions cause more severe perceptual and attentional difficulties than lesions of their left-sided counterpart. This match between anatomical asymmetry and right-sided functional dominance suggests that the correspondence between size and dominance of regions is a general principle of cerebral lateralization that is not confined to left-hemisphere dominance.

Asymmetries of white matter distribution

The idea that the functional importance of a cerebral region corresponds with its size is intellectually not very appealing. It is reminiscent of Franz Gall's "craniology" that laid the first grounds of localizing cerebral functions in the early nineteenth century but had been rejected as too simplistic already by the associationists (Liepmann, 1909). Further research investigating the micro-anatomical underpinning of the macro-anatomical size differences painted a more differentiated picture of the asymmetries between corresponding regions of both hemispheres. It turned out that the larger areas differed from their counterparts not by a greater number of neurons but by a greater proportion of white matter. Scrutiny of the distribution of white matter asymmetries in unselected samples of subjects or, respectively, brains, confirmed that the proportion of white matter rather than the volume of the region are decisive for functional dominance (Anderson et al., 1999; Hutsler & Galuske, 2003;

Smiley et al., 2012). Thus, the seminal study of Geschwind and Levitsky reported asymmetry of the superior temporal region in favor of a left side in 65% of the brains, while in 10% the right side was larger, and in the remaining 25% there was no asymmetry. Their study did not consider the handedness of the subjects, but even with allowance for right-sided speech dominance in a substantial proportion of left-handers, left-sided dominance for speech would have been expected in more than 90% of their unselected sample of brains. Consequently there must have been a considerable number of subjects in whom left-hemisphere dominance was not associated with corresponding anatomical asymmetry. Using advanced methods of magnetic resonance imaging for examining both total volume of regions and the proportions of white matter within them, Pujol et al. (2002) replicated the incidence of 65% for greater volumes of left than right temporal lobes, but found that the proportion of white matter was higher on the left side in 91% of subjects and thus came much closer to the expected incidence of left-hemisphere dominance for speech than by considering only differences of cortical volume (Knecht et al., 2000).

Linking anatomy to function

If you leaf through the following pages you will note that the book is approaching the end. At this stage I will put aside the skepticism toward theories that postulate congruence between anatomy and function and present a speculation as to how structural properties of the cerebral cortex could bring forward the functional properties of segmentation and combination that putatively underlie the lateralization of core manifestations of apraxia. In contrast to the classical diagrams depicting the posterior to anterior stream of action control (see Chapter 4), my speculation looks for the correspondence with function not at the macro but at the micro level of neuronal anatomy.

Cortical neurons are organized in columns that are arranged perpendicularly to the surface.[1] Their "backbones" are pyramidal cells. They have numerous short extensions, the dendrites, and one or few long extensions, the axons. Synapses transmit excitatory or inhibitory signals between dendrites of adjacent neurons or between axons and dendrites of distant neurons. The main constituents of white matter are myelin sheets covering the axons. Myelin sheets speeds up the transduction of signals through the axons. The thicker they are, the faster is transduction speed. Speed of transduction is particularly important when axons connect widely distant neuronal columns. Consequently, a greater proportion of white matter is correlated with a higher speed of signal transduction and longer maximal ranges between connected columns. To make space for the thickly myelinated fibers distances between adjacent neuronal columns are wider.

Speculation about the correspondence between these anatomical and physiological features and lateralization of functions can be classified according to which of these three properties they emphasize.

[1] This is a very abbreviated and simplified overview of cortical anatomy which serves only to enable understanding of the following speculations.

Speed of transduction is crucial for the proposal that thicker myelination of left superior temporal cortex allows fast processing of acoustic signals. This enables fine-grained temporal resolution of rapid changes in the flow of acoustic information which is necessary for the distinction of speech sounds (Anderson et al., 1999; Hutsler, 2003; Zatorre, 2003). This proposal concentrates on left-hemisphere dominance for speech. It has been extended into the hypothesis that the ability to process rapid temporal variations is a general property of regions with high proportions of white matter (Golestani et al., 2002), but the application of this hypothesis to apraxia is not convincing, because speed of processing does not appear as a crucial factor for the genesis of apraxia. Brain damage may slow down the planning and execution of movements ipsilateral to the lesioned hemisphere, but this slowing varies independently from the presence and severity of apraxia (see Chapter 13).

The longer maximal distances between connected neuronal columns are the basis of the hypothesis that thicker myelination enables efficient cooperation in large intrahemispheric neuronal networks. Again, the major example is language, but for this hypothesis the important feature of language concerns the anatomy of the perisylvian language areas. Multiple aspects of linguistic abilities are supported by multiple interconnected regions of perisylvian temporal, parietal, and frontal regions (Hervé et al., 2006). High-speed transmission of signals between them is necessary to integrate the different aspects of language. Application of this hypothesis to apraxia is possible. We will come back to it when discussing the different contributions of frontal, parietal, and temporal areas to the core manifestations of apraxia.

A hypothesis that is particularly apt to provide an anatomical basis for segmentation and combination of features combines the wider distance between adjacent neuronal columns with the heightened efficiency of connections between more widely spaced neuronal columns (Buxhoeveden & Casanova, 2000; Galuske et al., 2000; Jung-Beeman, 2005). Narrow spacing of neuronal columns results in interdigitation and synaptic contact between neurons of adjacent columns, whereas wider spacing reduces direct contact between neighboring columns. On the assumption that single columns code single features of perceptions or actions, wider spacing may correspond to clear separation between distinct features whereas closer overlap between columns would support a more continuous coding with no sharp separation between related features or concepts. The combination of the representation of features in distinct non-overlapping neural columns with the fast fibers' capacity to make rapid connection between widely spaced columns provides a convincing neuronal analog to the segmentation and combination of features that we have identified as the crucial property of the core manifestations of apraxia.

Frontal, parietal, and temporal contributions to apraxia

My further speculations on correspondence between anatomy and function concern the macro anatomy of apraxia. They presuppose that the micro-anatomical principles of lateralized functions apply to all of the core manifestations of apraxia. However, lesions affecting individual core manifestations are located in different parts of the left hemisphere. In particular, imitation of hand postures and tool use depend heavily on integrity of inferior parietal regions, whereas imitation of finger postures and pantomime of tool use are more sensitive to inferior frontal lesions.[2] I propose that these differences can at least partly be referred to different weights of the two components of lateralized function, segmentation and combination. The proposal says that segmentation of perceived visual entities into their significant features and probably also the temporary storage of these features in working memory is accomplished by parietal regions. In a previous paper I suggested calling this function of left parietal lobe categorical apprehension of spatial relationships (Goldenberg, 2009).

The role of the left inferior frontal region is more difficult to define. Its contribution seems to be needed when significant features must be selected out of several candidates. In contrast to the role of inferior parietal regions the emphasis here is on the selection between features rather than on the segmentation of compounds into their features. We have exemplified this difference in the discussion of the neural substrates of imitation of hand and finger postures (see Chapter 7). The importance of the inferior frontal contribution may be enhanced when selection and combination of features must obey more or less arbitrary constraints, as is the case for pantomime of tool use where crucial features of the tool and its use must be expressed by a continuous sequence of manual actions that also occur in actual use.

A further difference between parietal and frontal contributions might be that the inferior parietal region is concerned exclusively with the analysis of external spatial relationships whereas the left inferior frontal region is also involved in retrieval from semantic memory (Thompson-Schill, 2005). This aspect is particularly important for pantomime of tool use. Presumably it necessitates connection of the left inferior frontal region to the lateral temporal lobe which is a main repository of semantic memory including functional knowledge about tools (Frey, 2007; Whitney et al., 2012) (see Chapter 8).

With a possible exception of imitation of hand postures which seem to depend quite exclusively on parietal lobe integrity (see Chapter 7), the neural substrates of the core manifestations of apraxia are thus distributed across different regions of the left hemisphere. I assume that all regions involved share the general micro-anatomical properties of lateralized functions. Among them is the rapid transmission of signals to distant but functionally closely related regions. The wide distances between the frontal, parietal, and temporal regions contributing to the core manifestations of apraxia makes this consequence of the micro anatomy of lateralized function relevant for apraxia. This relevance is borne out by observations of core symptoms of apraxia resulting from subcortical lesions that interrupt transmission of neural signals through fiber tracts connecting the cortical areas supporting imitation, pantomime, and actual tool use (Agostini et al., 1983; Kertesz & Ferro, 1984; Poncet et al., 1987; Hanna-Pladdy et al., 2001b).

---

[2] Defective imitation of finger postures has not been included into the core manifestations of apraxia because it can also result from right-hemisphere lesions, but this does not exclude that the left-hemisphere variant is caused by the same mechanisms as the core manifestations.

The cognitive side of motor control

I have now presented a hypothesis concerning the anatomical correlates of apraxia. Endorsement or rejection of this hypothesis calls for empirical research. For example, a testable prediction would be that regions whose lesion cause core symptoms of apraxia have high cortical thickness and a high proportion of white matter.

At the end of Chapter 5 I argued that research and theorizing on apraxia is ultimately driven by the opposition between the high and low levels of motor control, and that this opposition ultimately refers to a mind–body dichotomy. I promised to look for the high- versus low-level dichotomy on both sides of scientific reports, that is, in the observations and results on the one side, and in the authors' preferences for high- or low-level explanations of these results on the other. Of course, this applies also to my own theoretical proposal. In the final paragraphs of this chapter I will try to analyze how both aspects of the dichotomy appear in it.

Concerning the contents of my proposal, the dichotomy appears quite prominently. Segmentation and combination are identified as the basic elements of cognition, and their central role for apraxia as a high-level cognitive intervention on motor control. In the discussion of anatomy the interaction between lateralized and bilateral neural substrates of motor control is conceptualized as intervention of high-level upon low-level mechanisms of neural motor control. Opposition between high and low levels of motor control thus formed part of the contents of the theory.

The assignment of my theoretical stance to preferences for high, cognitive, and mental, or low, motor and body, explanations is less unequivocal. I proposed that segmentation and combination are grounded in the anatomical structure of the brain. This proposal explains properties of the mind by properties of the brain. It thus qualifies it as a low-level account. However, the properties that are being explained are core constituents of high-level cognitive functions. Arguably, it is this ambiguity which makes the hypothesis that core manifestations of apraxia are manifestations of segmentation and combination and that segmentation and combination depend on the anatomical properties of strictly lateralized brain regions, attractive. It confirms their cognitive character but suggests an explanation as to how this cognitive side of motor control emerges from structural properties of the brain.

Chapter 16

Levels of therapy

Throughout this book there has been a strong emphasis on clinical observations as a major source of insight into the nature of apraxia. Clinical experience doubtlessly includes successes and failures of therapy, but until now we have neglected this ecologically important aspect. There are two excuses for this neglect. First, the number of studies exploring therapy of apraxia is smaller by far than those treating other clinical issues. It seems to me a fair estimate that the number of patients who participated in therapy studies is close to hundredfold smaller than of those who contributed data to diagnostic and experimental studies of apraxia. Secondly, therapy studies are methodically notoriously problematic. Discussions of discrepant results are always in danger of ending up in disputes about statistical pitfalls rather than about theoretical implications of results.

I nonetheless decided to add a chapter on therapy but I will avoid extensive discussions of methodical problems and concentrate on two issues that are of theoretical interest for the general theme of this book, the opposition of high- versus low-level approaches to apraxia. The first of these issues is the question of whether successes obtained by treating one manifestation of apraxia generalize to other manifestations. The second concerns the efficacy of task-specific versus general approaches to therapy of apraxia.

Generalization of therapeutic successes

As we discussed extensively throughout this book, apraxia is not a unitary disorder. There is a common thread that comes to the fore most conspicuously in the core manifestations, but there is also heterogeneity and dissociation between different manifestations of apraxia. This makes it a priori very unlikely that a therapy addressing one manifestation of apraxia will have the same impact on all of its manifestations.

Indeed, virtually all therapy studies concentrated on only one aspect of apraxia. They addressed either the use of tools and objects or the production of communicative gestures. Imitation was included very rarely (Barbarulo et al., 2008), presumably because its ecological relevance was not considered sufficient for justifying the time and costs of therapeutic trials.

There is one exception to the rule that therapeutic trials concentrate either on tool and object use or on communicative gestures and consequently look for generalization of progress only within that domain of actions. This study (Smania et al., 2000, 2006) included aphasic patients who had been classified as apraxic either for the use of single conventional tools (De Renzi & Lucchelli, 1988) or for imitation of a mixture of meaningful and meaningless gestures (De Renzi et al., 1980) or for both. The training program taught patients to produce pantomimes of tool use and emblematic gestures on command and to imitate meaningless gestures. Surprisingly, this training led to significant improvement not only of imitation of gestures but also of single tool use and, in a second study with the same design, even of the caregivers' estimate of the patients' independency for activities of daily living (Smania et al., 2006).

It is difficult to reconcile such a pervasive generalization of therapeutic successes across all manifestations of apraxia with the heterogeneity of apraxia that I have defended throughout this book. It has, however, until now remained a singular finding. In the following sections I will discuss evidence for generalization separately for the therapy of tool and object use and of communicative gestures.

Use of tools and objects

As we discussed in Chapters 8 and 9, everyday use of tools and objects is usually embedded in multistep actions with multiple tools and objects. Training of naturalistic actions that are necessary for independence in daily living is a regular part of occupational therapy after stroke or other brain damage (Legg et al., 2006). Apraxia is only one out of many possible problems that such training must address. Studies exploring specifically the efficacy of therapy for apraxia of tool and object use have also concentrated on ecologically significant multistep actions like dressing, grooming, or preparing food and beverages (Miller, 1986; van Heugten et al., 1998, 2000; Goldenberg & Hagmann, 1998a; Donkervoort et al., 2001; Goldenberg et al., 2001a; Geusgens et al., 2006; Sunderland et al., 2006; Buxbaum et al., 2008).

The question of whether therapeutic successes generalize from trained to non-trained tasks received controversial responses. Geusgens et al. (2006) re-analyzed data from a large Dutch multicenter study that compared "strategy training" (see later) and "conventional occupational therapy" for restituting independence on activities of daily living in patients with left brain damage. Independence was assessed for four activities of daily living, such as washing the face and upper body or putting on a shirt. Training tasks were selected from these four tasks individually, according to the patient's needs and preferences, so that on average two tasks were trained and two were not. Strategy training led to a significant improvement of independence and this improvement was the same for trained and non-trained tasks. Indeed, inspection of the data reveals that it was even somewhat stronger for non-trained tasks.

While this study suggests an optimistic outlook on the generalization to non-trained activities of daily living, two studies from our group supported a more critical attitude. The first of them (Goldenberg & Hagmann, 1998a) included patients with left-hemisphere stroke who were aphasic and hemiplegic and failed on at least two out of the three activities of brushing their teeth, putting on a T-shirt, and buttering a slice of bread. Independence on these three activities was assessed every week. Between two assessments, one of the three activities was trained whereas maximal support but no therapeutic advice was given when the patients had to perform the other activities in their daily routine. In the following week another activity was trained, and in the third week the remaining activity.

The cycle was repeated until the patients could complete all three activities. Comparison between the development of independence during periods with and without therapy yielded clear-cut results: independence improved during periods of training. On average two weeks of training were necessary for attaining full independence on one trained activity. By contrast, independency on the same activities did not change during weeks without therapy. The few instances of improvement during a week without therapy were balanced by instances of deterioration during such weeks. Since the course of non-trained activities was observed in parallel to that of the trained activities, this absence of improvement indicated absence of generalization of improvement from trained to non-trained activities.

Our second study included patients with left brain damage, aphasia, and apraxia for tool use, who had already acquired independence in basic activities of daily living (Goldenberg et al., 2001a). Accordingly, the therapy addressed more complex multistep actions with multiple tools and objects including technical devices like making coffee with a drop coffee maker or fixing a tape recorder (see Chapter 9). The study design was similar to that of the previous study. There were four tasks divided in two pairs. The need for assistance and number of errors were assessed for all of them in regular intervals. After two intervals without therapy which served as a control for the effects of repeated testing, one pair was subjected to training during two intervals, while the other pair received no therapy. Then the other pair was trained for two intervals. Again, the results were straightforward: apart from some improvement during the first baseline period, error rates diminished only when the respective tasks were trained. There was no generalization of improvement to the simultaneously non-trained tasks.

After completion of the whole therapy program we repeated the final testing with slightly different variants of the tools and devices used during training. For example, the tape recorder was replaced by a Walkman and the electric outlet for connecting the coffee maker was replaced by a mobile socket. These modifications led to an increase of the error rate, though not to a return to their height at the beginning of therapy. Apparently they had been sufficient to scratch at the limits of generalization from trained to non-trained naturalistic actions.

Communicative gesture

Giving an overview of generalization of therapeutic successes for the training of communicative gestures is more difficult than for training of tool and object use. On the one hand, the number of therapy studies is higher, but on the other hand the number of patients included in them is lower and some of them are based on only one or two cases (Code & Gaunt, 1986; Coelho & Duffy, 1990; Cubelli et al., 1991; Maher & Ochipa, 1997). All of these studies were conducted with aphasic patients who could potentially benefit from developing gesture as an alternative channel for communication.

In all of these studies patients were able to acquire the production of meaningful gestures on command which was, however, usually not given verbally but by presentation of a picture of the object that was to be indicated by a gesture. Generalization of this success to non-trained gestures varied widely. At the one extreme there is one group (Schlanger & Freimann, 1979) and one single case study (Cubelli et al., 1991) of patients whose improvement on producing comprehensible pantomimes of tool use was virtually the same for trained and non-trained pantomimes, while at the other extreme a group study reported a significant deterioration of the production of successfully trained gestures when they were elicited with different pictures of objects than those used during training, suggesting restriction of therapeutic success not only to trained gestures but also to minor details of the training setup (Coelho & Duffy, 1987). Between these extremes there are several studies that found improvement of non-trained gestures significant but inferior to that of trained gestures (Code & Gaunt, 1986; Maher & Ochipa, 1997; Daumüller & Goldenberg, 2010)

We used the same basic paradigm as in our studies of naturalistic actions for exploring efficacy and generalization of gesture training for patients with severe aphasia (Daumüller & Goldenberg, 2010). A set of 24 communicative gestures were divided into three sets of eight. Within each set six gestures referred to objects and their use (e.g., put on glasses, watching TV) and two conveyed messages that do not indicate a distinct object (eg., yes, no, being married). The gestures were pragmatic combinations of pantomimes, pictographs (e.g., drawing the outlines of the glasses before the eyes), deictics (e.g., pointing to the ring finger for indicating marriage), and emblems (e.g., thumbs up for yes). Production of all gestures to command was probed at intervals of two weeks. Scoring of

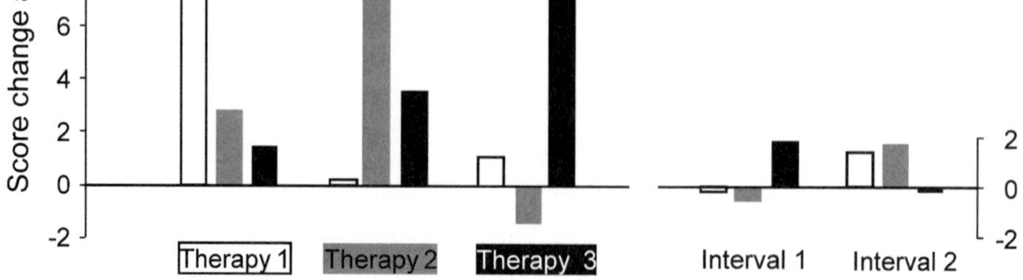

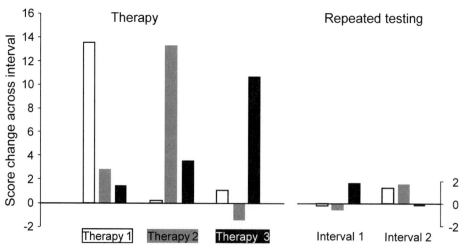

Figure 16.1 Design and results of our gesture therapy study. Left: Increases of scores from start to end of a therapy period for trained and non-trained gestures. The shades of the x-labels correspond with the shades of the gesture sets that were trained during the labeled period. Thus, the white bar in the first period indicates the improvement of the gestures that were trained in the white period while the gray and the black bars show the simultaneous development of the non-trained gestures. Right: Changes of scores across intervals with no therapy were assessed in a second study with a comparable group of patients.

gestures considered their accuracy and the need for assistance. During each interval one set of gestures was trained. There was no baseline condition in the therapy study itself, but in a second study a comparable group of aphasic patients was tested three times in weekly intervals without interpolated training to control for the effects of repeated testing.

Figure 16.1 demonstrates the results of both parts of the study. Improvement of trained gestures was massively higher than simultaneous improvement of non-trained gestures, but there was also statistically significant improvement of the non-trained gestures, and this improvement was higher than the improvement brought forward by mere repetition of testing in the second part of the study. It thus seems that there was indeed some generalization from gesture training to the production of non-trained gestures. We will come back to possible mechanisms underlying this generalization when we discuss the efficacy of task-specific and general approaches to therapy.

Task-specific versus general approaches to therapy

In the preceding section we have discussed whether therapeutic alleviation of apraxia remains item specific or generalizes to non-trained items and tasks. In this section we will discuss the same basic dichotomy for the choice of therapeutic methods, opposing approaches that concentrate on selected items or tasks to approaches that aim at restoring general aptitudes. Again, we will do this separately for use of tool and objects, and for communicative gestures.

Use of tools and objects

The Dutch group who reported generalization of improvement to non-trained activities classified their approach as "strategy training" because it was intended to teach patients "strategies to compensate for the apraxic impairment during the performance of activities of daily living" (van Heugten et al., 1998; Donkervoort et al., 2001; Geusgens et al., 2006). Examples of such strategies are "self-verbalization to support the performance and writing down or showing pictures of the proper sequence of activities" (Donkervoort et al., 2001, p. 553). Presumably this approach combines task-specific elements (e.g., pictures of the proper sequence) with generally applicable methods (e.g., self-verbalization). Similar approaches were proposed by Miller (1986) and Sunderland et al. (2006).

In our second therapy study we explicitly compared a task-specific approach aiming at acquisition and consolidation of routine performance with one aimed at gaining insight into the functional relationships between the tools and objects and enhancing the general capacity of mechanical problems solving. We named them "direct training" and "exploration training." In direct training the patient was led to carry out the entire activity with a minimum of errors. Support was given at all critical stages and was reduced only at the measure of the patients' increasing competence. Performance of the whole activity was sometimes interrupted for rehearsal of a critical passage but was completed after repeated performance of the critical actions. Only actions or objects involved in the activity were employed for training.

During exploration training the objects involved in the activities were explored, but the activities themselves were not carried out. The therapist tried to direct the patient's attention to functionally significant details of the objects. Patients were led to palpate and to draw the objects with particular emphasis on critical details, and the objects were compared with other objects subserving either the same or different purposes. Emphasis on critical details was also stressed by matching objects with photographs of exemplars which differed in the arrangement of functionally significant details such as, for example, several tape recorders differing in the location of the play button.

I already mentioned that in this second therapy of tool and object use study we had two intervals of training for each pair of activities. During the first of them patients had exploration training, and during the second interval direct training of the same pair of activities. The results were a drawback for our expectation that exploration training would enable patients to apply mechanical problem solving for solving both trained and non-trained tasks. Exploration training had no significant effect on either of them. Improvement on trained tasks was brought forward exclusively by direct training and did not generalize to untrained activities. We concluded that therapy can establish routines for performing trained tasks but cannot restore the general abilities necessary for coping with novel instances of tool and object use.

Communicative gestures

On scrutinizing the method section of papers reporting therapy of communicative gestures one can discern two elements that are present in most of them. The first is a stepwise isolation of the gesture as an independent means of communication. For example, training of the pantomime of drinking from a glass starts with actual execution of this act. Then, the action of use is dissociated from its purpose in that the empty glass is led to the mouth and tilted as if it contained fluid. The next step is an empty-handed repetition of the action immediately after performing it with the object. Then, the pantomime is requested on sight of the object and, in a further step, on sight of various pictures of it (Maher & Ochipa, 1997; Daumüller et al., 2010). For emblematic or pictographic gestures, appreciation of the gesture as an independent carrier of meaning can be based on variable combinations with other expressions of the same meaning. For example, patients may be asked to imitate a gesture simultaneously with the presentation of pictures or words indicating its meaning, or they may be asked to select matching pictures or words to gestures that are presented by the therapist (Code & Gaunt, 1986; Coelho & Duffy, 1990).

The second element of gesture therapy concerns the shape of the gesture. Since patients are apraxic their gestures are frequently ill-formed or amorphous and lack distinctive features. Therapists may direct attention to crucial features by verbal instruction, by demonstration of the differences between the patient's gestures and correct gestures, by

[1] Note that in this context defective imitation gains ecological significance as a hindrance for gesture training. It is, however, questionable whether a dedicated training of imitation would be helpful. Again, the efficacy would depend on transfer from trained hand and finger postures to the specific gestures needed for communication.

leading patients to imitate the correct gesture,[1] or by passive molding of the patient's hand (Maher & Ochipa, 1997).

Possibly, these two elements of gesture training contribute differentially to the generalization of success from trained to non-trained gestures. Insight into the independent communicative value of gestures is not item-specific but concerns the production of any communicative gestures. In Chapter 11 we discussed that for efficient gestural communication patients must overcome the lifelong habit of producing gestures that accompany and illustrate speech in favor of producing gestures that replace speech. When patients succeed in gaining this insight they will become more likely to try a gesture when they cannot express their opinions or desires verbally, and the mere act of trying will also lead to some improvement for production of non-trained gestures.

By contrast, the production of well-formed gestures is hindered by apraxia. In order to find out the correct shape of untrained gestures, patients must select and combine distinct features of their content, but their inability to do so is a core deficit of apraxia. Apparently therapy cannot overcome the core of apraxia. Patients can be taught to produce the correct shape of single gestures but they remain unable to generate the correct shapes of non-trained gestures.

Levels of therapy

The empirical fundament of the available therapy studies is too weak to allow definite conclusions, but their tendency is rather supportive of a skeptical attitude toward generalization of therapy success. Several studies demonstrate that improvement are task or even item specific, and therapeutic approaches that aimed at restitution of general aptitudes were less efficient than approaches that concentrated on practice and rehearsal of concrete tasks. We have identified the inability to cope with novel actions as one of the criteria for a high-level disturbance in apraxia. The lack of generalization is equivalent to an inability to cope with novel actions. We may conclude that therapy fails to restore the high-level components of apraxia or, said in another way, the cognitive side of motor control.

References

Abler, W. L. (1989). On the particulate principle of self-diversifying systems. *Journal of Social and Biological Structures, 12*, 1–13.

Adie, W. J. & Critchley, M. (1927). Forced grasping and groping. *Brain, 50*, 142–70.

Agostini, E., Coletti, A., Orlando, G., & Tredici, G. (1983). Apraxia in deep cerebral lesions. *Journal of Neurology, Neurosurgery, and Psychiatry, 46*, 804–8.

Akelaitis, A. J. (1945). Studies on the corpus callosum IV: Diagonistic dyspraxia following partial and complete section of the corpus callosum. *American Journal of Psychiatry, 101*, 954–9.

Akelaitis, A. J., Risteem, W. A., Herren, R. Y., & Van Wagenen, W. P. (1942). Studies on the corpus callosum III: A contribution to the study of dyspraxia and apraxia following partial and complete section of the corpus callosum. *Archives of Neurology and Psychiatry, 47*, 971–1008.

Alajouanine, T. & Lhermitte, F. (1960). Les troubles des activités expressives du langage dans l'aphasie Leurs relations aves les apraxies. *Revue Neurologique, 102*, 604–29.

Alexander, M. P. & Annet, M. (1996). Crossed aphasia and related anomalies of cerebral organization: Case reports and a genetic hypothesis. *Brain and Language, 55*, 213–39.

Alexander, M. P., Baker, E., Naeser, M. A., Kaplan, E., & Palumbo, C. (1992). Neuropsychological and neuroanatomic dimensions of ideomotor apraxia. *Brain, 115*, 87–107.

Alivisatos, B. & Petrides, M. (1997). Functional activation of the human brain during mental rotation. *Neuropsychologia, 35*, 111–18.

Ambrosoni, E., Della Sala, S., Motto, C., Oddo, S., & Spinnler, H. (2006). Gesture imitation with lower limbs following left hemisphere stroke. *Archives of Clinical Neuropsychology, 21*, 349–58.

Andersen, S. W., Damasio, H., & Tranel, D. (1990). Neuropsychological impairments associated with lesions caused by tumor or stroke. *Archives of Neurology, 47*, 397–405.

Anderson, B., Southern, B. S., & Powers, R. E. (1999). Anatomic asymmetries of the posterior superior temporal lobes: A postmortem study. *Neuropsychiatry, Neuropsychology, and Behavioural Neurology, 12*, 247–54.

Anema, H. A., Kessels, R. P. C., De Haan, E. H. F., Kappelle, L. J., Leijten, F. S., van Zandvoort, M. J. E., *et al.* (2008). Differences in finger localistion performance of patients with finger agnosia. *NeuroReport, 19*, 1429–33.

Aouka, N., Goldenberg, G., & Nadel, J. (2003). Exploring children's body knowledge via imitation of meaningless gestures. *XIth European Conference on Developmental Psychology, 17-3*, 259.

Archibald, Y. M. (1987). Persisting apraxia in two left-handed, aphasic patients with right-hemisphere lesions. *Brain and Cognition, 6*, 412–28.

Assal, G. & Butters, J. (1973). Troubles du schéma corporel lors des atteintes hémisphériques gauches. *Schweizer Medizinische Rundschau, 62*, 172–9.

Assal, G., Perentes, E., & Deruaz, J. (1981). Crossed aphasia in a right-handed patients. *Archives of Neurology, 38*, 455–8.

Aziz-Zadeh, L., Maeda, F., Zaidel, E., Mazziotta, J. C., & Iacoboni, M. (2002). Lateralization in motor facilitation during action observation: a TMS study. *Experimental Brain Research, 144*, 127–31.

Baldo, J. V. & Dronkers, N. F. (2006). The role of inferior parietal and inferior frontal cortex in working memory. *Neuropsychology, 20*, 529–38.

Barbarulo, A. M., Pappatà, S., Puoti, G., Prinster, A., Grossi, D., Cotrufo, R., *et al.* (2008). Rehabilitation of gesture imitation: A case study with fMRI. *Neurocase, 14*, 293–306.

Barbieri, C. & De Renzi, E. (1988). The executive and ideational components of apraxia. *Cortex, 24*, 535–44.

Bartha, L., Marien, P., Poewe, W., & Benke, T. (2004). Linguistic and neuropsychological deficits in crossed conduction aphasia. Report of three cases. *Brain and Language, 88*, 83–95.

Bartolo, A., Cubelli, R., Della Sala, S., Drei, S., & Marchetti, C. (2001). Double dissociation between meaningful and meaningless gesture reproduction in apraxia. *Cortex, 37*, 696–9.

Basso, A., Capitani, E., Laiacona, M., & Zanobio, M. E. (1985). Crossed aphasia: One or more syndromes? *Cortex, 21*, 25–45.

Beaton, A. A. (2003). The nature and determinants of handedness. In K. Hugdahl & R. J. Davidson (Eds.), *The asymmetrical brain* (pp. 105–58). Cambridge, MA: MIT Press.

Behrmann, M. & Penn, C. (1984). Non-verbal communication of aphasic patients. *British Journal of Disorders of Communication, 19*, 155–68.

Bekkering, H., Brass, M., Woschina, S., & Jacobs, A. M. (2005). Goal-directed imitation in patients with ideomotor apraxia. *Cognitive Neuropsychology, 22*, 419–32.

Bekkering, H., Wohlschläger, A., & Gattis, M. (2000). Imitation of gestures in children is goal-directed. *Quarterly Journal of Experimental Psychology, 53A*, 153–64.

Bell, B. D. (1994). Pantomime recognition impairment in aphasia: An analysis of error types. *Brain and Language, 47*, 269–78.

Bellugi, U., Poizner, H., & Klima, E. S. (1989). Language, modality and the brain. *Trends in Neuroscience, 12*, 380–8.

Benton, A. L. (1961). The fiction of the "Gerstmann Syndrome". *Journal of Neurology, Neurosurgery, and Psychiatry, 24*, 176–81.

Binkofski, F., Amunts, K., Stephan, K. M., Posse, S., Schormann, T., Freund, H. J., *et al.* (2000). Broca's region subserves imagery of motion: A combined cytoarchitectonic and fMRI study. *Human Brain Mapping, 11*, 273–85.

Binkofski, F., Buccino, G., Dohle, C., Seitz, R. J., & Freund, H. J. (1999). Mirror agnosia and mirror ataxia constitute different parietal lobe disorders. *Annals of Neurology, 46*, 51–61.

Bizzozero, I., Costato, D., Della Sala, S., Papagno, C., Spinnler, H., & Venneri, A. (2000). Upper and lower face apraxia: role of the right hemisphere. *Brain, 123*, 2213–30.

Bleuler, E. (1893). Ein Fall von aphasischen Symptomen, Hemianopsie, amnestischer Farbenblindheit und Seelenlähmung. *Archiv für Psychiatrie und Nervenkrankheiten, 25*, 32–73.

Bogen, J. E. (1993). The callosal syndromes. In K. M. Heilman & E. Valenstein (Eds.), *Clinical neuropsychology* (3rd edn, pp. 337–407). New York, NY: Oxford University Press.

Bogen, J. E. & Gazzaniga, M. S. (1965). Cerebral commisurotomy in man. Minor hemisphere dominance for certain visuospatial functions. *Journal of Neurosurgery, 23*, 394–9.

Boldrini, P., Zanella, R., Cantaglio, A., & Basaglia, N. (1992). Partial hemispheric disconnection syndrome of traumatic origin. *Cortex, 28*, 135–44.

Bonhoeffer, K. (1914). Klinischer und anatomischer Befund zur Lehre von der Apraxie und der "motorischen Sprachbahn". *Monatschrift für Psychiatrie und Neurologie, 35*, 113–28.

Borod, J. C., Fitzpatrick, P. M., Helm-Estabrooks, N., & Goodglass, H. (1989). The relationship between limb apraxia and the spontaneous use of communicative gesture in aphasia. *Brain and Cognition, 10*, 121–31.

Boronat, C. B., Buxbaum, L. J., Coslett, H. B., Tang, K., Saffran, E. M., Kimberg, D. Y., *et al.* (2005). Distinctions between manipulation and function knowledge of objects: evidence from functional magnetic resonance imaging. *Cognitive Brain Research, 23*, 361–73.

Bourneville, D. M. & Regnarde, P. (1879). *Iconographie photographic de la Salpétrière, première partie.* Paris: V.A. Delhaye & Lecroinier, Editeurs.

Bozeat, S., Patterson, K., & Hodges, J. R. (2002). When objects lose their meaning: What happens to their use? *Cognitive, Affective & Behavioral Neuroscience, 2*, 236–51.

Brain, R. (1961). Henry Head: The man and his ideas. *Brain, 84*, 561–9.

Brain, W. R. (1941). Visual disorientation with special reference to lesions of the right cerebral hemisphere. *Brain, 64*, 244–73.

Brainin, M., Seiser, A., & Matz, K. (2008). The mirror world of motor inhibition: The alien hand syndrome in chronic stroke. *Journal of Neurology, Neurosurgery, and Psychiatry, 79*, 246–52.

Brass, M. & Heyes, C. (2005). Imitation: is cognitive neuroscience solving the correspondence problem? *Trends in Cognitive Sciences, 9*, 489–95.

Brion, S. & Jedynak, C. P. (1972). Troubles de transfert interhémisphérique (callosal disconnection). A propos de trois observations de tumeurs du corps calleux. Le signe de la main étrangère. *Revue Neurologique, 126*, 257–66.

Broca, P. (1861). Perte de la parole, ramollissement chronique et destruction partielle du lobe antérieur gauche du cerveau. *Communication Société d'Anthropologie, Séance du 18 avril 1861.*

Broca, P. (1865). Du siège de la faculté du langage articulé dans l'hemisphere gauche du cerveau. *Bulletin de la Société d'Anthopologie, 6*, 377–93.

Broca, P. (2006). Comments regarding the seat of the faculty of spoken language, followed by an observation of aphemia (loss of speech) [Remarques sur le Siége de la Faculté du Langage Articulé, Suivies d'une Observation d'aphemie; Bulletin de la Société Anatomique de Paris: 330–357, 1861]. In Y. Grodzinsky & K. Amunts (Eds.), *Broca's region* (pp. 291–304). Oxford: Oxford University Press.

Brooks, V. B. (1986). Controlled variables. In V. B. Brooks (Ed.), *The neural basis of motor control* (pp. 129–48). Oxford: Oxford University Press.

Bruns, L. (1897). Ueber Seelenlähmung. In *Festschrift anlässlich des fünfzigjährigen Bestehens der Provinzial-Irrenanstalt zu Nietleben bei Halle* (pp. 376–95). Leipzig: F. C. W. Vogel.

Buccino, G., Binkofski, F., Fink, G. R., Fadiga, L., Fogassi, L., Gallese, V., *et al.* (2001). Action observation activates premotor and parietal areas in a somatotopic manner: an fMRI study. *European Journal of Neuroscience, 13*, 400–4.

Buck, R. & Duffy, R. J. (1980). Nonverbal communication of affect in brain-damaged patients. *Cortex, 16*, 351–62.

Buck, R. & VanLear, C. A. (2002). Verbal and nonverbal communication: Distinguishing symbolic, spontaneous, and pseudo-spontaneous nonverbal behavior. *Journal of Communication, 52*, 522–42.

Buckingham, H. W. (1984). Early development of association theory in psychology as a forerunner to connection theory. *Brain and Cognition, 3*, 19–34.

Buxbaum, L. J. (2001). Ideomotor apraxia: a call to action. *Neurocase, 7*, 445–58.

Buxbaum, L. J. & Coslett, H. B. (2001). Specialised structural descriptions for human body parts: Evidence from autotopagnosia. *Cognitive Neuropsychology, 18*, 289–306.

Buxbaum, L. J., Haaland, K. Y., Hallett, M., Wheaton, L., Heilman, K. M., Rodriguez, A., *et al.* (2008). Treatment of limb apraxia. Moving forward to improved action. *American Journal of Physical Medicine and Rehabilitation, 87*, 149–61.

Buxbaum, L. J., Kyle, K., Grossman, M., & Coslett, H. B. (2007). Left inferior parietal representations for skilled hand-object interactions: evidence from stroke and corticobasal degeneration. *Cortex, 43*, 411–23.

Buxbaum, L. J., Kyle, K. M., & Menon, R. (2005). On beyond mirror neurons: Internal representations subserving imitation and recognition of skilled object-related actions in humans. *Cognitive Brain Research, 25*, 226–39.

Buxbaum, L. J. & Saffran, E. M. (2002). Knowledge of object manipulation and object function: dissociations in apraxic and nonapraxic patients. *Brain and Language, 82*, 179–99.

Buxbaum, L. J., Schwartz, M. F., & Carew, T. G. (1997). The role of semantic memory in object use. *Cognitive Neuropsychology, 14*, 219–54.

Buxbaum, L. J., Schwartz, M. F., Coslett, H. B., & Carew, T. G. (1995). Naturalistic action and praxis in callosal apraxia. *Neurocase, 1*, 3–17.

Buxbaum, L. J., Schwartz, M. F., & Montgomery, M. W. (1998). Ideational apraxia and naturalistic action. *Cognitive Neuropsychology, 15*, 617–44.

Buxhoeveden, D. & Casanova, M. (2000). Comparative lateralisation patterns in the language area of human, chimpanzee, and rhesus monkey brains. *Laterality, 5*, 315–30.

Cabeza, R. & Nyberg, L. (2000). Imagining cognition II: An empirical review of 275 PET and fMRI studies. *Journal of Cognitive Neuroscience, 12*, 1–47.

Canessa, N., Borgo, F., Cappa, S. F., Perani, D., Falini, A., Buccino, G., *et al.* (2008). The different neural correlates of action and functional knowledge in semantic memory: An fMRI study. *Cerebral Cortex, 18*, 740–51.

Caplan, D. (1987). *Neurolinguistics and linguistic aphasiology*. Cambridge: Cambridge University Press.

Carlesimo, G. A., Fadda, L., & Caltagirone, C. (1993). Basic mechanisms of constructional apraxia in unilateral brain-damaged patients: Role of visuo-perceptual and executive disorders. *Journal of Clinical and Experimental Neuropsychology, 15*, 342–58.

Carmo, J. C. & Rumiati, R. I. (2009). Imitation of transitive and intransitive actions in healthy individuals. *Brain and Cognition, 69*, 460–4.

Catani, M. & ffytche, D. H. (2005). The rises and falls of disconnection syndromes. *Brain, 128*, 2224–39.

Cermak, S. A., Coster, W., & Drake, C. (1980). Representational and nonrepresentational gestures in boys with learning disabilities. *The American Journal of Occupational Therapy, 34*, 19–26.

Chen, R., Cohen, L. G., & Hallet, M. (1997). Role of the ipsilateral motor cortex in voluntary movement. *Canadian Journal of Neurological Science, 24*, 284–91.

Chomsky, N. (1957). *Syntactic structures*. Berlin: Mouton de Gruyter.

Cicone, M., Wapner, W., Foldi, N., Zurif, E., & Gardner, H. (1979). The relation between gesture and language in aphasic communication. *Brain and Language, 8*, 324–49.

Clark, M., Merians, A. S., Kothari, A., Poizner, H., Macauley, B., Rothi, L. J. G., *et al.* (1994). Spatial planning deficits in limb apraxia. *Brain, 117*, 1093–106.

Clark, S., Tremblay, F., & Ste-Marie, D. (2004). Different modulation of corticospinal excitability during observation, mental imagery and imitation of hand actions. *Neuropsychologia, 42*, 105–12.

Coccia, M., Bartolini, M., Luzzi, S., Provinciali, L., & Lambon Ralph, M. A. (2004). Semantic memory is an amodal, dynamic system: Evidence from the interaction of naming and object use in semantic dementia. *Cognitive Neuropsychology, 21*, 513–27.

Cocks, N., Hird, K., & Kirsner, K. (2007). The relationship between right hemisphere damage and gesture in spontaneous discourse. *Aphasiology, 21*, 299–319.

Code, C. & Gaunt, C. (1986). Treating severe speech and limb apraxia in a case of aphasia. *British Journal of Disorders of Communication, 21*, 11–20.

Coelho, C. A. & Duffy, R. J. (1987). The relationship of the acquisition of manual signs to severity of aphasia: a training study. *Brain and Language, 31*, 328–45.

Coelho, C. A. & Duffy, R. J. (1990). Sign acquisition in two aphasic subjects with limb apraxia. *Aphasiology, 4*, 1–8.

Cooper, R. & Shallice, T. (2000). Contention scheduling and the control of routine activities. *Cognitive Neuropsychology, 17*, 297–338.

Cooper, R. P. (2007). Tool use and related errors in ideational apraxia: The quantitative simulation of patient error profiles. *Cortex*, *43*, 319–37.

Cooper, R. P., Schwartz, M. F., Yule, P., & Shallice, T. (2005). The simulation of action disorganisation in complex activities of daily living. *Cognitive Neuropsychology*, *22*, 959–1004.

Corballis, M. C. (1991). *The lopsided ape*. New York, NY: Oxford University Press.

Corballis, M. C. & Sergent, J. (1989). Hemispheric specialization for mental rotation. *Cortex*, *25*, 15–25.

Coulthard, E., Rudd, A., & Husain, M. (2008). Motor neglect associated with loss of action inhibition. *Journal of Neurology, Neurosurgery, and Psychiatry*, *79*, 1401–4.

Critchley, M. (1930). The anterior cerebral artery and its syndromes. *Brain*, *53*, 120–65.

Critchley, M. (1953). *The parietal lobes*. New York, NY: Hafner Publishing Company.

Cubelli, R., Marchetti, C., Boscolo, G., & Della Sala, S. (2000). Cognition in action: testing a model of limb apraxia. *Brain and Cognition*, *44*, 144–65.

Cubelli, R., Trentini, P., & Montagna, C. G. (1991). Re-education of gestural communication in a case of chronic global aphasia and limb apraxia. *Cognitive Neuropsychology*, *8*, 369–80.

Dabis, C., Kleinman, J. T., Newhart, M., Gingis, L., Pawlak, M., & Hillis, A. E. (2008). Speech and language functions that require a functioning Broca's area. *Brain and Language*, *105*, 50–8.

Damasio, A. R. (1989). Time-locked multiregional retroactivation: A systems-level proposal for the neural substrates of recall and recognition. *Cognition*, *33*, 25–62.

Daumüller, M. & Goldenberg, G. (2010). Therapy to improve gestural expression in aphasia: a controlled clinical trial. *Clinical Rehabilitation*, *24*, 55–65.

Davis, G. A. & Wilcox, M. J. (1985). *Adult aphasia rehabilitation: Applied pragmatics*. San Diego, CA: College-Hill Press.

Dawson, A. M., Buxbaum, L. J., & Duff, S. V. (2010). The impact of left hemisphere stroke on force control with familiar and novel objects: Neuroanatomic substrates and relationship to apraxia. *Brain Research*, *1317*, 124–36.

De Ajuriaguerra, J. & Hécaen, H. (1960). Les apraxies: Varietes cliniques et lateralisation lesionelle. *Revue Neurologique*, *102*, 566–91.

De Ajuriaguerra, J. & Tissot, R. (1969). The apraxias. In P. J. Vinken & G. W. Bruyn (Eds.), *Handbook of clinical neurology, Vol. 4* (pp. 48–66). Amsterdam: North Holland.

de Buck, D. (1899). Les parakinésies. *Journal de Neurologie (Société Belge de Neurologie)*, *4*, 361–74.

Delis, D. C., Knight, R. T., & Simpson, G. (1983). Reversed hemispheric organization in a left-hander. *Neuropsychologia*, *21*, 13–24.

Della Sala, S., Faglioni, P., Motto, C., & Spinnler, H. (2006a). Hemisphere asymmetry for imitation of hand and finger movements, Goldenberg's hypothesis reworked. *Neuropsychologia*, *44*, 1496–500.

Della Sala, S., Maistrello, B., Motto, C., & Spinnler, H. (2006b). A new account of face apraxia based on a longitudinal study. *Neuropsychologia*, *44*, 1159–65.

Della Sala, S., Marchetti, C., & Spinnler, H. (1991). Right-sided anarchic (alien) hand: a longitudinal study. *Neuropsychologia*, *29*, 1113–28.

Della Sala, S., Marchetti, C., & Spinnler, H. (1994). The anarchic hand: a fronto-mesial sign. In F. Boller & J. Grafman (Eds.), *Handbook of Clinical Neuropsychology, Volume 9* (pp. 233–55). Amsterdam: Elsevier Science B. V.

Della Sala, S., Spinnler, H., & Venneri, A. (2004). Walking difficulties in patients with Alzheimer's disease might originate from gait apraxia. *Journal of Neurology, Neurosurgery, and Psychiatry*, *75*, 196–201.

Denes, G., Cappelletti, J. Y., Zilli, T., Dallaporta, F., & Gallana, A. (2000). A category-specific deficit of spatial representation: the case of autotopagnosia. *Neuropsychologia*, *38*, 345–50.

Denny-Brown, D. (1958). The nature of apraxia. *Journal of Nervous and Mental Disease*, *126*, 9–32.

De Renzi, E. (1990). Apraxia. In F. Boller & J. Grafman (Eds.), *Handbook of clinical neuropsychology Vol. 2* (pp. 245–63). Amsterdam: Elsevier.

De Renzi, E. & Barbieri, C. (1992). The incidence of the grasp reflex following hemispheric lesions and its relation to frontal damage. *Brain, 115*, 293–313.

De Renzi, E., Cavalleri, F., & Facchini, S. (1996). Imitation and utilisation behaviour. *Journal of Neurology, Neurosurgery, and Psychiatry, 61*, 396–400.

De Renzi, E., Faglioni, P., & Sorgato, P. (1982). Modality-specific and supramodal mechanisms of apraxia. *Brain, 105*, 301–12.

De Renzi, E. & Lucchelli, F. (1988). Ideational apraxia. *Brain, 111*, 1173–85.

De Renzi, E., Motti, F., & Nichelli, P. (1980). Imitating gestures—A quantitative approach to ideomotor apraxia. *Archives of Neurology, 37*, 6–10.

De Renzi, E., Pieczuro, A., & Vignolo, L. A. (1966). Oral apraxia and aphasia. *Cortex, 2*, 50–73.

De Renzi, E., Pieczuro, A., & Vignolo, L. A. (1968). Ideational apraxia: a quantitative study. *Neuropsychologia, 6*, 41–55.

De Renzi, E. & Scotti, G. (1970). Autotopagnosia: fiction or reality? *Archives of Neurology, 23*, 221–7.

De Renzi, E., Scotti, G., & Spinnler, H. (1969). Perceptual and associative disorders of visual recognition. *Neurology, 19*, 634–42.

de Vignemont, F. (2010). Body schema and body image—Pros and cons. *Neuropsychologia, 48*, 669–80.

de Vignemont, F., Majid, A., Jola, C., & Haggard, P. (2009). Segmenting the body into parts: Evidence from biases in tactile perception. *Quarterly Journal of Experimental Psychology, 62*, 500–12.

de Vignemont, F., Tsakiris, M., & Haggard, P. (2006). Body mereology. In G. Knoblich, I. M. Thornton, M. Grosjean, & M. Shiffrar (Eds.), *Human body perception from the inside out* (pp. 147–70). New York, NY: Oxford University Press.

Di Pellegrino, G., Fadiga, L., Fogassi, L., Gallese, V., & Rizzolatti, G. (1992). Understanding motor events: a neurophysiological study. *Experimental Brain Research, 91*, 176–80.

Didi-Huberman, G. (1982). *Invention de l'hystérie. Charcot et l'iconographie photographic de la Salpétrière*. Paris: Edition Macula.

Donaghey, C. L., McMillan, T. M., & O'Neill, B. (2010). Errorless learning is superior to trial and error when learning a practical skill in rehabilitation: a randomized controlled trial. *Clinical Rehabilitation, 24*, 195–201.

Donkervoort, M., Dekker, J., Stehmann-Saris, J. C., & Deelman, B. G. (2001). Efficacy of strategy training in left hemisphere stroke with apraxia: A randomised clinical trial. *Neuropsychological Rehabilitation, 11*, 549–66.

Dovern, A., Fink, G., Saliger, J., Karbe, H., Koch, I., & Weiss, P. (2011). Apraxia impairs intentional retrieval of incidentally acquired motor knowledge. *Journal of Neuroscience, 31*, 8102–8.

Dronkers, N. F., Plaisant, O., Iba-Zizen, M. T., & Cabanis, E. A. (2007). Paul Broca's historic cases: high resolution MR imaging of the brains of Leborgne and Lelong. *Brain, 130*, 1432–41.

Duensing, F. (1953). Raumagnostische und ideatorisch-apraktische Störung des gestaltenden Handelns. *Deutsche Zeitschrift für Nervenheilkunde, 170*, 72–94.

Duffy, R. J. & Buck, R. (1979). A study of the relationship between propositional (pantomime) and subpropositional (facial expression) extraverbal behaviors in aphasics. *Folia phoniatrica, 31*, 129–36.

Duffy, R. J. & Duffy, J. R. (1981). Three studies of deficits in pantomimic expression and pantomimic recognition in aphasia. *Journal of Speech and Hearing Research, 14*, 70–84.

Duffy, R. J. & Duffy, J. R. (1989). An investigation of body part as object (BPO) responses in normal and brain-damaged people. *Brain and Cognition, 10*, 220–36.

Duffy, R. J., Duffy, J. R., & Pearson, K. L. (1975). Pantomime recognition in aphasics. *Journal of Speech and Hearing Disorders, 18*, 116–32.

Duffy, R. J., Watt, J. H., & Duffy, J. R. (1994). Testing causal theories of pantomimic deficits in aphasia using path analysis. *Aphasiology*, *8*, 361–79.

Dumont, C., Ska, B., & Schiavetto, A. (1999). Selective impairment of transitive gestures: an unusual case of apraxia. *Neurocase*, *5*, 447–58.

Edwards, B. (1979). *Drawing on the right side of the brain—How to unlock your hidden artistic talent.* Glasgow: William Collins Sons & Co Ltd.

Ehrsson, H. H., Geyer, S., & Naito, E. (2006). Imagery of voluntary movements of fingers, toes, and tongue activates corresponding body-part-specific motor representations. *Journal of Neurophysiology*, *90*, 3304–16.

Ekman, P. & Friesen, W. V. (1969). The repertoire of nonverbal behavior: categories, origins, usage, and coding. *Semiotica*, *1*, 49–89.

Eling, P. (2006). The psycholinguistic approach to aphasia of Chajm Steinthal. *Aphasiology*, *20*, 1072–84.

Eling, P. (2011). Lichtheim's golden shot. *Cortex*, *47*, 501–8.

Enfield, N. J., Majid, A., & van Staden, M. (2006). Cross-linguistic categorisation of the body: Introduction. *Language Sciences*, *28*, 137–47.

Fadiga, L., Fogassi, L., Pavesi, G., & Rizzolatti, G. (1995). Motor facilitation during action observation: A magnetic stimulation study. *Journal of Neurophysiology*, *73*, 2608–11.

Fazio, P., Cantagallo, A., Craighero, L., D'Ausilio, A., Roy, A. C., Pozzo, T., *et al.* (2009). Encoding of human action in Broca's area. *Brain*, *132*, 1980–8.

Felician, O., Ceccaldi, M., Didic, M., Thinus-Blanc, C., & Poncet, M. (2003). Pointing to body parts: a double dissociation study. *Neuropsychologia*, *41*, 1307–16.

Ferrari, P. F., Rozzi, S., & Fogassi, L. (2005). Mirror neurons responding to observation of actions made with tools in monkey ventral premotor cortex. *Journal of Cognitive Neuroscience*, *17*, 212–26.

Ferro, J. M., Mariano, G., & Castro-Caldas, A. (1983). CT-scan correlates of gesture recognition. *Journal of Neurology, Neurosurgery, and Psychiatry*, *46*, 943–52.

Fex, B. & Mansson, A. C. (1998). The use of gestures as a compensatory strategy in adults with acquired aphasia compared to children with specific language impairment (SLI). *Journal of Neurolinguistics*, *11*, 191–206.

Feyereisen, P., Barter, D., Goossens, M., & Clerebaut, N. (1988). Gestures and speech in referential communication by aphasic subjects: channel use and efficiency. *Aphasiology*, *2*, 21–32.

Feyereisen, P., Gendron, M., & Seron, X. (1999). Disorders of everyday actions in subjects suffering from senile dementia of the Alzheimer's type: An analysis of dressing performance. *Neuropsychological Rehabilitation*, *9*, 169–88.

Feyereisen, P., Seron, X., & De Macar, M. (1981). L'interpretation de differentes categories de gestes chez des sujets aphasiques. *Neuropsychologia*, *19*, 515–21.

ffytche, D. H. & Catani, M. (2005). Beyond localization: from hodology to function. *Philosophical Transactions of the Royal Society of London, B*, *360*, 767–79.

Finger, S. (2000). *Minds behind the brain. A history of the pioneers and their discoveries.* Oxford: Oxford University Press.

Fink, G. R., Manjaly, Z. M., Stephan, K. M., Gurd, J. M., Zilles, K., Amunts, K., *et al.* (2006). A role for Broca's area beyond language processing. Evidence from neuropsychology and fMRI. In Y. Grodzinsky & K. Amunts (Eds.), *Broca's region* (pp. 254–70). Oxford: Oxford University Press.

Finkelnburg, C. M. (1870). Sitzung der Niederrheinischen Gesellschaft in Bonn. Medizinische Section. *Berliner Klinische Wochenschrift*, *7*, 449–50, 460–2.

Fitts, P. M. (1954). The information capacity of the human motor system in controlling the amplitude of movement. *Journal of Experimental Psychology*, *47*, 381–91.

Fodor, J. A. & Pylyshyn, Z. W. (1988). Connectionism and cognitive architecture: A critical analysis. *Cognition*, *28*, 3–72.

Fogassi, L. & Luppino, G. (2005). Motor functions of the parietal lobe. *Current Opinion in Neurobiology*, *15*, 626–31.

Foix, C. (1916). Contribution a l'étude de l'apraxie ideomotrice, de son anatomie pathologique et de ses rapports avec les syndromes qui ordinairment l'accompagnent. *Revue Neurologique*, *29*, 283–98.

Forde, E. M. E., Humphreys, G. W., & Remoundou, M. (2004). Disordered knowledge of action order in action disorganisation syndrome. *Neurocase*, *10*, 19–28.

Franz, E. A., Ford, S., & Werner, S. (2007). Brain and cognitive processes of imitation in bimanual situations: Making inferences about mirror neuron systems. *Brain Research*, *1145*, 138–49.

Freund, H. J. (1987). Abnormalities of motor behavior after cortical lesions in humans. In V. B. Mountcastle, F. Plum, & S. R. Geiger (Eds.), *Handbook of physiology section 1: The nervous system volume 5: Higher functions of the brain part 2* (pp. 763–810). Bethesda, MD: American Physiological Society.

Frey, S. H. (2007). What puts the how in where? Tool use and the divided visual streams hypothesis. *Cortex*, *43*, 368–75.

Friedmann, N. (2006). Speech production in Broca's agrammatic aphasia: Syntactic tree pruning. In Y. Grodzinsky & K. Amunts (Eds.), *Broca's region* (pp. 63–82). Oxford: Oxford University Press.

Fritsch, G. & Hitzig, E. (1870). Ueber die elektrische Erregbarkeit des Großhirns. *Archiv für Anatomie, Physiologie und wissenschaftliche Medizin*, *37*, 300–32.

Fukutate, T. (2008). Apraxia of tool use: An autopsy case of biparietal infarction. *European Neurology*, *49*, 45–52.

Gainotti, G. (1985). Constructional apraxia. In J. A. M. Frederiks (Ed.), *Handbook of clinical neurology, second series, vol. 1 (45): Clinical neuropsychology* (pp. 491–506). Amsterdam: Elsevier.

Gainotti, G., Cianchetti, C., & Tiacci, C. (1972). The influence of the hemispheric side of lesion on non verbal tasks of finger localization. *Cortex*, *8*, 364–81.

Gainotti, G. & Lemmo, M. A. (1976). Comprehension of symbolic gestures in aphasia. *Brain and Language*, *3*, 451–60.

Galaburda, A. M. (1985). Norman Geschwind 1926–1984. *Neuropsychologia*, *23*, 297–304.

Gallagher, S. (1986). Body image and body schema: a conceptual clarification. *The Journal of Mind and Behavior*, *7*, 541–54.

Galuske, R. A. W., Schlote, W., Bratzke, H., & Singer, W. (2000). Interhemispheric asymmetries of the modular structure in human temporal cortex. *Science*, *289*, 1946–9.

Garrod, S. & Pickering, M. J. (2004). Why is conversation so easy? *Trends in Cognitive Sciences*, *8*, 8–11.

Gattis, M., Bekkering, H., & Wohlschläger, A. (2002). Goal-directed imitation. In A. N. Meltzoff & W. Prinz (Eds.), *The imitative mind. Development, evolution, and brain bases* (pp. 183–205). Cambridge: Cambridge University Press.

Gazzaniga, M. (1970). *The bisected brain*. New York, NY: Appleton-Century-Crofts.

Gazzaniga, M. (2000). Cerebral specialization and interhemispheric communication. Does the corpus callosum enable the human condition? *Brain*, *123*, 1293–326.

Gazzaniga, M. S., Bogen, J. E., & Sperry, R. W. (1967). Dyspraxia following division of the cerebral commissures. *Archives of Neurology*, *16*, 606–12.

Gerstmann, J. (1924). Fingeragnosie—eine umschriebene Störung der Orientierung am eigenen Körper. *Wiener Klinische Wochenschrift*, *37*, 1010–12.

Gerstmann, J. (1942). Problems of imperception of disease and of impaired body territories with organic lesions. Relation to body scheme and its disorders. *Archives of Neurology and Psychiatry*, *48*, 890–913.

Gerstmann, J. & Schilder, P. (1926). Ueber eine besondere Gangstoerung bei Stirnhirnserkrankungen. *Wiener Medizinische Wochenschrift*, *76*, 97–102.

Geschwind, N. (1963). Carl Wernicke, the Breslau School and the history of aphasia. In E. C. Carterette (Ed.), *Brain function, volume III: Speech, language, and communication* (pp. 1–16). Berkeley, CA: University of California Press.

Geschwind, N. (1965). Disconnexion syndromes in animal and man. *Brain*, *88*, 237–94, 585–644.

Geschwind, N. (1975). The apraxias: Neural mechanisms of disorders of learned movements. *American Scientist*, *63*, 188–95.

Geschwind, N. & Damasio, A. R. (1985). Apraxia. In J. A. M. Frederiks (Ed.), *Handbook of clinical neurology, Vol. 1 (49): Clinical neuropsychology* (pp. 423–32). Amsterdam New York, NY: Elsevier.

Geschwind, N. & Kaplan, E. (1962). A human cerebral deconnection syndrome. *Neurology*, *12*, 675–85.

Geschwind, N. & Levitsky, W. (1968). Human brain: Left-right asymmetries in temporal speech region. *Science*, *161*, 186–7.

Geusgens, C., van Heugten, C. M., Donkervoort, M., van den Ende, E., Jolles, J., & van den Heuvel, W. (2006). Transfer of training effects in stroke patients with apraxia: An exploratory study. *Neuropsychological Rehabilitation*, *16*, 213–29.

Giovannetti, T., Libon, D. J., Buxbaum, L. J., & Schwartz, M. F. (2002). Naturalistic action impairment in dementia. *Neuropsychologia*, *40*, 1220–32.

Giroud, M. & Dumas, R. (1995). Clinical and topographical range of callosal infarction: a clinical and radiological correlation study. *Journal of Neurology, Neurosurgery, and Psychiatry*, *59*, 238–42.

Glindemann, R., Klintwort, D., Ziegler, W., & Goldenberg, G. (2002). *Bogenhausener Semantik-Untersuchung BOSU*. München: Urban & Fischer.

Glosser, G., Wiener, M., & Kaplan, E. (1986). Communicative gestures in aphasia. *Brain and Language*, *27*, 345–59.

Glosser, G., Wiley, M. J., & Barnoski, E. J. (1998). Gestural communication in Alzheimer's disease. *Journal of Clinical and Experimental Neuropsychology*, *20*, 1–13.

Gold, B. T. & Buckner, R. L. (2002). Common prefrontal regions coactivate with dissociable posterior regions during controlled semantic and phonological tasks. *Neuron*, *35*, 803–12.

Goldberg, G., Mayer, N. H., & Toglia, J. U. (1981). Medial frontal cortex infarction and the alien hand sign. *Archives of Neurology*, *38*, 683–6.

Goldenberg, G. (1989). The ability of patients with brain damage to generate mental visual images. *Brain*, *112*, 305–25.

Goldenberg, G. (1995). Imitating gestures and manipulating a mannikin—the representation of the human body in ideomotor apraxia. *Neuropsychologia*, *33*, 63–72.

Goldenberg, G. (1996). Defective imitation of gestures in patients with damage in the left or right hemisphere. *Journal of Neurology, Neurosurgery, and Psychiatry*, *61*, 176–80.

Goldenberg, G. (1999). Matching and imitation of hand and finger postures in patients with damage in the left or right hemisphere. *Neuropsychologia*, *37*, 559–66.

Goldenberg, G. (2001). Imitation and matching of hand and finger postures. *Neuroimage*, *14*, S132–6.

Goldenberg, G. (2002). Goldstein and Gelb's case Schn.—a classic case in neuropsychology? In C. Code, C. W. Wallesch, Y. Joanette, & A. Roch-Lecours (Eds.), *Classic cases in neuropsychology*, *Vol. 2* (pp. 281–99). Hove: Psychology Press.

Goldenberg, G. (2003a). Apraxia and beyond—life and works of Hugo Karl Liepmann. *Cortex*, *39*, 509–25.

Goldenberg, G. (2003b). Pantomime of object use: a challenge to cerebral localization of cognitive function. *Neuroimage*, *20*, S101–6.

Goldenberg, G. (2003c). The neuropsychological assessment and treatment of disorders of voluntary movement. In P. Halligan, U. Kischka, & J. C. Marshall (Eds.), *Handbook of clinical neuropsychology* (pp. 340–52). Oxford: Oxford University Press.

Goldenberg, G. (2005). Body image and the self. In T. E. Feinberg & J. P. Keenan (Eds.), *The lost self: Pathologies of the brain and identity* (pp. 81–99). San Francisco, CA: Oxford University Press.

Goldenberg, G. (2007). *Neuropsychologie—Grundlagen, Klinik, Rehabilitation. 4. Auflage.* München: Elsevier, Urban & Fischer.

Goldenberg, G. (2009). Apraxia and the parietal lobes. *Neuropsychologia, 47*, 1449–59.

Goldenberg, G., Daumüller, M., & Hagmann, S. (2001a). Assessment and therapy of complex ADL in apraxia. *Neuropsychological Rehabilitation, 11*, 147–68.

Goldenberg, G. & Hagmann, S. (1997). The meaning of meaningless gestures: A study of visuo-imitative apraxia. *Neuropsychologia, 35*, 333–41.

Goldenberg, G. & Hagmann, S. (1998a). Therapy of activities of daily living in patients with apraxia. *Neuropsychological Rehabilitation, 8*, 123–42.

Goldenberg, G. & Hagmann, S. (1998b). Tool use and mechanical problem solving in apraxia. *Neuropsychologia, 36*, 581–9.

Goldenberg, G., Hartmann, K., & Schlott, I. (2003). Defective pantomime of object use in left brain damage: apraxia or asymbolia? *Neuropsychologia, 41*, 1565–73.

Goldenberg, G., Hartmann-Schmid, K., Sürer, F., Daumüller, M., & Hermsdörfer, J. (2007a). The impact of dysexecutive syndrome on use of tools and technical equipment. *Cortex, 43*, 424–35.

Goldenberg, G., Hentze, S., & Hermsdörfer, J. (2004). The effect of tactile feedback on pantomime of object use in apraxia. *Neurology, 63*, 1863–7.

Goldenberg, G., Hermsdörfer, J., Glindemann, R., Rorden, C., & Karnath, H. O. (2007b). Pantomime of tool use depends on integrity of left inferior frontal cortex. *Cerebral Cortex, 17*, 2769–76.

Goldenberg, G., Hermsdörfer, J., & Laimgruber, K. (2001b). Imitation of gestures by disconnected hemispheres. *Neuropsychologia, 39*, 1432–43.

Goldenberg, G. & Iriki, A. (2007). From sticks to coffee-maker: Mastery of tools and technology by human and non-human primates. *Cortex, 43*, 285–8.

Goldenberg, G. & Karnath, H. O. (2006). The neural basis of imitation is body-part specific. *Journal of Neuroscience, 26*, 6282–7.

Goldenberg, G., Münsinger, U., & Karnath, H. O. (2009). Severity of neglect predicts accuracy of imitation in patients with right hemisphere lesions. *Neuropsychologia, 47*, 2948–52.

Goldenberg, G. & Spatt, J. (2009). The neural basis of tool use. *Brain, 132*, 1645–55.

Goldenberg, G. & Strauss, S. (2002). Hemisphere asymmetries for imitation of novel gestures. *Neurology, 59*, 893–7.

Goldenberg, G., Wimmer, A., Holzner, F., & Wessely, P. (1985). Apraxia of the left limbs in a case of callosal disconnection: The contribution of medial frontal lobe damage. *Cortex, 21*, 135–48.

Goldin-Meadow, S. (2005). *The resilience of language. What gestures in deaf children can tell us about how all children learn language.* New York, NY: Psychology Press.

Goldstein, K. (1908). Zur Lehre von der motorischen Apraxie. *Journal of Psychology and Neurology, 11*, 169–87, 270–83.

Goldstein, K. (1909). Der makroskopische Hirnbefund in meinem Fall von linksseitiger Apraxie. *Neurologisches Centralblatt, 28*, 898–906.

Goldstein, K. (1928). Beobachtungen über die Veränderungen des Gesamtverhaltens bei Gehirnschädigung. *Monatschrift für Psychiatrie und Neurologie, 68*, 217–42.

Goldstein, K. (1948). *Language and language disturbances.* New York, NY: Grune and Stratton.

Goldstein, K. (1995). *The organism—a holistic approach to biology derived from pathological data in man (Deutsche Originalausgabe: Der Organismus, Amsterdam 1934, englische Originalausgabe New York 1993).* New York, NY: Zone Books.

Golestani, N., Paus, T., & Zatorre, R. J. (2002). Anatomical correlates of learning novel speech sounds. *Neuron, 35*, 997–1010.

Goodale, M. A., Jakobson, L. S., & Keillor, J. M. (1994). Differences in the visual control of pantomimed and natural grasping movements. *Neuropsychologia, 32*, 1159–78.

Goodale, M. A. & Milner, A. D. (1992). Separate visual pathways for perception and action. *Trends in Neuroscience, 15*, 20–5.

Goodglass, H. & Kaplan, E. (1963). Disturbance of gesture and pantomime in aphasia. *Brain, 86*, 703–20.

Goodwin, C. (2000). Gesture, aphasia, and interaction. In D. McNeill (Ed.), *Language and gesture* (pp. 84–98). Cambridge: Cambridge University Press.

Gordon, H. (1922). Hand and ear tests. *British Journal of Psychology, 13*, 283–300.

Graff-Radford, N. R., Welsh, K., & Godersky, J. (1987). Callosal apraxia. *Neurology, 37*, 100–5.

Graham, N. L., Zeman, A., Young, A. W., Patterson, K., & Hodges, J. R. (1999). Dyspraxia in a patient with corticobasal degeneration: the role of visual and tactile inputs to action. *Journal of Neurology, Neurosurgery, and Psychiatry, 67*, 334–44.

Grünbaum, A. A. (1930). Über Apraxia. *Zentralblatt für die gesamte Neurologie und Psychiatrie, 55*, 788–92.

Grünbaum, A. S. F. & Sherrington, C. S. (1901). Observation on the physiology of the cerebral cortex of some of the higher apes. *Proceedings of the Royal Society of London, 69*, 206–9.

Haaland, K. Y. (1984). The relationship of limb apraxia severity to motor and language deficits. *Brain and Cognition, 3*, 307–16.

Haaland, K. Y. & Delaney, H. D. (1981). Motor deficits after left or right hemisphere damage due to stroke or tumor. *Neuropsychologia, 19*, 17–27.

Haaland, K. Y. & Flaherty, D. (1984). The different types of limb apraxia errors made by patients with left versus right hemisphere damage. *Brain and Cognition, 3*, 370–84.

Haaland, K. Y. & Harrington, D. L. (1994). Limb-sequencing deficits after left but not right hemisphere damage. *Brain and Cognition, 24*, 104–22.

Haaland, K. Y., Harrington, D. L., & Knight, R. T. (1999). Spatial deficits in ideomotor limb apraxia—a kinematic analysis of aiming movements. *Brain, 122*, 1169–82.

Haaland, K. Y., Harrington, D. L., & Knight, R. T. (2000). Neural representations of skilled movement. *Brain, 123*, 2306–13.

Haaland, K. Y., Harrington, D. L., & Yeo, R. (1987). The effects of task complexity on motor performance in left and right CVA patients. *Neuropsychologia, 25*, 783–94.

Haaland, K. Y., Porch, B. E., & Delaney, H. D. (1980). Limb apraxia and motor performance. *Brain and Language, 9*, 315–23.

Haaland, K. Y., Prestopnik, J. L., Knight, R. T., & Lee, R. R. (2004). Hemispheric asymmetries for kinematic and positional aspects of reaching. *Brain, 127*, 1145–58.

Hadar, U., Burstein, A., Krauss, R., & Soroker, N. (1998). Ideational gestures and speech in brain-damaged subjects. *Language and Cognitive Processes, 13*, 59–76.

Halligan, P. W. & Marshall, J. C. (1994). Towards a principled explanation of unilateral neglect. *Cognitive Neuropsychology, 11*, 167–206.

Hanlon, R. E., Mattson, D., Demery, J. A., & Dromerick, A. W. (1998). Axial movements are relatively preserved with respect to limb movements in aphasic patients. *Cortex, 34*, 731–42.

Hanna-Pladdy, B., Daniels, S. K., Fieselman, M. A., Thompson, K., Vasterling, J. J., Heilman, K. M., *et al.* (2001a). Praxis lateralization: errors in right and left hemisphere stroke. *Cortex, 37*, 219–30.

Hanna-Pladdy, B., Heilman, K. M., & Foundas, A. L. (2001b). Cortical and subcortical contributions to ideomotor apraxia—Analysis of task demands and error types. *Brain, 124*, 2513–77.

Hanna-Pladdy, B., Mendoza, J. E., Apostolos, G. T., & Heilman, K. M. (2002). Lateralised motor control: hemispheric damage and the loss of deftness. *Journal of Neurology, Neurosurgery, and Psychiatry, 73*, 574–7.

Harrington, A. (1987). *Medicine, mind, and the double brain—a study in nineteenth-century thought.* Princeton, NJ: Princeton University Press.

Harrington, A. (1996). *Reenchanted science—Holism in German culture from Wilhelm II to Hitler.* Princeton, NJ: Princeton University Press.

Harrington, D. L. & Haaland, K. Y. (1992). Motor sequencing with left hemisphere damage—are some cognitive deficits specific to limb apraxia? *Brain, 115*, 857–74.

Hartmann, F. (1907). Beitraege zur Apraxielehre. *Monatschrift für Psychiatrie und Neurologie, 21*, 97–118, 248–70.

Hartmann, K., Goldenberg, G., Daumüller, M., & Hermsdörfer, J. (2005). It takes the whole brain to make a cup of coffee: The neuropsychology of naturalistic actions involving technical devices. *Neuropsychologia, 43*, 625–37.

Hay, J. C., Pick, H. I., & Ikeda, K. (1965). Visual capture produced by prism spectacles. *Psychonomic Science, 2*, 215–16.

Hayakawa, Y., Yamadori, A., Fujii, T., Suzuki, K., & Tobita, M. (2000). Apraxia of single tool use. *European Neurology, 43*, 76–81.

He, S. (2008). Holes, objects, and the left hemisphere. *Proceedings of the National Academy of Sciences of the United States of America, 105*, 1103–4.

Head, H. (1920). Aphasia and kindred disorders of speech. *Brain, 43*, 87–165.

Head, H. (1921). Aphasia: An historical review. *Brain, 43*, 390–411.

Head, H. (1926). *Aphasia and kindred disorders of speech.* London: Cambridge University Press.

Heath, M., Roy, E. A., Black, S. E., & Westwood, D. A. (2001). Intransitive limb gestures and apraxia following unilateral stroke. *Journal of Clinical and Experimental Neuropsychology, 23*, 628–42.

Hécaen, H. (1984). *Les Gauchers.* Paris: Presse Universitaire de France.

Hécaen, H., De Agostini, M., & Monzon.-Montes, A. (1981). Cerebral organization in left handers. *Brain and Language, 12*, 261–84.

Hécaen, H. & De Ajuriaguerra, J. (1945). L'apraxie de l'habillage: ses rapports avec la planotopolinésie et les troubles de la somatognosie. *Encéphale, 35*, 113–43.

Hécaen, H. & Gimeno-Alava, A. (1960). L'apraxie unilaterale gauche. *Revue Neurologique, 102*, 648–53.

Hegarty, M. (2004). Mechanical reasoning by mental simulation. *Trends in Cognitive Sciences, 8*, 280–5.

Heilbronner, K. (1905). Zur Frage der motorischen Asymbolie (Apraxie). *Zeitschrift für Psychologie und Physiologie der Sinnesorgane, 39*, 161–205.

Heilman, K. M. (1975). A tapping test in apraxia. *Cortex, 11*, 259–63.

Heilman, K. M. (1979). Apraxia. In K. M. Heilman & E. Valenstein (Eds.), *Clinical Neuropsychology* (pp. 159–85). New York, NY: Oxford University Press.

Heilman, K. M., Coyle, J. M., Gonyea, E. F., & Geschwind, N. (1973). Apraxia and agraphia in a left-hander. *Brain, 96*, 21–8.

Heilman, K. M., Maher, L. M., Greenwald, M. L., & Rothi, L. J. G. (1997). Conceptual apraxia from lateralized lesions. *Neurology, 49*, 457–64.

Heilman, K. M. & Rothi, L. J. G. (1993). Apraxia. In K. M. Heilman & E. Valenstein (Eds.), *Clinical neuropsychology* (pp. 141–64). New York, NY: Oxford University Press.

Heilman, K. M., Rothie, L. J., & Valenstein, E. (1982). Two forms of ideomotor apraxia. *Neurology, 32*, 342–6.

Heilman, K. M., Schwartz, H. D., & Watson, R. T. (1978). Hypoarousal in patients with the neglect syndrome and emotional indifference. *Neurology, 28*, 229–32.

Heilman, K. M. & Van Den Abell, T. (1980). Right hemisphere dominance for attention: The mechanism underlying hemispheric asymmetries of attention (neglect). *Neurology, 30*, 327–30.

Hermsdörfer, J., Blankenfeld, H., & Goldenberg, G. (2003). The dependence of ipsilesional aiming on task demands, lesioned hemisphere, and apraxia. *Neuropsychologia, 41*, 1628–43.

Hermsdörfer, J. & Goldenberg, G. (2002). Ipsilesional deficits during fast diadocokinetic hand movements following unilateral brain damage. *Neuropsychologia, 40*, 2100–15.

Hermsdörfer, J., Laimgruber, K., Kerkhoff, G., Mai, N., & Goldenberg, G. (1999a). Effects of unilateral brain damage on grip selection, coordination, and kinematics of ipsilesional prehension. *Experimental Brain Research, 128*, 41–51.

Hermsdörfer, J., Li, Y., Randerath, J., Goldenberg, G., & Johannsen, L. (2012). Tool use without a tool: kinematic characteristics of pantomiming as compared to actual use and the effect of brain damage. *Experimental Brain Research, 218*, 201–14.

Hermsdörfer, J., Mai, N., Spatt, J., Marquardt, C., Veltkamp, R., & Goldenberg, G. (1996). Kinematic analysis of movement imitation in apraxia. *Brain, 119*, 1575–86.

Hermsdörfer, J., Terlinden, G., Mühlau, M., Goldenberg, G., & Wohlschläger, A. M. (2007). Neural representation of pantomime and actual tool use: Evidence from an event-related fMRI study. *Neuroimage*, 36, T109–18.

Hermsdörfer, J., Ulrich, S., Marquardt, C., Goldenberg, G., & Mai, N. (1999b). Prehension with the ipsilesional hand after unilateral brain damage. *Cortex, 35*, 139–62.

Herrmann, M., Reichle, T., Lucius-Hoene, G., Wallesch, C. W., & Johannsen-Horbach, H. (1988). Nonverbal communication as a compensative strategy for severely nonfluent aphasics?—a quantitative approach. *Brain and Language, 33*, 41–54.

Hervé, P., Crivello, F., Perchey, G., Mazoyer, B., & Tzourio-Mazoyer, N. (2006). Handedness and cerebral anatomical asymmetries in young adult males. *Neuroimage, 29*, 1066–79.

Hitzig, E., Westphal, C. F. O., Steinthal, H., Lazarus, M., & Virchow, R. (1874). Discussion über Aphasie. *Verhandlungen der Berliner Gesellschaft für Anthropologie, Ethnologie und Urgeschichte, 1874*, 130–40.

Hodges, J. R., Bozeat, S., Lambon Ralph, M. A., Patterson, K., & Spatt, J. (2000). The role of conceptual knowledge in object use—evidence from semantic dementia. *Brain, 123*, 1913–25.

Hodges, J. R., Patterson, K., Graham, N., & Dawson, K. (1996). Naming and knowing in dementia of Alzheimer's type. *Brain and Language, 54*, 302–25.

Hodges, J. R., Spatt, J., & Patterson, K. (1999). "What" and "how": Evidence for the dissociation of object knowledge and mechanical problem-solving skills in the human brain. *Proceedings of the National Academy of Sciences of the United States of America, 96*, 9444–8.

Hoff, F. (1931). Balkentumor mit linksseitiger Astereognosis und Apraxie. *Deutsche Zeitschrift für Nervenheilkunde, 123*, 89–100.

Hogrefe, K., Ziegler, W., & Goldenberg, G. (2011). Measuring the formal diversity of hand gestures by their hamming distance. In G. Stam & M. Ishino (Eds.), *Integrating gestures. The interdisciplinary nature of gesture* (pp. 75–88). Amsterdam: John Benjamins Publishing Company.

Hogrefe, K., Ziegler, W., Weidinger, N., & Goldenberg, G. (2012). Non-verbal communication in severe aphasia: Influence of aphasia, apraxia, or semantic processing? *Cortex, 48*, 952–62.

Hoppe, K. D. (1977). Split brain and psychoanalysis. *Psychoanalitic Quarterly, 46*, 220–44.

Howes, D. H. (1988). Ideomotor apraxia: evidence for the preservation of axial commands. *Journal of Neurology, Neurosurgery, and Psychiatry, 51*, 593–8.

Huber, W., Poeck, K., Weniger, D., & Willmes, K. (1983). *Aachener aphasie test*. Goettingen: Hogreve.

Huber, W., Poeck, K., & Willmes, K. (1984). The Aachen Aphasia Test. In F. C. Rose (Ed.), *Advances in neurology, Vol. 42: Progress in aphasiology* (pp. 291–303). New York, NY: Raven Press.

Humphreys, G. W. & Forde, E. M. E. (1998). Disordered action schema and action disorganisation syndrome. *Cognitive Neuropsychology, 15*, 771–812.

Husain, M. & Rorden, C. (2003). Non-spatially lateralized mechanisms in hemispatial neglect. *Nature Review Neuroscience, 4*, 26–36.

Hutsler, J. (2003). The specialized structure of human language cortex: Pyramidal cell size asymmetries within auditory and language-associated regions of the temporal lobes. *Brain and Language, 86*, 226–42.

Hutsler, J. & Galuske, R. A. W. (2003). Hemispheric asymmetries in cerebral cortical networks. *Trends in Neuroscience, 26*, 429–35.

Iacoboni, M., Woods, R. P., Brass, M., Bekkering, H., Mazziotta, J. C., & Rizzolatti, G. (1999). Cortical mechanisms of human imitation. *Science, 286*, 2526–8.

Iestwaart, M., Carey, D. P., & Della Sala, S. (2006). Tapping, grasping and aiming in ideomotor apraxia. *Neuropsychologia, 44*, 1175–84.

Iestwaart, M., Carey, D. P., Della Sala, S., & Dijkhuizen, R. S. (2001). Memory-driven movements in limb apraxia: is there evidence for impaired communication between the dorsal and the ventral streams?*Neuropsychologia, 39*, 950–61.

Jackson, J. H. (1932a). On the nature of the duality of the brain. In J. Taylor, G. Holmes, & F. M. R. Walshe (Eds.), *Selected writings of John Hughlings Jackson. Vol. 2* (pp. 129–45). London: Hodder and Stoughton. (Original work published 1874.)

Jackson, J. H. (1932b). Remarks on non-protrusion of the tongue in some cases of aphasia. In J. Taylor, G. Holmes, & F. M. R. Walshe (Eds.), *Selected writings of John Hughlings Jackson. Vol. 2* (pp. 153–4). London: Hodder and Stoughton. (Original work published 1878.)

Jackson, J. H. (1932c). Case of large cerebral tumour without optic neuritis and with left hemiplegia and imperception. In J. Taylor, G. Holmes, & F. M. R. Walshe (Eds.), *Selected writings, Vol. 2* (pp. 146–52). Nijmegen: Arts & Boeve.

Jacobs, S., Bussel, B., Combeaud, M., & Roby-Brami, A. (2009). The use of a tool requires its incorporation into the movement: Evidence from stick-pointing in apraxia. *Cortex, 45*, 444–55.

Jacyna, L. S. (1999). The 1874 aphasia debate in the Berliner Gesellschaft für Anthropologie. *Brain and Language, 69*, 5–15.

Jacyna, L. S. (2000). *Lost words. Narratives of language and the brain 1825–1926.* Princeton, NJ: Princeton University Press.

Jager, G. & Postma, A. (2003). On the hemispheric specialization for categorical and coordinate spatial relations: a review of the current evidence. *Neuropsychologia, 41*, 504–15.

Jakobson, R. (1976). *Six lecons sur le son et le sens.* Paris: Les editions de minuit.

Jansen, P. & Heil, M. (2010). Gender differences in mental rotation across adulthood. *Experimental Aging Research, 36*, 94–104.

Jason, G. W. (1983a). Hemispheric asymmetries in motor functions: I. Left hemisphere specialization for memory but not for performance. *Neuropsychologia, 21*, 35–46.

Jason, G. W. (1983b). Hemispheric asymmetries in motor functions: II. Ordering does not contribute to left-hemisphere specialization. *Neuropsychologia, 21*, 47–58.

Jason, G. W. & Pajurkova, E. M. (1992). Failure of metacontrol: breakdown in behavioural unity after lesion of the corpus callosum and infero-medial frontal lobes. *Cortex, 28*, 241–60.

Jeannerod, M. (1986). The formation of finger grip during prehension. A cortically mediated visuomotor pattern. *Behavioural Brain Research, 19*, 99–116.

Jeannerod, M. (1988). *The neural and behavioural organization of goal-directed movements*. Oxford: Clarendon Press.

Johnson-Frey, S. H., Newman-Norlund, R., & Grafton, S. T. (2005). A distributed left hemisphere network active during planning of everyday tool use skills. *Cerebral Cortex, 15*, 681–95.

Jones, G. A. & Jones, J. M. (2000). *Information and Coding Theory*. London: Springer.

Jung-Beeman, M. (2005). Bilateral brain processes for comprehending natural language. *Trends in Cognitive Sciences, 9*, 512–8.

Kalénine, S., Buxbaum, L. J., & Coslett, H. B. (2010). Critical brain regions for action recognition: lesion symptom mapping in left hemisphere stroke. *Brain, 133*, 3269–80.

Kazui, S. & Sawada, T. (1993). Callosal apraxia without agraphia. *Annals of Neurology, 33*, 401–3.

Kazui, S., Sawada, T., Naritomi, H., Kuriyama, Y., & Yamaguchi, T. (1992). Left unilateral ideomotor apraxia in ischemic stroke within the territory of the anterior cerebral artery. *Cerebrovascular Diseases, 2*, 35–9.

Kean, M. L. (1994). Introduction to selection from the work of Norman Geschwind. In P. Eling (Ed.), *Readers in the history of aphasia* (pp. 355–9). Amsterdam: John Benjamins Publishing Company.

Kellenbach, M. L., Brett, M., & Patterson, K. (2003). Actions speak louder than functions: The importance of manipulability and action in tool representation. *Journal of Cognitive Neuroscience, 15*, 30–46.

Kendon, A. (1981). Geography of gesture. *Semiotica, 37*, 129–63.

Kendon, A. (2004). *Gesture—visible action as utterance*. Cambridge: Cambridge University Press.

Kertesz, A. & Ferro, J. M. (1984). Lesion size and location in ideomotor apraxia. *Brain, 107*, 921–33.

Kertesz, A., Ferro, J. M., & Shewan, C. M. (1984). Apraxia and aphasia: the functional-anatomical basis for their dissociation. *Neurology, 34*, 40–7.

Kertesz, A. & Hooper, P. (1982). Praxis and language: The extent and variety of apraxia in aphasia. *Neuropsychologia, 20*, 275–84.

Keysers, C. & Perrett, D. I. (2004). Demystifying social cognition: a Hebbian perspective. *Trends in Cognitive Sciences, 8*, 501–7.

Kimura, D. (1977). Aquisition of a motor skill after left-hemisphere damage. *Brain, 100*, 527–42.

Kimura, D. (1982). Left-hemisphere control of oral and brachial movements and their relation to communication. *Philosophical Transactions of the Royal Society of London, B, 298*, 135–49.

Kimura, D. (1983a). *Neuromotor mechanisms in human communication*. New York, NY: Oxford University Press, Clarendon Press.

Kimura, D. (1983b). Speech representation in an unbiased sample of left-handers. *Human Neurobiology, 2*, 147–54.

Kimura, D. & Archibald, Y. (1974). Motor functions of the left hemisphere. *Brain, 97*, 337–50.

Kinsbourne, M. & Warrington, E. K. (1962). A study of finger agnosia. *Brain, 85*, 47–66.

Kleist, K. (1934). *Gehirnpathologie*. Leipzig: Johann Ambrosius Barth.

Kleist, K. (1937). Bericht über die Gehirnpathologie in ihrer Bedeutung für Neurologie und Psychiatrie. *Zeitschrift für die gesamte Neurologie und Psychiatrie, 158*, 159–93.

Klippi, A. (2003). Collaborating in aphasic group conversation: striving for mutual understanding. In C. Goodwin (Ed.), *Conversation and brain damage* (pp. 117–43). Oxford: Oxford University Press.

Knecht, S., Dräger, B., Deppe, M., Bobe, L., Lohmann, H., Flöel, E. B., *et al.* (2000). Handedness and hemispheric language dominance in healthy humans. *Brain, 123*, 2512–8.

Kolb, B. & Milner, B. (1981). Performance of complex arm and facial movements after focal brain lesions. *Neuropsychologia, 19*, 491–503.

Kosslyn, S. M., Flynn, R. A., Amsterdam, J. B., & Wang, G. (1990). Components of high-level vision: A cognitive neuroscience analysis and accounts of neurological syndromes. *Cognition, 34*, 203–77.

Kritikos, A., Breen, N., & Mattingley, J. B. (2005). Anarchic hand syndrome: bimanual coordination and sensitivity to irrelevant information in unimanual reaches. *Cognitive Brain Research, 24*, 634–47.

Kroll, M. (1910). Beiträge zum Studium der Apraxie. *Zeitschrift für die gesamte Neurologie und Psychiatrie, 23*, 315–45.

Kussmaul, A. (1885). *Die Störungen der Sprache. Versuch einer Pathologie der Sprache*. Leipzig: F. C. W. Vogel.

Laeng, B. (2006). Constructional apraxia after left or right unilateral stroke. *Neuropsychologia, 44*, 1595–606.

Laeng, B., Chabris, C. F., & Kosslyn, S. M. (2003). Asymmetries in encoding spatial relations. In K. Hugdahl & R. J. Davidson (Eds.), *The asymmetrical brain* (pp. 303–40). Cambridge, MA: MIT Press.

Laimgruber, K., Goldenberg, G., & Hermsdörfer, J. (2005). Manual and hemispheric asymmetries in the execution of actual and pantomimed prehension. *Neuropsychologia, 43*, 682–92.

Lambon Ralph, M. A., Cipolotti, L., Manes, F., & Patterson, K. (2010). Taking both sides: do unilateral anterior temporal lobe lesions disrupt semantic memory? *Brain, 133*, 3242–55.

Laplane, D. & Degos, J. D. (1983). Motor neglect. *Journal of Neurology, Neurosurgery, and Psychiatry, 46*, 152–8.

Laquer, L. (1888). Zur Localisation der sensorischen Aphasie. *Neurologisches Centralblatt, 7*, 337–51.

Latour, B. (1993). *Petites lecons de sociologie des sciences*. Paris: Éditions la Découverte.

Lauro-Grotto, R., Piccini, C., & Shallice, T. (1997). Modality-specific operations in dementia. *Cortex, 33*, 593–622.

Lausberg, H. & Cruz, R. F. (2004). Hemispheric specialisation for imitation of hand-head positions and finger configurations: a controlled study in patients with complete callosotomy. *Neuropsychologia, 42*, 320–34.

Lausberg, H., Cruz, R. F., Kita, S., Zaidel, E., & Ptito, A. (2003). Pantomime to visual presentation of objects: left hand dyspraxia in patients with complete callosotomy. *Brain, 126*, 343–60.

Lausberg, H., Göttert, R., Münβinger, U., Boegner, F., & Marx, P. (1999). Callosal disconnection syndrome in a left-handed patient due to infarction of the total length of the corpus callosum. *Neuropsychologia, 37*, 253–66.

Lausberg, H., Zaidel, E., Cruz, R. F., & Ptito, A. (2007). Speech-independent production of communicative gestures: Evidence from patients with complete callosal disconnection. *Neuropsychologia, 45*, 3092–104.

Lavados, M., Carrasco, X., Pena, M., Zaidel, E., Zaidel, D., & Aboitiz, F. (2002). A new sign of callosal disconnection syndrome: agonistic dyspraxia. A case study. *Neurocase, 8*, 480–3.

Le May, A., David, R., & Thomas, A. P. (1988). The use of spontaneous gesture by aphasic patients. *Aphasiology, 2*, 137–45.

Legg, L. A., Drummond, A. E., & Langhorne, P. (2006). Occupational therapy for patients with problems in activities of daily living after stroke (Review). *Cochrane Database of Systematic Reviews*, 1–35.

Lehmkuhl, G., Poeck, K., & Willmes, K. (1983). Ideomotor apraxia and aphasia: An examination of types and manifestations of apraxic symptoms. *Neuropsychologia, 21*, 199–212.

Lent, D. (1896). Dr. Ferd. Carl Maria Finkelnburg. *Centralblatt für allgemeine Gesundheitspflege, 15*, 185–9.

Lepine, R. (1897). Sur un cas particulier de cécité psychique. Default de reconnaissance de certain objects. Apraxie sans aphasie. *Revue de Medicine, 17*, 452–63.

Lewis, J. W. (2006). Cortical networks related to human use of tools. *The Neuroscientist, 12*, 211–31.

Lhermitte, F. (1983). "Utilization behaviour" and its relation to lesions of the frontal lobes. *Brain, 106*, 237–55.

Lhermitte, J., de Massary, J., & Kyriaco, N. (1928). Le role de la pensée spatiale dans l'apraxie. *Revue Neurologique*, *41*, 895–903.

Lhermitte, J. & Trelles, J. O. (1933). Sur l'apraxie pure constructive. Les troubles de la pensée spatiale et de la somatognosie dans l'apraxie. *L'Encephale*, *28*, 413–44.

Li, Y., Randerath, J., Goldenberg, G., & Hermsdörfer, J. (2011). Size-weight illusion and anticipatory grip force scaling following unilateral cortical brain lesion. *Neuropsychologia*, *49*, 914–23.

Liberman, A. M., Cooper, F. S., Shankweiler, D. P., & Studdert-Kennedy, M. (1967). Perception of the speech code. *Psychological Review*, *74*, 431–61.

Liepmann, H. (1900). Das Krankheitsbild der Apraxie (motorische Asymbolie) auf Grund eines Falles von einseitiger Apraxie. *Monatschrift für Psychiatrie und Neurologie*, *8*, 15–44, 102–32, 182–97.

Liepmann, H. (1905a). Der weitere Krankheitsverlauf bei dem einseitig Apraktischen und der Gehirnbefund auf Grund von Serienschnitten. 1. *Monatschrift für Psychiatrie und Neurologie*, *17*, 289–311.

Liepmann, H. (1905b). *Ueber Störungen des Handelns bei Gehirnkranken*. Berlin: Karger.

Liepmann, H. (1906). Der weitere Krankheitsverlauf bei dem einseitig Apraktischen und der Gehirnbefund auf Grund von Serienschnitten. 2. *Monatschrift für Psychiatrie und Neurologie*, *17*, 217–43.

Liepmann, H. (1908). *Drei Aufsätze aus dem Apraxiegebiet*. Berlin: Karger.

Liepmann, H. (1909). Franz Joseph Gall. *Deutsche Medizinische Wochenschrift*, *35*, 979–80.

Liepmann, H. (1913). Motorische Aphasie und Apraxie. *Monatschrift für Psychiatrie und Neurologie*, *34*, 485–94.

Liepmann, H. (1920). Apraxie. In H. Brugsch (Ed.), *Ergebnisse der gesamten Medizin* (pp. 516–43). Wien Berlin: Urban & Schwarzenberg.

Liepmann, H. (1929). Klinische und psychologische Untersuchung und anatomischer Befund bei einem Fall von Dyspraxie und Agraphie [posthumous publication]. *Monatschrift für Psychiatrie und Neurologie*, *71*, 169–214.

Liepmann, H. & Maas, O. (1907). Fall von linksseitiger Agraphie und Apraxie bei rechtsseitiger Laehmung. *Journal für Psychologie und Neurology*, *10*, 214–27.

Lissauer, H. (1890). Ein Fall von Seelenblindheit nebst einem Beitrag zur Theorie derselben. *Archiv für Psychiatrie und Nervenkrankheiten*, *21*, 222–70.

Lupyan, G., Rakison, D. H., & McClelland, J. L. (2007). Language is not just for talking. Redundant labels facilitate learning of novel categories. *Psychological Science*, *18*, 1077–83.

Luria, A. R. (1980). *Higher cortical functions in man* (Basil Haigh, Trans., 2nd edn revised and expanded). New York, NY: Basic Books.

Maas, O. (1907). Ein Fall von linksseitiger Apraxie und Agraphie. *Neurologisches Centralblatt*, *26*, 789–92.

Maas, O. (1910). Fall von linksseitiger Apraxie mit bemerkenswerter Sensibilitaetsstoerung. *Neurologisches Centralblatt*, *29*, 962–7.

Maas, O. & Sittig, O. (1929). Zur Frage der Verteilung der motorischen Apraxie auf die Körperteile. *Monatschrift für Psychiatrie und Neurologie*, *73*, 40–51.

Maher, L. M. & Ochipa, C. (1997). Management and treatment of limb apraxia. In L. J. G. Rothi & K. M. Heilman (Eds.), *Apraxia—the neuropsychology of action* (pp. 75–92). Hove: Psychology Press.

Makuuchi, M. (2005). Is Broca's area crucial for imitation? *Cerebral Cortex*, *15*, 563–70.

Manuel, A., Radman, N., Mesot, D., Chouiter, L., Clarke, S., Annoni, J. M., *et al.* (2012). Inter-and intra-hemispheric dissociations in ideomotor apraxia: a large-scale lesion-symptom mapping study in subacute brain-damaged patients. *Cerebral Cortex*, Sep 17. [Epub ahead of print]

Marangolo, P., De Renzi, E., Di Pace, E., Ciurli, P., & Castriota-Skanderberg, A. (1998). Let not thy left hand know what thy right hand knoweth. The case of a patient with an infarct involving the callosal pathways. *Brain, 121*, 1459–67.

Marchetti, C. & Della Sala, S. (1998). Disentangling the alien and anarchic hand. *Cognitive Neuropsychiatry, 3*, 191–207.

Margolin, D. I. (1980). Right hemisphere dominance for praxis and left hemisphere dominance for speech in a left-hander. *Neuropsychologia, 18*, 715–19.

Marie, P. (1906a). Revision de la question de l'aphasie: la troisiem circonvolution frontale gauche je joue aucun ròle spécial dans la fonction du langage. *La Semaine Medicale, 26*, 241–7.

Marie, P. (1906b). Revision de la question de l'aphasie: que faut-il penser des aphasies sous-corticales (aphasies pures)? *La Semaine Medicale, 26*, 493–500.

Marie, P., Bouttier, H., & Bailey, P. (1922). La planotopokinésie. Étude sur les erreurs d'exécution de certains mouvements dans leurs rapports avec la représentation spatiale. *Revue Neurologique, 38*, 505–12.

Marie, P. & Foix, C. (1914). Phénomènes dits apraxiques, avec lésion du lobe pariétotemporal gauche. *Revue Neurologique, 27*, 275–7.

Marshall, J., Atkinson, J., Smulovitch, E., Thacker, A., & Woll, B. (2004). Aphasia in a user of British Sign Language: dissociation between sign and gesture. *Cognitive Neuropsychology, 21*, 537–54.

Matthews, M. S., Linskey, M. E., & Binder, D. K. (2008). William P. van Wagenen and the first corpus callosotomies for epilepsy. *Journal of Neurosurgery, 108*, 608–14.

Mayer, E., Martory, M. D., Pegna, A. J., Landis, T., Delavelle, J., & Annoni, J. M. (1999). A pure case of Gerstmann syndrome with a subangular lesion. *Brain, 122*, 1107–20.

Mayer-Gross, W. (1935). Some observations on apraxia. *Proceedings of the Royal Society of Medicine, 28*, 1203–12.

Mayer-Gross, W. (1936). Further observations on apraxia. *Journal of Mental Science, 82*, 744–62.

McClelland, J. L., Rumelhart, D. E., & Hinton, G. E. (1986). The appeal of parallel distributed processing. In D. E. Rumelhart & J. L. McClelland (Eds.), *Parallel distributed processing—Explorations in the microstructure of cognition, Volume 1: Foundations* (pp. 3–44). Cambridge, MA: MIT Press.

McCloskey, M. (1983). Intuitive physics. *Scientific American, 248*, 122–30.

McFie, J. & Zangwill, O. L. (1960). Visual-constructive disabilities associated with lesions of the left cerebral hemisphere. *Brain, 83*, 243–60.

McNabb, A. W., Carroll, W. M., & Mastaglia, F. L. (1988). "Alien hand" and loss of bimanual coordination after dominant anterior cerebral artery territory infarction. *Journal of Neurology, Neurosurgery, and Psychiatry, 51*, 218–22.

McNeill, D. (1985). So you think gestures are nonverbal? *Psychological Review, 92*, 350–71.

McNeill, D. (1992). *Hand and mind.* Chicago, IL: The University of Chicago Press.

Mehler, M. F. (1987). Visuo-imitative apraxia. *Neurology, 37*(Suppl 1), 129.

Meyer, D. E., Smith, J. E. K., Kornblum, S., Abrams, R. A., & Wright, C. E. (1990). Speed-accuracy tradeoffs in aimed movements: towards a theory of rapid voluntary action. In M. Jeannerod (Ed.), *Attention and Performance XII* (pp. 173–226). Hillsdale, NJ: Lawrence Erlbaum Associates.

Meynert, T. (1874). *Zur Mechanik des Gehirnbaues.* Wien: Wilhelm Braumüller.

Meynert, T. (1884). *Psychiatrie. Klinik der Erkrankungen des Vorderhirns begründet auf dessen Bau, Leistung und Ernährung.* Wien: Braumüller.

Meynert, T. (1889). *Klinische Vorlesungen über Psychiatrie auf wissenschaftlichen Grundlagen für Studirende und Aerzte, Juristen und Psychologen.* Wien: Wilhelm Braumüller.

Miller, N. (1986). *Dyspraxia and its management.* London: Croom Helm.

Mishkin, M., Ungerleider, L. G., & Macko, K. A. (1983). Object vision and spatial vision: Two visual pathways. *Trends in Neuroscience, 6*, 414–7.

Moll, J., de Oliveira-Souza, R., Passman, L. J., Cimini Cunha, F., Souza-Lima, F., & Andreiuolo, P. A. (2000). Functional MRI correlates of real and imagined tool-use pantomimes. *Neurology, 54*, 1331–6.

Moore, D. S. & Johnson, S. P. (2008). Mental rotation in human infants. *Psychological Science, 19*, 1063–6.

Morlaas, J. (1928). *Contribution à l'étude de l'apraxie*. Paris: Amédée Legrand.

Moro, V., Pernigo, S., Urgesi, C., Zapparoli, P., & Aglioti, S. M. (2008). Finger recognition and gesture imitation in Gerstmann's syndrome. *Neurocase, 15*, 13–23.

Morris, D., Collett, P., Marsch, P., & O'Shaughnessy, M. (1979). *Gestures. Their origins and distribution*. London: Jonathan Cape Ltd.

Motomura, N. & Yamadori, A. (1994). A case of ideational apraxia with impairment of object use and preservation of object pantomime. *Cortex, 30*, 167–70.

Mozaz, M., Gonzales-Rothi, L., Anderson, J. M., Crucian, G. P., & Heilman, K. M. (2002). Postural knowledge of transitive pantomimes and intransitive gestures. *Journal of the International Neuropsychological Society, 8*, 958–62.

Munari, B. (2005). *Speak Italian. The fine art of the gesture*. San Francisco, CA: Chronicle Books.

Munk, H. (1877). Zur Physiologie der Grosshirnrinde. *Berliner Klinische Wochenschrift, 14*, 505–6.

Munk, H. (1878). Weitere Mitteilungen zur Physiologie der Grosshirnrinde. *Archiv für Anatomie und Physiologie / Physiologische Abteilung, 2*, 162–78.

Munk, H. (1881). *Über die Funktionen der Großhirnrinde. Gesammelte Mitteilungen aus den Jahren 1877–1880*. Berlin: August Hirschwald.

Mutha, P. K., Sainburg, R. L., & Haaland, K. Y. (2010). Coordination deficits in ideomotor apraxia during visually targeted reaching reflect impaired visuomotor transformations. *Neuropsychologia, 48*, 3855–67.

Mutha, P. K., Sainburg, R. L., & Haaland, K. Y. (2011). Left parietal regions are critical for adaptive visuomotor control. *Journal of Neuroscience, 31*, 6972–81.

Nathan, P. W. (1947). Facial apraxia and apraxic dysarthria. *Brain, 70*, 449–78.

Negri, G. A., Lunardelli, A., Reverberi, C., Gigli, G. L., & Rumiati, R. I. (2007a). Degraded semantic knowledge and accurate object use. *Cortex, 43*, 376–88.

Negri, G. A. L., Rumiati, R. I., Zadini, A., Ukmar, M., Mahon, B. Z., & Caramazza, A. (2007b). What is the role of motor simulation in action and object recognition? Evidence from apraxia. *Cognitive Neuropsychology, 24*, 795–816.

Neumärker, K. J. & Bartsch, A. J. (2003). Karl Kleist (1879–1960)—A pioneer of neuropsychiatry. *History of Psychiatry, 14*, 411–58.

Njiokiktjien, C., Verschoor, C. A., Vranken, M., & Vroklage, L. M. (2000). Development of ideomotor praxis representation. *Developmental Medicine & Child Neurology, 42*, 253–7.

Norman, D. A. (1989). *The design of everyday things*. New York, NY: Currency Doubleday.

Norman, D. A. (1993). *Things that make us smart: defending human attributes in the age of the machine*. Reading, MA: Perseus Books.

Nothnagel, H. (1887). Über die Lokalisation der Gehirnkrankheiten. Neurologisches vom VI. Congress für innere Medicin. *Neurologisches Centralblatt, 6*, 213–16.

Ochipa, C., Rothi, J. G., & Heilman, K. M. (1989). Ideational apraxia: A deficit in tool selection and use. *Annals of Neurology, 25*, 190–3.

Ochipa, C., Rothi, L. F. G., & Heilman, K. M. (1992). Conceptual apraxia in Alzheimer's disease. *Brain, 115*, 1061–71.

Ogden, J. A. (1985). Autotopagnosia. Occurence in a patient without nominal aphasia and with an intact ability to point to parts of animals and objects. *Brain, 108*, 1009–22.

O'Reilly, A. W. (1995). Using representations: Comprehension and production of actions with imagined objects. *Child Development*, *66*, 999–1010.

Osiurak, F., Aubin, G., Allain, P., Jarry, C., Etcharry-Bouyx, F., Richard, I., *et al.* (2008a). Different constraints on grip selection in brain-damaged patients: Object use versus object transport. *Neuropsychologia*, *46*, 2431–4.

Osiurak, F., Aubin, G., Allain, P., Jarry, C., Richard, I., & Le Gall, D. (2008b). Object utilization and object usage. A single-case study. *Neurocase*, *14*, 169–83.

Osiurak, F., Jarry, C., Aubin, G., Allain, P., Etcharry-Bouyx, F., Richard, I., *et al.* (2009). Unusual use of objects after unilateral brain damage. The technical reasoning model. *Cortex*, *45*, 769–83.

Osiurak, F., Jarry, C., & Le Gall, D. (2011). Re-examining the gesture engram hypothesis. New perspectives on apraxia of tool use. *Neuropsychologia*, *49*, 299–312.

Paterson, A. & Zangwill, O. L. (1944). Disorders of visual space perception associated with lesions of the right cerebral hemisphere. *Brain*, *67*, 331–58.

Peigneux, P., Van der Linden, M., Andres-Benito, P., Sadzot, B., Franck, G., & Salmon, E. (2000). Exploration neuropsychologique et par imagerie fonctionelle cérébrale d'une apraxie visuo-imitative. *Revue Neurologique*, *156*, 459–72.

Pelgrims, B., Olivier, E., & Andres, M. (2011). Dissociation between manipulation and conceptual knowledge of object use in the supramarginal gyrus. *Human Brain Mapping*, *32*, 1802–10.

Petreska, B., Billard, A. G., Hermsdörfer, J., & Goldenberg, G. (2010). Revisiting a study of callosal apraxia: The right hemisphere can imitate the orientation but not the position of the hand. *Neuropsychologia*, *48*, 2509–16.

Phillips, L. H., Wynn, V., Gilhooly, K. J., Della Sala, S., & Logie, R. H. (1999). The role of memory in the Tower of London task. *Memory*, *7*, 209–31.

Pick, A. (1898). Ueber Störungen der Identification (Asymbolie, Apraxie, Agnosie). In *Beiträge zur Pathologie und pathologischen Anatomie des Centralnervensystems mit Bemerkungen zur normalen Anatomie desselben* (pp. 1–14). Berlin: S. Karger.

Pick, A. (1902). Zur Psychologie der motorischen Apraxie. *Neurologisches Centralblatt*, 994–1000.

Pick, A. (1905a). *Studien zur motorischen Apraxia und ihr nahe stehenden Erscheinungen; ihre Bedeutung in der Symptomatologie psychopathischer Symptomenkomplexe*. Leipzig: Franz Deuticke.

Pick, A. (1905b). *Studien zur motorischen Apraxia und ihr nahestende Erscheinungen; ihre Bedeutung in der Symptomatologie psychopathischer Symptomenkomplexe*. Leipzig: Franz Deuticke.

Pick, A. (1922). Störung der Orientierung am eigenen Körper. Beitrag zur Lehre vom Bewußtsein des eigenen Körpers. *Psychologische Forschung*, *1*, 303–18.

Picket, L. W. (1974). An assessment of gestural and pantomimic deficit in aphasic patients. *Acta Symbolica*, *5*, 69–86.

Piercy, M., Hécaen, H., & De Ajuriaguerra, J. (1960). Constructional apraxia associated with unilateral cerebral lesions—left and right sided cases compared. *Brain*, *83*, 225–42.

Pineas, H. (1924). Ein Fall von linksseitiger motorischer Apraxie nach Balkenerweichung. *Monatschrift für Psychiatrie und Neurologie*, *56*, 43–6.

Poeck, K. (1969). Phantome nach Amputation und bei angeborenen Gliedmaβenmangel. *Deutsche Medizinische Wochenschrift*, *46*, 2367–74.

Poeck, K. (1982). The two types of motor apraxia. *Archives Italiennes de Biologie*, *120*, 361–9.

Poeck, K. & Kerschensteiner, M. (1971). Ideomotor apraxia following right-sided cerebral lesion in a left-handed subject. *Neuropsychologia*, *9*, 359–61.

Poeck, K. & Lehmkuhl, G. (1980). Ideatory apraxia in a left-handed patient with right-sided brain lesion. *Cortex*, *16*, 273–84.

Poeck, K., Lehmkuhl, G., & Willmes, K. (1982). Axial movements in ideomotor apraxia. *Journal of Neurology, Neurosurgery, and Psychiatry*, *45*, 1125–9.

Poeck, K. & Orgass, B. (1964). Die Entwicklung des Körperschemas bei Kindern im Alter von 4-10 Jahren. *Neuropsychologia, 2*, 109–30.

Poeck, K. & Orgass, B. (1966). Gerstmann's syndrome and aphasia. *Cortex, 2*, 421–37.

Poeck, K. & Orgass, B. (1969). An experimental investigation of finger agnosia. *Neurology, 19*, 801–7.

Poizner, H., Clark, M., Merians, A. S., Macauley, B., Rothi, L. J. G., & Heilman, K. M. (1995). Joint coordination deficits in limb apraxia. *Brain, 118*, 227–42.

Poizner, H., Mack, L., Verfaellie, M., Rothi, L. J. G., & Heilman, K. M. (1990). Three-dimensional computer graphic analysis of apraxia. *Brain, 113*, 85–101.

Poizner, H., Merians, A. S., Clark, M. A., Macauley, B., Rothi, L. J. G., & Heilman, K. M. (1998). Left hemisphere specialization for learned, skilled, and purposeful action. *Neuropsychology, 12*, 163–82.

Poncet, M., Ali-Cherif, A., Choux, M., Boudouresques, J., & Lhermitte, F. (1978). Etude neuropsychologique d'un syndrome de disconnexion calleuse totale avec hemianopsie laterale homonyme droite. *Revue Neurologique, 134*, 633–53.

Poncet, M., Habib, M., & Robillard, A. (1987). Deep left parietal lobe syndrome: conduction aphasia and other neurobehavioural disorders due to a small subcortical lesion. *Journal of Neurology, Neurosurgery, and Psychiatry, 50*, 709–13.

Poncet, M., Pellissier, J. F., Sebahoun, M., & Nasser, C. J. (1971). A propos d'un cas d'autotopagnosie secondaire à une lésion pariéto-occipitale de l'hémisphère majeur. *Encéphale, 61*, 1–14.

Poppelreuter, W. (1917). *Die psychischen Schäden durch Kopfschuß im Krieg 1914/16*. Leipzig: L. Voss.

Poppelreuter, W. (1990). *Disturbances of lower and higher visual capacities caused by occipital damage* (Trans. J. Zihl with the assistance of L. Weiskrantz). Oxford: Oxford University Press.

Povinelli, D. J. (2000). *Folk physics for apes—the chimpanzee's theory of how the world works*. Oxford: Oxford University Press.

Prillwitz, S., Leven, R., Zienert, H., Hanke, T., & Henning, J. (1989). *Hamburger Notationssystem für Gebärdensprachen. Eine Einführung*. Hamburg: Signum Verlag.

Prinz, W. (1987). Ideo-motor action. In H. Heuer & A. F. Sanders (Eds.), *Perspectives on perception and action* (pp. 47–76). Hillsdale, NJ: Lawrence Erlbaum.

Pujol, J., López-Sala, A., Deus, J., Cardonner, N., Sebastián-Gallés, N., Conesa, G., *et al.* (2002). The lateral asymmetry of the human brain studied by volumetric magnetic resonance imaging. *Neuroimage, 17*, 670–9.

Raade, A. S., Rothi, L. J. G., & Heilman, K. M. (1991). The relationship between buccofacial and limb apraxia. *Brain and Cognition, 16*, 130–46.

Randerath, J., Goldenberg, G., Spijkers, W., Li, Y., & Hermsdörfer, J. (2011). From pantomime to actual use: how affordances can facilitate actual tool—use. *Neuropsychologia, 49*, 2410–6.

Rapcsak, S. Z., Croswell, S. C., & Rubens, A. B. (1989). Apraxia in Alzheimer's disease. *Neurology, 39*, 664–8.

Rapcsak, S. Z., Ochipa, C., Beeson, P. M., & Rubens, A. B. (1993). Praxis and the right hemisphere. *Brain and Cognition, 23*, 181–202.

Rapcsak, S. Z., Rothi, L. J. G., & Heilman, K. M. (1987). Apraxia in a patient with atypical cerebral dominance. *Brain and Cognition, 6*, 450–63.

Raymer, A. M., Merians, A. S., Adair, J. C., Schwartz, R. L., Williamson, D. J. G., Rothi, L. J. G., *et al.* (1999). Crossed apraxia. *Cortex, 35*, 183–200.

Raymer, A. M. & Ochipa, C. (1997). Conceptual praxis. In L. J. G. Rothi & K. M. Heilman (Eds.), *Apraxia: The neuropsychology of action* (pp. 51–61). Hove: Psychology Press.

Rizzolatti, G., Fadiga, L., Fogassi, L., & Gallese, V. (2002). From mirror neurons to imitation: Facts and speculations. In A. N. Meltzoff & W. Prinz (Eds.), *The imitative mind. Development, evolution, and brain bases* (pp. 247–266). Cambridge: Cambridge University Press.

Rizzolatti, G. & Matelli, M. (2003). Two different streams form the dorsal visual system: anatomy and functions. *Experimental Brain Research, 153*, 146–57.

Rizzolatti, G. & Sinigaglia, C. (2008). *Mirrors in the brain. How our minds share actions and emotions.* Oxford: Oxford University Press.

Rizzolatti, G. & Sinigaglia, C. (2010). The functional role of the parieto-frontal mirror circuit: interpretations and misinterpretations. *Nature Review Neuroscience, 11*, 264–74.

Robertson, I. H. (1990). Digit span and visual neglect: a puzzling relationship. *Neuropsychologia, 28*, 217–22.

Robertson, S. I. (2001). *Problem solving.* Hove: Psychology Press.

Roeltgen, D. P., Sevush, S., & Heilman, K. M. (1983). Pure Gerstmann's syndrome from a focal lesion. *Archives of Neurology, 40*, 46–7.

Rorden, C. & Karnath, H. O. (2004). Using human brain lesions to infer function: a relic from a past era in the fMRI age? *Nature Review Neuroscience, 5*, 813–19.

Rorden, C., Karnath, H. O., & Bornilha, L. (2007). Improving lesion-symptom mapping. *Journal of Cognitive Neuroscience, 19*, 1081–8.

Rosenbaum, D. A., Marchak, F., Barnes, H. J., Vaughan, J., Slotta, J. D., & Jorgensen, M. J. (1990). Constraints for action selection: Overhand versus underhand grips. In M. Jeannerod (Ed.), *Attention and performance XIII: Motor representation and control* (pp. 321–42). Hillsdale, NJ: Lawrence Erlbaum.

Rossetti, Y., Rode, G., Pisella, L., Farnè, A., Boisson, D., & Perenin, M. T. (1998). Prism adaptation to a rightward optical deviation rehabilitates left hemispatial neglect. *Nature, 395*, 166–9.

Rothi, L. J. G., Heilman, K. M., & Watson, R. T. (1985). Pantomime comprehension and ideomotor apraxia. *Journal of Neurology, Neurosurgery, and Psychiatry, 48*, 207–10.

Rothi, L. J. G., Ochipa, C., & Heilman, K. M. (1991). A cognitive neuropsychological model of limb praxis. *Cognitive Neuropsychology, 8*, 443–58.

Rothi, L. J. G., Ochipa, C., & Heilman, K. M. (1997). A cognitive neuropsychological model of limb praxis and apraxia. In L. J. G. Rothi & K. M. Heilman (Eds.), *Apraxia—the neuropsychology of action* (pp. 29–50). Hove: Psychology Press.

Rowlands, M. (2003). *Externalism. Putting mind and world back together again.* Chesham: Acumen Publishing Limited.

Roy, E. A., Black, S. E., Blair, N., & Dimeck, P. T. (1998). Analysis of deficits in gestural pantomime. *Journal of Clinical and Experimental Neuropsychology, 20*, 628–43.

Roy, E. A. and Hall, C. (1992). Limb apraxia: A process approach. In L. Proteau and D. Elliott (Eds.), *Vision and Motor Control* (pp. 261–82). Amsterdam: Elsevier.

Roy, E. A. & Square, P. A. (1985). Common considerations in the study of limb, verbal and oral apraxia. In E. A. Roy (Ed.), *Neuropsychological studies of apraxia and related disorders* (pp. 111–62). Amsterdam: North-Holland.

Roy, E. A., Square-Storer, P., Hogg, S., & Adams, S. (1991). Analysis of task demands in apraxia. *International Journal of Neuroscience, 56*, 177–86.

Rumiati, R. I., Weiss, P. H., Shallice, T., Ottoboni, G., Noth, J., Zilles, K., *et al.* (2004). Neural basis of pantomiming the use of visually presented objects. *Neuroimage, 21*, 1224–31.

Rumiati, R. I., Zanini, S., Vorano, L., & Shallice, T. (2001). A form of ideatonal apraxia as a selective deficit of contention scheduling. *Cognitive Neuropsychology, 18*, 617–42.

Rusconi, E., Pinel, P., Dehaene, S., & Kleinschmidt, A. (2010). The enigma of Gerstmann's syndrome revisited: a telling tale of the vicissitudes of neuropsychology. *Brain, 133*, 320–32.

Sauguet, J., Benton, A. L., & Hécaen, H. (1971). Disturbances of the body schema in relation to language impairment and hemispheric locus of lesion. *Journal of Neurology, Neurosurgery, and Psychiatry, 34*, 496–501.

Saygin, A. P., Wilson, S. M., Dronkers, N. F., & Bates, E. (2004). Action comprehension in aphasia: linguistic and non-linguistic deficits and their lesion correlates. *Neuropsychologia, 42*, 1788–804.

Schaefer, S. Y., Haaland, K. Y., & Sainburg, R. L. (2007). Ipsilesional motor deficits following stroke reflect hemispheric specializations for movment control. *Brain, 130*, 2146–58.

Schaefer, S. Y., Haaland, K. Y., & Sainburg, R. L. (2009). Hemispheric specialition and functional impact of ipsilesional deficits in movement coordination and accuracy. *Neuropsychologia, 47*, 2953–66.

Schank, R. C. & Abelson, R. P. (1977). *Scripts, plans, goals and understanding. An inquiry into human knowledge structures.* Hillsdale, NJ: Lawrence Erlbaum Associates.

Schilder, P. (1935). *The image and appearance of the human body.* London: Kegan Paul.

Schlanger, P. & Freimann, R. (1979). Pantomime therapy with aphasics. *Aphasia Apraxia Agnosia, 1*, 34–9.

Schlesinger, B. (1928). Zur Auffassung der optischen und konstruktiven Apraxie. *Zeitschrift für die gesamte Neurologie und Psychiatrie, 117*, 649–97.

Schofield, W. N. (1976). Do children find movements which cross the body midline difficult? *Quarterly Journal of Experimental Psychology, 28*, 571–82.

Schwartz, M. F. & Buxbaum, L. J. (1997). Naturalistic action. In L. J. G. Rothi & K. M. Heilman (Eds.), *Apraxia—the neuropsychology of action* (pp. 269–90). Hove: Psychology Press.

Schwartz, M. F., Buxbaum, L. J., Montgomery, M. W., Fitzpatrick-DeSalme, E. J., Hart, T., Ferraro, M., *et al.* (1999). Naturalistic action production following right hemisphere stroke. *Neuropsychologia, 37*, 51–66.

Schwartz, M. F., Lee, S. S., Coslett, H. B., Montgomery, M. W., Buxbaum, L. J., Carew, T. G., *et al.* (1998). Naturalistic action impairment in closed head injury. *Neuropsychology, 12*, 13–28.

Schwartz, M. F., Montgomery, M. W., Fitzpatrick-DeSalme, E. J., Ochipa, C., Coslett, H. B., & Mayer, N. H. (1995). Analysis of a disorder of everyday action. *Cognitive Neuropsychology, 12*, 863–92.

Selnes, O. A., Pestronk, A., Hart, J., & Gordon, B. (1991). Limb apraxia without aphasia from a left sided lesion in a right handed patient. *Journal of Neurology, Neurosurgery, and Psychiatry, 54*, 734–7.

Semenza, C. (1988). Impairment of localization of body parts following brain damage. *Cortex, 24*, 443–50.

Seron, X., van der Kaa, M. A., Remitz, A., & Van der Linden, M. (1979). Pantomime interpretation and aphasia. *Neuropsychologia, 17*, 661–8.

Shallice, T. (1982). Specific impairments of planning. *Philosophical Transactions of the Royal Society of London, B, 298*, 199–209.

Shallice, T. (1988). *From neuropsychology to mental structure.* Cambridge: Cambridge University Press.

Shallice, T., Burgess, P. W., Schon, F., & Baxter, D. M. (1989). The origins of utilization behaviour. *Brain, 112*, 1587–98.

Silveri, M. C. & Ciccarelli, N. (2009). Semantic memory in object use. *Neuropsychologia, 47*, 2634–41.

Sirigu, A., Cohen, L., Duhamel, J. R., Pillon, B., Dubois, B., & Agid, Y. (1995). A selective impairment of hand posture for object utilization in apraxia. *Cortex, 31*, 41–56.

Sirigu, A., Duhamel, J. R., & Poncet, M. (1991a). The role of sensorimotor experience in object recognition—a case of multimodal agnosia. *Brain, 114*, 2555–73.

Sirigu, A., Grafman, J., Bressler, K., & Sunderland, T. (1991b). Multiple representations contribute to body knowledge processing. *Brain, 114*, 629–42.

Sittig, O. (1928). *Über Apraxie—Eine klinische Studie.* Berlin: S. Karger.

Smania, N., Aglioti, S. M., Girardi, F., Tinazzi, M., Fiaschi, A., Cosentino, A., *et al.* (2006). Rehabilitation of limb apraxia improves daily life activities in patients with stroke. *Neurology, 67*, 2050–2.

Smania, N., Girardi, F., Domenicali, C., & Aglioti, S. (2000). The rehabilitation of limb apraxia: A study in left-brain-damaged patients. *Archives of Physical Medicine and Rehabilitation, 81*, 379–88.

Smiley, J. F., Konnova, K., & Bleiwas, C. (2012). Cortical thickness, neuron density and size in the inferior parietal lobe in schizophrenia. *Schizophrenia Research*, *136*, 43–50.

Spatt, J., Bak, T., Bozeat, S., Patterson, K., & Hodges, J. R. (2002). Apraxia, mechanical problem solving and semantic knowledge—contributions to object usage in corticobasal degeneration. *Journal of Neurology*, *249*, 601–8.

Sperry, R. W. (1961). Cerebral organization and behavior. *Science*, *133*, 1749–57.

Squire, L. R., Knowlton, B., & Musen, G. (1993). The structure and organization of memory. *Annual Review of Psychology*, *44*, 453–95.

Stamenova, V., Roy, E. A., & Black, S. E. (2010). Associations and dissociations of transitive and intransitive gestures in left and right hemisphere stroke patients. *Brain and Cognition*, *72*, 483–90.

Starr, A. (1888). Apraxia and aphasia: their varieties, and the methods of examination for their detection. *Medical Record*. (Cited in Wilson, S. A. K. (1908). A contribution to the study of apraxia with a review of the literature. *Brain*, *31*, 164–216.)

Steinthal, H. (1871). *Abriss der Sprachwissenschaft*. Berlin: Ferd. Dümmlers Verlagsbuchhandlung Harrwitz und Gossmann.

Steinthal, H. (1874). Diskussion von Hitzigs Vortrag über Localisation psychischer Centren in der Hirnrinde. *Verhandlungen der Berliner Gesellschaft für Anthropologie, Ethnologie und Urgeschichte*, *1874*, 47–50.

Steinthal, H. (1881). *Abriss der Sprachwissenschaft* (2nd edn). Berlin: Ferd. Dümmlers Verlagsbuchhandlung Harrwitz und Gossmann.

Stengel, E. (1944). Loss of spatial orientation, constructional apraxia and Gerstmann's syndrome. *Journal of Mental Science*, *90*, 753–60.

Stiles, A. (2006). Robert Louis Stevenson's Jekyll and Hyde and the double brain. *SEL Studies in English Literature 1500-1900*, *46*, 879–900.

Strauss, H. (1922). Über konstruktive Apraxie. *Monatschrift für Psychiatrie und Neurologie*, *56*, 65–124.

Subiaul, F., Cantlon, J. F., Holloway, R. L., & Terrace, H. C. (2004). Cognitive imitation in Rhesus macaques. *Science*, *305*, 407–10.

Sunderland, A. (2007). Impaired imitation of meaningless gestures in ideomotor apraxia: A conceptual problem not a disorder of action control? A single case investigation. *Neuropsychologia*, *45*, 1621–31.

Sunderland, A., Walker, C. M., & Walker, M. F. (2006). Action errors and dressing disability after stroke: An ecological approach to neuropsychological assessment and intervention. *Neuropsychological Rehabilitation*, *16*, 666–83.

Takashi, M. (2003). Action models and verbal descriptions in object representations given through gestures by preschool children. *Psychological Report*, *93*, 1295–306.

Tanaka, S. & Inui, T. (2002). Cortical involvement for action imitation of hand/arm postures versus finger configurations: an fMRI study. *NeuroReport*, *13*, 1599–602.

Tanaka, Y., Iwasa, H., & Obayashi, T. (1990a). Right hand agraphia and left hand apraxia following callosal damage in a right-hander. *Cortex*, *26*, 665–71.

Tanaka, Y., Iwasa, H., & Yoshida, M. (1990b). Diagonistic apraxia: Case report and movement-related potentials. *Neurology*, *40*, 657–61.

Tanaka, Y., Yoshida, A., Kawahata, N., Hashimoto, R., & Obayashi, T. (1996). Diagonistic dyspraxia: Clinical characteristics, responsible lesion and possible underlying mechanism. *Brain*, *119*, 859–73.

Tessari, A., Canessa, N., Ukmar, M., & Rumiati, R. I. (2007). Neuropsychological evidence for a strategic control of multiple routes in imitation. *Brain*, *130*, 1111–26.

Tessari, A. & Rumiati, R. I. (2004). The strategic control of multiple routes in imitation of action. *Journal of Experimental Psychology: Human Perception and Performance*, *30*, 1107–16.

Thompson-Schill, S. L. (2005). Dissecting the language organ: A new look at the role of Broca's area in language processing. In A. Cutler (Ed.), *Twenty first century psycholinguistics. Four cornerstones* (pp. 173–89). Mahwah, NJ: Lawrence Erlbaum Associates.

Thompson-Schill, S. L., Swick, D., Farah, M. J., D'Esposito, M., Kan, I. P., & Knight, R. T. (1998). Verb generation in patients with focal frontal lesions: A neuropsychological test of neuroimaging findings. *Proceedings of the National Academy of Sciences of the United States of America, 95*, 15855–60.

Tognola, G. & Vignolo, L. A. (1980). Brain lesions associated with oral apraxia in stroke patients: A clinico-neuroradiological investigation with the CT scan. *Neuropsychologia, 18*, 257–72.

Tranel, D., Kemmerer, D., Adolphs, R., Damasio, H., & Damasio, A. R. (2003). Neural correlates of conceptual knowledge for actions. *Cognitive Neuropsychology, 20*, 409–32.

Tretriluxana, J., Gordon, J., Fisher, B. E., & Winstein, C. J. (2009). Hemisphere specific impairments in reach-to-grasp control after stroke: effects of object size. *Neurorehabilitation and Neural Repair, 23*, 679–91.

Trojano, L. & Conson, M. (2008). Visuospatial and visuoconstructive deficits. In G. Goldenberg & B.Miller (Eds.), *Handbook of clinical neurology, 3rd series, Vol. 88: Neuropsychology and behavioral neurology* (pp. 373–92). Edinburgh: Elsevier.

Tucha, O., Steup, O., Smely, C., & Lange, K. W. (1997). Toe agnosia in Gerstmann syndrome. *Journal of Neurology, Neurosurgery, and Psychiatry, 63*, 399–403.

Tulving, E. (1985). How many memory systems are there? *American Psychologist, 40*, 385–98.

Tzourio-Mazoyer, N., Josse, G., Crivello, F., & Mazoyer, B. (2004). Interindividual variability in the hemispheric organization for speech. *Neuroimage, 21*, 422–35.

Unterrainer, J. M., Rahm, B., Leonhart, R., Ruff, C. C., & Halsband, U. (2003). The Tower of London: the impact of instructions, cueing, and learning on planning abilities. *Cognitive Brain Research, 17*, 675–83.

Vaina, L. M. & Jaulent, M. C. (1991). Object structure and action requirements: A compatibility model for functional recognition. *International Journal of Intelligent Systems, 6*, 313–36.

Valenstein, E. & Heilman, K. M. (1979). Apraxic agraphia with neglect-induced paragraphia. *Archives of Neurology, 36*, 506–8.

van der Horst, L. (1934). Constructive apraxia. Psychological views on the conception of space. *The Journal of Nervous and Mental Diseases, 80*, 645–50.

van Heugten, C. M., Dekker, J., Deelman, B. G., Stehmann-Saris, J. C., & Kinebanian, A. (2000). Rehabilitation of stroke patients with apraxia: the role of additional cognitive and motor impairments. *Disability and Rehabilitation, 22*, 547–54.

van Heugten, C. M., Dekker, J., Deelman, B. G., van Dijk, A. J., Stehmann-Saris, J. C., & Kinebanian, A. (1998). Outcome of strategy training in stroke patients with apraxia: a phase-II study. *Clinical Rehabilitation, 12*, 294–303.

van Staden, M. & Majid, A. (2006). Body colouring task. *Language Sciences, 28*, 158–61.

Van Vleuten, C. F. (1907). Linksseitige motorische Apraxie—Ein Beitrag zur Physiologie des Balkens. *Zeitschrift für Psychiatrie, 64*, 203–39, 389.

Varney, N. R. (1978). Linguistic correlates of pantomime recognition in aphasic patients. *Journal of Neurology, Neurosurgery, and Psychiatry, 41*, 564–8.

Varney, N. R. & Damasio, H. (1987). Locus of lesion in impaired pantomime recognition. *Cortex, 23*, 699–704.

Verstichel, P., Cambier, J., Masson, C., Masson, M., & Robine, B. (1994). Apraxie et autotopagnosie sans aphasie ni agraphie, mais avec activité compulsive de langage au cours d'une lésion hémisphérique droite. *Revue Neurologique, 150*, 274–81.

Verstynen, T., Diedrichsen, J., Albert, N., Aparicio, P., & Ivry, R. B. (2004). Ipsilateral motor cortex activity during unimanual hand movements relates to task complexity. *Journal of Neurophysiology, 93*, 1209–22.

Vignolo, L. A. (1990). Non-verbal conceptual impairment in aphasia. In F. Boller & J. Grafman (Eds.), *Handbook of clinical neuropsychology* (pp. 185–206). Amsterdam: Elsevier.

Vingerhoets, G., Acke, F., Alderweireldt, A., Nys, J., Vandemaele, P., & Achten, E. (2012). Cerebral lateralization of praxis in right- and left-handedness: Same pattern, different strength. *Human Brain Mapping, 33*, 763–77.

Vingerhoets, G., Vandekerckhove, E., Honoré, P., Vandemaele, P., & Achten, E. (2011). Neural correlates of pantomiming familiar and unfamiliar tools: Action semantics versus mechanical problem solving. *Human Brain Mapping, 32*, 905–18.

Volpe, B. T., Sidtis, J. J., Holtzmann, J. D., Wilson, D. H., & Gazzaniga, M. S. (1982). Cortical mechanisms involved in praxis: Observations following partial and complete section of the corpus callosum in man. *Neurology, 32*, 645–50.

von Monakow, C. (1914). *Die Lokalisation im Grosshirn und der Abbau der Funktion durch kortikale Herde*. Wiesbaden: J. F. Bergmann.

Wada, Y., Nakagawa, Y., Nishikawa, T., Aso, N., Inokowa, M., Kashiwagi, A., *et al.* (2000). Role of somatosensory feedback from tools in realizing movements by patients with ideomotor apraxia. *European Neurology, 41*, 73–8.

Wang, B., Zhou, T. G., Zhuo, Y., & Chen, L. (2007). Global topological dominance in the left hemisphere. *Proceedings of the National Academy of Sciences of the United States of America, 104*, 21014–19.

Wang, L. & Goodglass, H. (1992). Pantomime, praxis, and aphasia. *Brain and Language, 42*, 402–18.

Watkins, T. E., Strafella, A. P., & Paus, T. (2003). Seeing and hearing speech excites the motor system involved in speech production. *Neuropsychologia, 41*, 989–94.

Watson, R. T. & Heilman, K. M. (1983). Callosal apraxia. *Brain, 106*, 391–403.

Werner, H. (1952). *The acquisition of word meaning—a developmental study*. Evanston, IL: Child Development Publications.

Wernicke, C. (1874). *Der aphasische Symptomenkomplex—eine psychologische Studie auf anatomischer Basis*. Breslau: Max Cohn & Weigert.

Whitney, C., Kirk, M., O'Sullivan, J., Lambon Ralph, M. A., & Jefferies, E. (2012). The neural organization of semantic control: TMS evidence for a distributed network in left inferior frontal and posterior middle temporal gyrus. *Cerebral Cortex, 21*, 1066–75.

Wigan, A. L. (1844). *A new view of insanity: The duality of the mind proved by the structure, functions and diseases of the brain*. Whitefish, MT: Kessinger Publishing's Rare Reprints.

Wilson, B. A., Baddeley, A., Evans, J., & Shiel, A. (1994). Errorless learning in the rehabilitation of memory impaired people. *Neuropsychological Rehabilitation, 4*, 307–26.

Wilson, S. A. K. (1908). A contribution to the study of apraxia with a review of the literature. *Brain, 31*, 164–216.

Winstein, C. J. & Pohl, P. S. (1995). Effects of unilateral brain damage on the control of goal- directed hand movements. *Experimental Brain Research, 105*, 163–74.

Woodworth, R. S. (1899). The accuracy of voluntary movement. *Psychological Review, 3*, 1–114.

Young, R. M. (1990). *Mind, brain, and adaptation in the nineteenth century*. New York, NY: Oxford University Press.

Zago, M. & Lacquanti, F. (2005). Cognitive, perceptual and action-oriented representations of falling objects. *Neuropsychologia, 43*, 178–88.

Zaidel, D. & Sperry, R. W. (1977). Some long term motor effects of cerebral commissurotomy in man. *Neuropsychologia, 15*, 193–204.

Zangwill, O. L. (1960). Le probleme de l'apraxie ideatoire. *Revue Neurologique, 102*, 595–633.

Zatorre, R. J. (2003). Hemispheric asymmetries in the processing of tonal stimuli. In K. Hugdahl & R. J. Davidson (Eds.), *The asymmetrical brain* (pp. 411–40). Cambridge, MA: MIT Press.

Zhang, J. (1997). The nature of external representations in problem solving. *Cognitive Science*, *21*, 179–217.

Zhang, J. X., Feng, C. M., Fox, P. T., Gao, J. H., & Tan, L. H. (2004). Is left inferior frontal gyrus a general mechanism for selection? *Neuroimage*, *23*, 596–603.

Ziemann, U., Ishii, K., Borgheseri, A., Yaseen, Z., Battaglia, F., Hallet, M., *et al.* (1999). Dissociation of the pathways mediating ipsilateral and contralateral motor-evoked potentials in human hand and arm muscles. *Journal of Physiology*, *518*, 895–906.

Subject Index

Note: page numbers in *italics* refer to figures and tables. References to footnotes are indicated by the suffix 'n' followed by the footnote number, for example 141n2.

Author Index

Note: page numbers in *italics* refer to figures and tables. References to footnotes are indicated by the suffix 'n', followed by the footnote number, for example 187n1.